62343

THE ANATOMY
OF THE
NERVOUS SYSTEM

Its Development and Function

By

STEPHEN WALTER RANSON, M.D., Ph.D.

*Late Professor of Neurology and Director of Neurological
Institute, Northwestern University Medical School, Chicago*

Revised by

SAM LILLARD CLARK, M.D., Ph.D.

*Late Professor and Chairman of the Department of Anatomy,
The Vanderbilt University School of Medicine, Nashville*

TENTH EDITION, 434 Illustrations, 11 in Color

W. B. SAUNDERS COMPANY
PHILADELPHIA AND LONDON

The Library of Congress has cataloged this book as follows:

Ranson, Stephen Walter, 1880–1942. The anatomy of the **nervous system;** its development and
   function. Revised by Sam Lillard Clark. 10th ed. Philadelphia, Saunders, 1959. 622 p. illus.
   25 cm. Includes bibliography. 1. Nervous system. i. Clark, Sam Lillard, 1898– ed. ii. Title.
   QM451.R3 1959 611.8 59–5080 ‡

Preface to the Tenth Edition

Form and function in biological systems, where survival is often the test of fitness, are inseparable attributes to be considered together for better understanding. In the study of the nervous system, where cells once formed survive as functional entities, sometimes for a century, the significance of structural details is obviously great. Although this text is primarily an anatomical one it has the same aim as that of the student using it, that is, to examine not only how the nervous system is made up but as far as possible how it works.

In the preparation of this revision, inclusions and alterations have been made with the hope that they will aid the student in understanding. As in the former editions, the references to the literature that have been included are not meant to be exhaustive but are provided as suggestions for further reading as well as to record newer information.

The terminology adopted by the International Anatomical Nomenclature Committee in 1955 has been used wherever possible. Many neuroanatomical terms, however, were not included in that list and the accepted practise has been generally the guide. Terms for parts of the cerebellum have been varied from the list of the IANC to include studies by Larsell and others from a comparative and embryologic point of view.

Additions and modifications of the text and illustrations have been made in many cases as the results of suggestions from teachers and students who have observed needs as the text was used and have graciously pointed them out. To each of them I am distinctly grateful. It is a pleasure to express my appreciation for certain new illustrations by Miss Susan Wilkes, who blended with her art a keen knowledge of anatomy. To Dr. Sarah Luse, I am indebted for the figures based on electron micrographs, which she prepared. Sincere appreciation is felt for the constant patience and care shown by Mrs. Margaret Martin in the preparation of the manuscript and in other phases of the work of revision.

The publishers have been generous with time and advice and I am grateful to them. The memories of my association with Dr. Ranson and his work are always pleasant, and they constantly affected the preparation of this revision of the text he originally created.

SAM L. CLARK

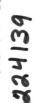

Contents

Chapter III

Chapter IV

Chapter XIII

Chapter XIV

Chapter XXI

the simplest reflex arc. Stimulation of the sensory cell causes nerve impulses to travel through its fiber to the neuropil, thence to a motor cell, and finally along a process of the latter to the muscle. In other words, there is a receptor, conductor, center, another conductor, and finally an effector; all of which bring the muscle fiber under the influence of such environmental changes as are able to *stimulate* the sensitive receptor.

In addition to the primary sensory and motor elements just enumerated, the ganglia contain nerve cells, the fibers of which run from one ganglion to another and serve to associate these in coordinated activity. These internuncial elements serve to establish functional connections among the different parts of the ganglionated nerve cord that constitutes the central nervous apparatus; and they lie entirely within this central organ. The slow waves of contraction that pass from head to tail as the worm creeps forward may be spread from segment to segment by such internuncial or association elements.

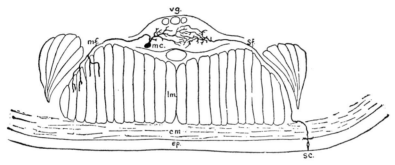

FIGURE 4.   Transverse section of the ventral chain and surrounding structures of an earthworm: *cm*, Circular muscles; *ep*, epidermis; *lm*, longitudinal muscles; *mc*, motor cell body; *mf*, motor nerve fiber; *sc*, sensory cell body; *sf*, sensory nerve fiber; *vg*, ventral ganglion. (Parker.)

The nervous system of the earthworm differs from that of the coelenterate in many ways, but the fundamental difference is one of centralization, since in the worm the greater part of it has separated from the skin and become concentrated in a series of interconnected ganglia which serve as a *central nervous system*. These ganglia receive nerve fibers, coming from the sense organs, and give off others, going to the muscles; and both types of fibers are brought together and grouped into nerves for convenience of passage between remote parts of the organism. The neuropil within a ganglion offers a variety of pathways to each incoming impulse which may accordingly find its way out along one or more of several motor fibers. The spreading of nerve impulses through the chain of ganglia is facilitated by the presence of the association fibers already mentioned. Nevertheless, conduction is not diffuse as in the nerve net of the medusa, but occurs along definite and more or less restricted lines related to the symmetry of the animal's form. The earthworm, like higher forms of animal life, has an anterior end which is thrust forward into new environment in normal locomotion as the animal seeks and consumes food. The specialization of the anterior end for feeding and exploring is reflected in even this lowly form in modification of the anterior part of the nervous system, and the brain of higher forms is forecast. In general, incoming impulses tend to be conducted antero-posteriorly. It is stated that, if a crawling earthworm is quickly chopped in two, the anterior part continues to crawl forward in coordinated fashion while the posterior part is thrown into incoordinate wiggles, as a result of the excessive stimuli arising at the cut, but conducted predominantly caudalward.

Pattern of the Vertebrate Nervous System. The vertebrate nervous system has much in common with that of the earthworm. The central nervous system of the annelid is split off from the ectoderm by a process of delamination, as will be seen by comparing the ventral nervous cord of the marine worm, Sigalion, with that of the earthworm (Figs. 4, 5). Through a comparable process of

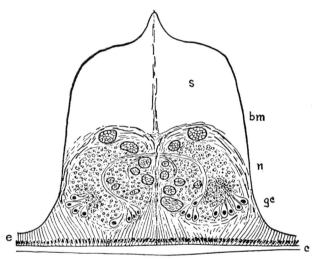

FIGURE 5. Transverse section of the ventral nervous cord of Sigalion: *bm*, basement membrane; *c*, cuticula; *e*, epidermis; *gc*, ganglion cells; *n*, nerve fibers and neuropil; *s*, space occupied by vacu-olated supporting tissue. (Parker, Hatschek.)

infolding of the ectoderm to form a neural tube, there is developed the central nervous system of the vertebrate (Fig. 12). The dorsal position of the neural tube in vertebrates, as compared with the ventral position of the solid nerve cord of the annelid, offers some difficulty in explanation of their phylogenetic rela-tionship, and has led to ingenious theories. In primitive chordates, such as the amphioxus, there is already a simple, dorsally placed, neural tube associated with segmented nerves. In true vertebrates the anterior end of the neural tube becomes irregularly enlarged to form the brain, while the posterior part remains less highly but more uniformly developed and forms the spinal cord.

There is further similarity in the nervous systems of vertebrates and the higher invertebrates in the location of primary motor and sensory nerve cells. In both types the primary motor cells lie within the central nervous system and send axons through nerves to the muscles, while the primary sensory cells lie outside the central nervous system. In lower forms the sensory cells tend to lie in or near the covering epithelium. In vertebrates the primary sensory cells for smell are located in the olfactory epithelium, but all others have migrated centrally along the sensory fibers, and send one process toward the periphery and another into the central system. The relative positions of these cells in the annelid, mollusc, and vertebrate are illustrated in Fig. 6. In the last the sensory cells are aggregated into masses known as the cerebrospinal ganglia, which are associated with peripheral nerves and are usually placed near the point of origin

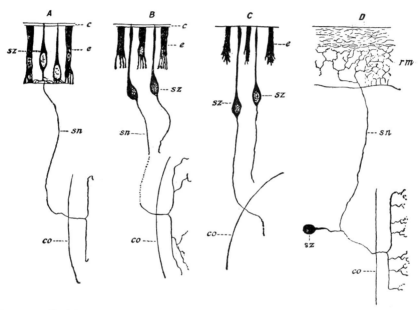

Figure 6. Peripheral sensory neurons of various animals: *A*, Oligochaetic worms (Lumbricus); *B*, polychaetic worms (Nereis); *C*, molluscs (Limax); *D*, vertebrates. The figure illustrates the gradual change in the position of the sensory cells in the phylogenetic series: *e*, Epithelial cells of sensory surface; *c*, cuticula; *sz*, cell body of peripheral sensory neuron; *rm*, rete Malpighii of epidermis; *sn*, axon; *co*, central nervous system. (Barker, Retzius.)

of these nerves from the brain or spinal cord. A comparison of Figs. 4 and 95 will show a striking similarity between the simple reflex arc in the earthworm and in man.

In higher animals with larger size of body and the acquisition of more complicated reactions, long lines of communication have been established between peripheral sense organs and muscle fibers, as well as other effectors, in widely separated parts of the body. The lines of communication constitute the nervous system, and through it messages started by sensory receptors in response to changes in the environment at a particular location reach more or less appropriate effectors and a response is produced. Environmental influences are internal as well as external to the animal, and an important part of the function of the nervous system is to transmit the impulses necessary for internal adjustments in bodily functions. In the adjustments, not only muscles, but glands,

certain pigmented cells (as chromatophores) and electric and phosphorescent
organs are involved as effectors.

Telencephalization. In higher forms as adaptation to environment occurred
and specialization of parts evolved, the head end, which meets first the changing
external environment, developed the special senses and special organs for captur-
ing and consuming food, for respiration, and, in air-breathing forms, for vocalization. Accompanying these regional developments the brain became more elaborate and the more complex parts of it developed at the anterior end. This process
of developing toward the anterior end of the brain an increasing number of
functions and nerve cells is a pattern observable through different species of
animals and has been termed *telencephalization*. Man's brain differs from that
of other mammals chiefly in the greater elaboration of cortical areas, as in the
temporal, parietal, and frontal lobes. This is especially notable in the frontal
lobes of the cerebrum where higher thought processes appear to focus. No doubt
new functions of the brain if they develop may be anticipated in this region, but
perhaps the capacity of man's frontal lobes has not yet been sufficiently
exploited.

To make somewhat clearer the arrangement of the human brain, which
becomes bent upon itself and convoluted on the surface, it is advantageous to
become acquainted with the parts of the brain of a vertebrate such as the dogfish
whose central nervous system is not bent, and in which relationship of parts
can be more clearly made out.

THE BRAIN OF THE DOGFISH—SQUALUS ACANTHIAS

The anatomical pattern of the central nervous system is common to all
vertebrates. It is essentially a tubular structure whose walls vary in thickness
and shape in different regions. The more posterior part, the spinal cord, has a
fairly uniform diameter; but the anterior part, the brain, is markedly modified in
thickness and form in its separate portions. The brain has three recognizable main subdivisions which, in order from the caudal to cranial end,
are hindbrain (rhombencephalon), midbrain (mesencephalon) and forebrain
(prosencephalon).

Rhombencephalon. The *medulla oblongata*, which together with the cerebellum forms the rhombencephalon, is continuous at the caudal extremity with
the cylindric spinal cord, and within it the central canal of the spinal cord
opens out into the fourth ventricle (Fig. 7). The medulla, which has somewhat
the shape of a truncated cone, is rostrally considerably larger than the cord, but
decreases in size as it is traced backward toward the point of junction with the
cord. In the mammal, a conspicuous transverse bundle of fibers associated with
the cerebellum is found on the ventral and lateral aspects of the metencephalic
portion of the medulla; and since this bundle appears to bridge between the
two sides of the hindbrain it was called the pons, a name that is sometimes used
to include the part of the metencephalon that is the direct continuation of the
myelencephalon. In the fish it is customary to consider as the medulla oblongata
all the axial part extending from the spinal cord to the mesencephalon. It forms
the ventral and lateral walls of the fourth ventricle; and when the roof of this

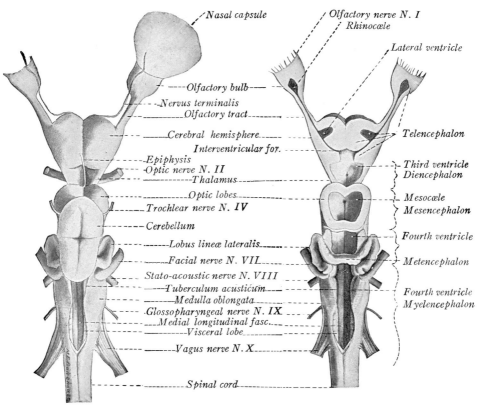

Nasal capsule

Olfactory nerve N. I
Rhinocœle

Lateral ventricle

Olfactory bulb

Nervus terminalis
Olfactory tract

Cerebral hemisphere
Interventricular for.

Telencephalon

Epiphysis
Optic nerve N. II
Thalamus

Third ventricle
Diencephalon

Optic lobes
Trochlear nerve N. IV

Mesocœle
Mesencephalon

Cerebellum

Lobus lineæ lateralis
Facial nerve N. VII
Stato-acoustic nerve N. VIII
Tuberculum acusticum
Medulla oblongata
Glossopharyngeal nerve N. IX
Medial longitudinal fasc.
Visceral lobe

Fourth ventricle

Metencephalon

Fourth ventricle
Myelencephalon

Vagus nerve N. X

Spinal cord

FIGURE 7. The brain of the dogfish, Squalus acanthias, dorsal view.

FIGURE 8. The brain of the dogfish, Squalus acanthias, with the ventricles opened, dorsal view.

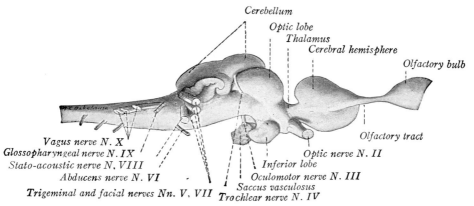

Cerebellum
Optic lobe
Thalamus
Cerebral hemisphere
Olfactory bulb

Olfactory tract

Vagus nerve N. X
Glossopharyngeal nerve N. IX
Stato-acoustic nerve N. VIII
Abducens nerve N. VI
Trigeminal and facial nerves Nn. V, VII

Optic nerve N. II
Inferior lobe
Oculomotor nerve N. III
Saccus vasculosus
Trochlear nerve N. IV

FIGURE 9. The brain of the dogfish, Squalus acanthias, lateral view.

cavity has been removed these walls are seen to surround a long and rather broad depression—the fossa rhomboidea or floor of the fourth ventricle—which tapers caudally like the point of a pen (Fig. 8).

The *cerebellum* forms an elongated mass attached dorsally to the medulla over which it projects caudally, while its rostral end overhangs the optic lobes of the mesencephalon (Fig. 7). Its dorsal surface is grooved by a pair of sulci arranged in the form of a cross. It contains a cavity, a part of the original rhombencephalic vesicle, which communicates with the fourth ventricle proper through a rather wide opening (Fig. 10). Behind the cerebellum, the fourth ventricle possesses a thin membranous roof which was torn away in the preparation from which Fig. 7 was drawn (Fig. 10).

Mesencephalon.   The *optic lobes* on the dorsal aspect of the mesencephalon are a pair of rounded masses separated by a median sagittal sulcus. They repre-

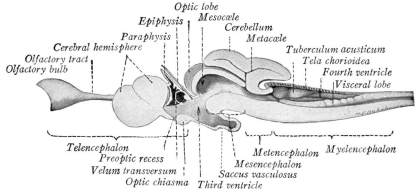

FIGURE 10.   The brain of the dogfish, Squalus acanthias, medial sagittal section.

sent the bulging roof of the mesencephalic cavity and are accordingly spoken of as the tectum mesencephali. Within this roof end the fibers which come from the retinae through the optic nerves. The floor of the cavity is formed by the ventral part of the mesencephalon. This appears like a direct continuation of the medulla oblongata, and in the mammal the crura cerebri are developed on its ventral surface. Emerging from the roof of the mesencephalon between the cerebellum and optic lobe is the fourth or *trochlear nerve*, and from the ventral aspect of this division of the brain arises the third or *oculomotor nerve*.

The Diencephalon.   The thin roof of the diencephalon, which can easily be torn away so as to expose the third ventricle (Figs. 9, 10), is attached by its caudal margin to a ridge containing a pair of knob-like thickenings, the *habenular nuclei*, and a commissure connecting the two. From a point just caudal to the middle of this commissure, there projects forward over the membranous roof of the ventricle a slender tube, the *epiphysis cerebri* or pineal body (Fig. 10), which comes in contact with the roof of the skull and ends in a slightly dilated extremity. The epiphysis and habenular nuclei belong to the *epithalamus*. The *thalamus* forms the thick lateral wall of the third ventricle and is traversed by the optic tracts on their way to the optic lobes. The *hypothalamus* is relatively large in the shark and presents, in addition to a pair of laterally placed oval masses, or inferior lobes, a thin-walled vascular outgrowth, the *saccus vasculosus* (Figs. 9, 10). Closely related to the ventral aspect of the hypothalamus is a glandular mass, derived by a process of evagination from the oral epithelium, and known as the *hypophysis*. On the ventral surface of the hypothalamus the optic nerves meet and cross in the *optic chiasma*.

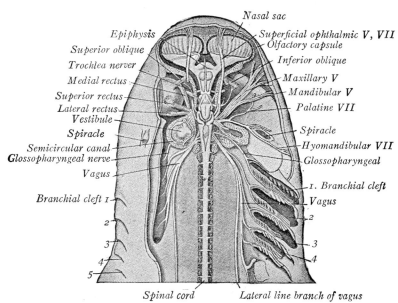

FIGURE 11. Dissection of the brain and cranial nerves of the dogfish, Scyllium catulus. The eye is shown on the left side, but has been removed on the right. (Marshall and Hurst, Parker and Haswell.)

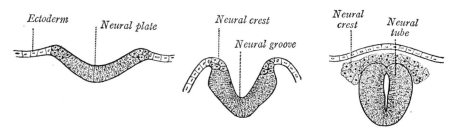

FIGURE 12. Development of neural tube and neural crest.

The **telencephalon** includes all of the brain in front of the velum *transversum*, a transverse fold projecting into the third ventricle from the membranous roof (Fig. 10), and consists of a median unpaired portion, and of the two *cerebral hemispheres* with their *olfactory bulbs*. The hemispheres are the evaginated portions of the telencephalon which, though partially separated from each other by a median sagittal fissure, are closely united by a massive plate that forms the medial walls of both lateral ventricles and enters into the boundary of each interventricular foramen (Fig. 8). From the lateral side of the rostral end of the hemisphere there projects forward the long and slender olfactory tract with a terminal enlargement, the *olfactory bulb*. This lies in contact with the nasal sac to which it gives off a number of fine nerve bundles, which together constitute the *olfactory* or *first cranial nerve*. At the rostral end of the brain, an additional nerve makes its exit from the hemisphere. It is known as the *nervus terminalis* and can be followed forward over the olfactory tract and bulb to the nasal sac (Fig. 7). A good idea of the shape and connections of the various brain ventricles and of the relation of the various parts of the brain to each other can be obtained from a study of Figs. 8 and 10.

The roof of the selachian forebrain presents a number of structures of great morphologic interest, two of which have already been mentioned, namely, the epiphysis and velum transversum. The former is an outpocketing of the roof of the diencephalon; the latter is an infolding and marks the line of separation between the two divisions of the prosencephalon. Rostral to the velum the roof of the telencephalon is evaginated to form a thin-walled sac, the *paraphysis*. The velum and paraphysis are readily identified in the mammalian embryo, but become obscured in the course of later development.

DEVELOPMENT OF THE NEURAL TUBE IN THE HUMAN EMBRYO

In its embryonic development the nervous system of man presents something like a synopsis of the early chapters of its phyletic history. Furthermore, so similarly do different species of vertebrates develop that it makes little difference whether the early stages of human or pig embryos are studied.

Each individual begins as a single celled structure, the fertilized ovum, which, after a series of cell divisions, forms a hollow ball of cells. Within this is a mass of cells which develops into the embryo proper. This inner cell mass develops by the formation of two adjacent hollow spheres of cells, one sphere being the ectoderm and the other entoderm. Along the line of fusion of these two structures is the primitive streak and primitive knot, and in the ectoderm extending anteriorly from the primitive knot a thickening appears by multiplication of its cells. This is the neural plate which, by modification of its shape, becomes the neural groove.

By the middle of the third week of development, when the human embryo is only about 1.5 mm. in length, the neural groove is indicated. The groove rapidly develops into a tube which in closing is associated with the formation of the neural crest, at first band-like, then segmented as ganglia are forecast. By the fourth week, when the embryo is about 5 mm. long, the neural tube is closed, the three primary brain vesicles are appearing, and nerves and ganglia are forming from neural crest cells (Fig. 12). The great significance of these early periods to the completeness of the mature brain is worth contemplating. The shifting of only a few cells in the wrong direction or the failure of a small part of the neural tube to close in an embryo less than half a centimeter in length could result in the death of the embryo, or serious malformation.

Except that it is flexed on itself, the brain of the *human embryo of five weeks* (Fig. 13) shows a marked resemblance to the diagram of a vertebrate brain without cerebral hemispheres (Fig. 15, *C, D*). The prosencephalic vesicle is divided by a constriction into the telencephalon and diencephalon with freely

intercommunicating cavities. The mesencephalon is well defined and presents
a sharp bend, the cephalic flexure. The rhombencephalon shows signs of separation into the metencephalon and myelencephalon and is bent at the pontile
flexure. Another curvature which develops at the junction of the brain and
spinal cord is known as the cervical flexure (Fig. 16). The pontile flexure later
straightens and is not found in the adult brain. The two others become less
pronounced as development progresses; the cervical flexure is nearly lost and
the cephalic flexure greatly reduced (Fig. 28).

From the walls of the prosencephalon there develop outpocketings on either
side, which form the optic cups and which are connected with the brain by the

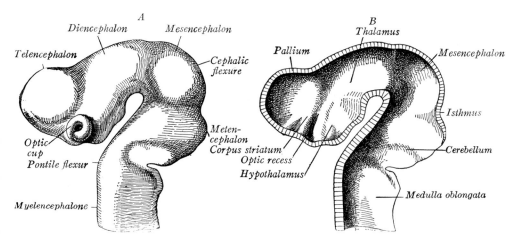

FIGURE 13.   Reconstructions of the brain of a 7 mm. embryo: *A*, Lateral view; *B*, in median sagittal
section. (His, Prentiss-Arey.)

optic stalks. From the cup develops the retina and through the stalk grow the
fibers of the optic nerve. These structures are, therefore, genetically parts of
the brain.

The Telencephalon of the Human Embryo.   By the time the embryo has
reached a length of 13 mm. the brain has passed into the stage represented by
diagrams *E, F, G* of Fig. 15. The lateral wall of the telencephalon, with the
corpus striatum and olfactory brain or *rhinencephalon*, has been evaginated on
either side to form paired structures, the cerebral hemispheres (Fig. 16). Except
for the corpus striatum and rhinencephalon the evaginated wall is relatively
thin, is known as the *pallium*, and develops into the cerebral cortex. The *lateral
ventricles* within the hemispheres represent portions of the original telencephalic
cavity and communicate with the third ventricle through the interventricular
foramina, which at this stage are relatively large. The lamina terminalis, connecting the two hemispheres in front of the third ventricle, represents the original anterior boundary of the telencephalon. Immediately behind this lamina
is a portion of the telencephalic cavity which forms the anterior part of the
third ventricle. The further development of these structures is readily traced

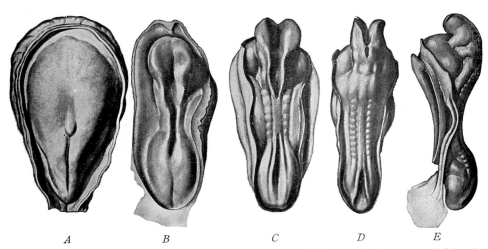

FIGURE 14.   Developmental stages of the human neural tube. Differences in size are masked by the greater enlargement of the younger embryos. (Streeter, Arey.)

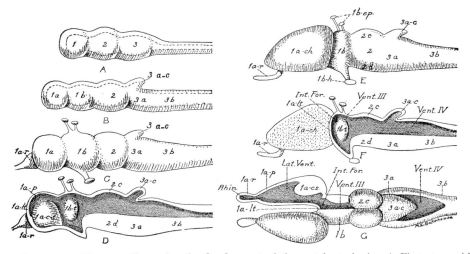

FIGURE 15.   Diagrams illustrating the development of the vertebrate brain: *A*, First stage, side view, the cavity indicated by dotted line; *B*, second stage; *C*, third stage, side view of a brain without cerebral hemispheres; *D*, the same in sagittal section; *E*, fourth stage, side view of a brain with cerebral hemispheres; *F*, the same in sagittal section; *G*, dorsal view of the same with the cavities exposed on the right side. *Rhin.*, rhinocoele; *Lat. Vent.*, lateral ventricle; *Int. For.*, interventricular foramen; *Vent. III*, third ventricle; *Vent. IV*, fourth ventricle. *1*, Prosencephalon; *1 a*, Telencephalon; *1 a-r*, Rhinencephalon; *1 a-p*, Pallium; *1 a-lt*, Lamina terminalis; *1 a-ch*, Cerebral hemisphere; *1 a-cs*, Corpus striatum; *1 b*, Diencephalon; *1 b-ep*, Epithalamus; *1 b-h*, Hypophysis; *1 b-t*, Thalamus; *2*, Mesencephalon; *2 c*, Optic lobes; *2 d*, Crura cerebri; *3*, Rhombencephalon; *3 a*, Metencephalon; *3 a-c*, Cerebellum; *3 b*, Myelencephalon.

in Fig. 17, which represents the brain of a human fetus of the third month. Comparing this figure with Fig. 28, in which the primary embryologic divisions of the brain are clearly labeled, it will be seen that the most striking feature of the development of the telencephalon is the great increase in size of the cerebral hemisphere.

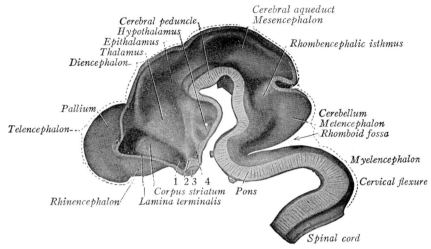

FIGURE 16.   A median section of the brain of a 13.6 mm. human embryo: 1, Optic recess; 2, ridge formed by optic chiasma; 3, optic chiasma; 4, infundibular recess. (His, Sobotta.)

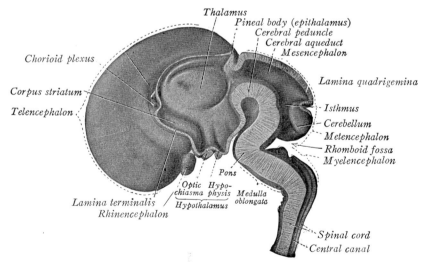

FIGURE 17.   The brain of a fetus of the third month in median sagittal section. (His, Sobotta.)

The Diencephalon.   The three principal divisions of the diencephalon—the *thalamus, epithalamus,* and *hypothalamus*—faintly indicated in an embryo of 13.6 mm., are well defined by the third month (Fig. 17). In transverse sections this division of the embryonic brain is seen to be composed of a pair of plates on either side, which with a roof and floor form the walls of the ventricle (Fig.

19). The more dorsal members of each pair of lateral plates become greatly thickened and form the thalamus, while the more ventral ones form the hypothalamus. On either side these plates meet at an angle, forming the hypothalamic sulcus.

The *hypothalamus* includes the *optic chiasma, tuber cinereum, posterior lobe of the hypophysis,* and the *mammillary bodies.* From the dorsal edge of the thalamic lamina, where this is attached to the thin roof plate, there is developed a thickened ridge, the *epithalamus,* which is transformed into the habenula and the pineal body. The roof plate of the diencephalon remains thin and forms the epithelial lining of the tela chorioidea or roof of the *third ventricle.* Because of the great growth of the thalamus this cavity becomes reduced to a vertical cleft, the walls of which ultimately fuse at one point to form the massa intermedia, a bridge of gray matter crossing the cavity (Fig. 30). The *metathalamus* is a convenient term which includes the medial and lateral geniculate bodies.

The Alar and Basal Lamina.   Each lateral half of the neural tube caudal to the prosencephalon consists of two plate-like longitudinally arranged columns separated by a groove known as the *sulcus limitans* (Fig. 18). Dorsal to this

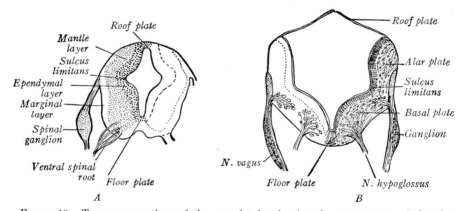

FIGURE 18.   Transverse sections of the neural tube showing the arrangement of the alar and basal lamina: *A,* Through the upper cervical region of the spinal cord in a 10 mm. human embryo (after Prentiss); *B,* through the myelencephalon of a 10.6 mm. human embryo (after His).

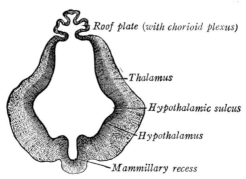

FIGURE 19.   Transverse section through the diencephalon of a 13.8 mm. embryo. (His, Prentiss-Arey.)

groove is the alar plate within which there are developed all the sensory centers of the brain stem and spinal cord. The basal plate lies ventral to the sulcus limitans and from it there are developed all the motor nuclei. The dorsal borders of the alar lamina are joined together by a roof plate and the ventral borders of the basal lamina are joined by a floor plate. It seems probable that the prosencephalon is formed exclusively from the alar plates (Schulte and Tilney, 1915, and Kingsbury, 1922).

Table Showing Subdivisions of the Neural Tube and Their Derivatives
(Modified from a Table in Keibel and Mall, Human Embryology)

	PRIMARY VESICLES	SUBDIVISIONS	DERIVATIVES	LUMEN
Brain....	Prosencephalon...	Telencephalon....	Cerebral cortex Corpora striata Rhinencephalon	Lateral ventricles Rostral portion of the third ventricle
		Diencephalon....	Epithalamus Thalamus Metathalamus Hypothalamus Optic chiasma Tuber cinereum Posterior lobe of hypophysis Mammillary bodies	The greater part of the third ventricle
	Mesencephalon	Mesencephalon...	Corpora quadrigemina Crura cerebri	Cerebral aqueduct
	Rhombencephalon	Metencephalon Myelencephalon	Cerebellum Pons Medulla oblongata	Fourth ventricle
Spinal cord			Spinal cord	Central canal

The Mesencephalon. The basal plate of the mesencephalon thickens to form the cerebral peduncles (Fig. 17); the alar plate forms the lamina quadrigemina in which are differentiated the quadrigeminal bodies; the cavity becomes the cerebral aqueduct.

The Rhombencephalon. The ventral part of the rhombencephalon, including both alar and basal plates, thickens to form the *pons* and *medulla oblongata* (Fig. 17). Most of the roof of this division remains thin and forms the epithelial lining of the tela chorioidea of the fourth ventricle (Fig. 18, *B*). But in the caudal portion of the myelencephalon the lumen of the neural tube becomes completely surrounded by thickened walls, forming the central canal of the closed portion of the medulla. The dorsal edge of the alar plate in the metencephalon becomes greatly thickened and, fusing across the median line with the similar structure of the opposite side, forms the anlage of the *cerebellum* (Figs. 17, 35).

To say various parts of the brain thicken to form this or that structure is to describe the change in gross external appearance of the developing brain, and this is the result of changes in the number, distribution, and form of the component cells and fibers which can best be appreciated through the microscopic study of the embryonic nervous system (Chap. IV).

In referring to the location of any portion of the nervous system of man, the term "anatomical position," that is, the erect extended position with palms

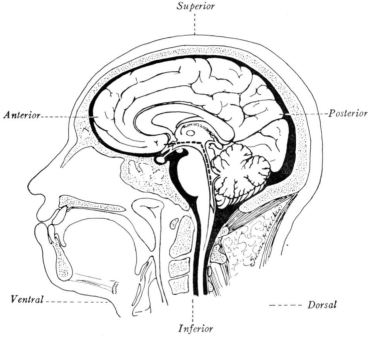

FIGURE 20. Sagittal section through the head to show relationship of brain to anatomical terms of direction. The dotted line indicates the bend in the original axis of the neural tube. Subarachnoid space is represented in black.

forward, is customarily used. In this position the terms of direction, anterior and posterior, as applied to the trunk are readily understood and are considered synonymous with ventral and dorsal. But the comparative anatomist uses the terms anterior and posterior to refer to the cranial and caudal ends of lower forms, which applies then to an axis at right angles to the anteroposterior axis of man. While this is clear in reference to the bodies of lower forms and man, the situation in the central nervous system of man requires additional attention. During development, the neural tube bends upon itself at the cranial end in forming the brain, and though there originally is more than one angle, the final result is to bring about an approximately 90° bend in the axis between the medulla and cerebrum.

As a result of this bending, the original dorsal aspect of the cranial part of the neural tube is referred to as upper or superior surface, while the original ventral aspect is the inferior or lower surface. In the case of a cerebral hemisphere the anterior end is the frontal pole and the posterior end the occipital pole. The terms dorsal and ventral can be used more readily if the original direction of the neural tube is kept in mind, and this can be visualized in the sagittal section of a brain, where the original anterior end of the neural tube is found as the lamina terminalis forming the anterior boundary of the third ventricle (Fig. 20).

CHAPTER II

Gross Anatomy
of the Nervous System

In the preceding pages the story of the progressive development of the nervous system from its relatively simple form in lower animals to its rather elaborate structure in vertebrates has been sketchily told, and the major chapters in the embryologic history of the nervous system in a species of vertebrates, man, have been briefly reviewed.

It is easy to see similarities in these phylogenetic and ontogenetic histories though they do not stand too close a comparison. Since the primary object of this text is to seek an understanding of the nervous system of man, the succeeding pages will be devoted to a discussion of its form and function.

The approach to the study of the detailed connections within the nervous system can be made in several ways. Whatever the approach, it is important to keep in mind that the fundamental structure is based upon the arrangement of nerve cells and their processes. Since the processes of nerve cells, the nerve fibers, extend great lengths in making connections, it is advantageous to become acquainted with the gross plan of the nervous system and the names of its various parts before attempting to follow the routes taken by nerve impulses over the contained paths. A study of morphology is usually secondary in interest to a study of function, but it is a necessary preliminary in the case of the nervous system.

As the morphologic picture is built up, the function of certain parts becomes obvious from the connections with other structures of known function. The function of some tracts and nerve cells not subjected to direct physiologic experiment must be surmised in this manner, although the function of many parts can be determined by observation of the effect of direct stimulation, or of alteration in function following damage to a part, or its destruction.

The shape taken by different parts of the nervous system is dependent upon accumulations of the bodies of nerve cells, referred to as *nuclei, ganglia* or *gray matter;* and bundles of nerve fibers referred to as *tracts, paths, funiculi, fasciculi, peduncles, commissures* or *white matter*, dependent upon their location and arrangement. The immediately following account will deal largely with the surface landmarks of the parts of the central nervous system in preparation for subsequent tracing of long paths in accounts of the internal structure.

Subdivisions of the Nervous System. It has been customary to subdivide the nervous system into parts for convenience of description, but there is no implication that these parts function separately. The nervous system is the integrator of bodily functions and all of its parts work together to this end. The usual subdivision emphasizes the location of different portions of the nervous system and is as follows:

> The central nervous system:
>   Brain
>   Spinal cord.
> The peripheral nervous system:
>   Cerebrospinal nerves:
>   Cranial nerves
>   Spinal nerves.
> The autonomic nervous system:
>   Sympathetic trunk
>   Visceral nerves
>   Peripheral ganglia.

The anatomic relationships of these subdivisions in man are illustrated in Fig. 21. The brain lies within and nearly fills the cranial cavity. It is continuous through the foramen magnum with the spinal cord, which occupies but does not fill the vertebral canal. From the brain arises a series of nerves usually enumerated as twelve pairs and known as cranial or cerebral nerves; while thirty-one pairs of segmentally arranged spinal nerves take origin from the spinal cord. The ganglionated sympathetic trunks lie parallel to the vertebral column. They are connected with each pair of spinal nerves and with nerves and ganglia of the viscera.

Branches of the cerebrospinal nerves reach most parts of the body. They are composed of *afferent fibers,* which receive and carry to the central nervous system inflowing impulses produced by external or internal stimuli, and of *efferent fibers,* which convey outgoing impulses to the organs of response. It is through the central nervous system that the incoming impulses find their way into the proper outgoing paths. To bring about this shunting of incoming impulses into the appropriate efferent paths requires the presence of untold numbers of central or association neurons, and it is of these that the central organs—brain and spinal cord—are chiefly composed. The greater the number of these association neurons in the nervous system of an animal, the greater the capacity of that species to vary the response to stimuli. Lowly forms with simple connections between afferent and efferent neurons are stereotyped in their responses to stimuli. Man with a large brain has great variety in his choice of responses.

THE SPINAL CORD

It is convenient to begin the study of the anatomy of the central nervous system with the spinal cord, which shows a segmental simplicity, and represents

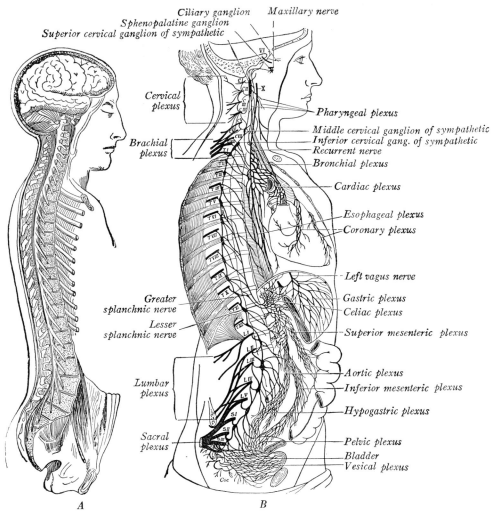

FIGURE 21. *A*, General view of the central nervous system, showing the brain and spinal cord
in situ. (Bourgery, Schwalbe, van Gehuchten.) *B*, Diagram of the autonomic nervous system and
its connections with the cerebrospinal nerves. (Schwalbe, Herrick.)

the pattern displayed in the original neural tube which, though recognizable in
the brain, is there much modified.

The spinal cord, or *medulla spinalis*, is a cylindric mass of nervous tissue
occupying the vertebral canal. It is 40 to 45 cm. in length, reaching from the
foramen magnum, where it is continuous with the *medulla oblongata*, to the
level of the first or second lumbar vertebra. Even above this level the vertebral
canal is by no means fully occupied by the cord (Fig. 21), which is surrounded
by protective membranes, while between these and the wall of the canal is a
rather thick cushion of adipose tissue containing a plexus of veins. Immediately

surrounding the brain and cord and adherent to them is the delicate, highly vascular *pia mater*. This is separated from the thick, fibrous *dura mater* by a membrane having the tenuity of a spider web, the *arachnoid*, which surrounds the *subarachnoid space*. This space is broken up by subarachnoid trabeculae and filled with *cerebrospinal fluid*. Between the arachnoid which, though thin, is a complete membrane, and the dura mater lies the *subdural space*, which contains only enough fluid normally to moisten the surfaces. There is no communication between the subarachnoid and subdural spaces. In spinal punctures the needle must traverse the subdural space to enter the subarachnoid space where the cerebrospinal fluid is found (Figs. 20, 22).

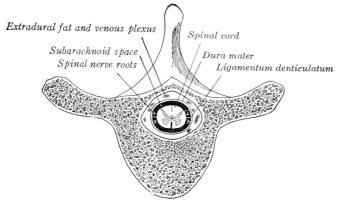

Extradural fat and venous plexus

Subarachnoid space
Spinal nerve roots

Spinal cord

Dura mater
Ligamentum denticulatum

FIGURE 22. Diagram showing the relation of the spinal cord to the vertebral column.

External Form. The spinal cord is not a perfect cylinder, but is somewhat flattened ventrodorsally, especially in the cervical region. Its diameter is not uniform throughout, being less in the thoracic than in the cervical and lumbar portions. That is to say, the cord presents two swellings (Fig. 23). The *cervical enlargement* (intumescentia cervicalis) comprises that portion of the cord from which the nerves of the brachial plexus arise, that is, the fourth cervical to the first thoracic segments inclusive. The *lumbar enlargement* (intumescentia lumbalis) is not quite so extensive and corresponds less accurately to the origin of the nerves innervating the lower extremity. At an early stage in the embryonic development of the spinal cord these enlargements are not present. In the time of their first appearance and in their subsequent growth they are directly related to the development of the limbs.

The enlargements are due to the greater quantity of nerve fibers entering and leaving the cord and the associated nerve cells, which are necessary to innervate the larger masses of tissue in the limbs. Animals with disproportionately large hind limbs, as the dinosaur, have lumbar enlargements of the cord with a diameter rivalling that of the brain. Animals like the whale, with great muscle masses rather evenly distributed through the trunk and minimal requirements for tissues of limbs, have a spinal cord of large diameter but with little tendency to local enlargement.

Below the lumbar enlargement, the spinal cord rapidly decreases in size and has a cone-shaped termination, the *conus medullaris*, from the end of which a slender filament, the *filum terminale*, is prolonged to the posterior surface of the coccyx (Fig. 25). This terminal filament descends in the middle line surrounded by the roots of the lumbar and sacral nerves, to the caudal end of the dural sac at the level of the second sacral vertebra. Here it perforates the dura mater, from which it receives an investment and then continues to the posterior surface of the coccyx. The last portion of the filament with its dural investment is often called the *filum of the spinal dura mater* (filum durae matris spinalis). The filum terminale is composed chiefly of pia mater; but in its rostral part it contains a prolongation of the central canal of the cord.

In some animals there occurs Reissner's fiber, which runs from the region of the epithalamus within the neural canal and terminates in the filum (Wislocki et al., 1956).

The spinal cord shows an obscure *segmentation*, in that it gives origin to thirty-one pairs of metameric nerves. These segments may be somewhat arbitrarily marked off from each other by imaginary planes passing through the highest root filaments of each successive spinal nerve. The highest of these planes, being just above the origin of the first cervical nerve, marks the separation of the spinal cord from the medulla oblongata. This is again an arbitrary line of separation, since both as to external form and internal structure the cord passes over into the medulla oblongata by insensible gradations. According to this method of subdivision there are in the cervical portion of the cord eight segments, in the thoracic twelve, in the lumbar five, and in the sacral five, while there is but one coccygeal segment.

Several *longitudinal furrows* are seen upon the surface of the cord (Fig. 23). Along the middle line of the ventral surface is the deep *anterior median fissure* (fissura mediana anterior). This extends into the cord to a depth amounting to nearly one-third of its anteroposterior diameter and contains a fold of pia mater. Along the middle line of the dorsal surface there is a shallow groove, the *posterior median sulcus* (sulcus medianus posterior). As may be seen in cross-sections the spinal cord is divided into approximately symmetric lateral halves by the two furrows just described and by the posterior median septum (Figs. 126, 127, 128). On either side, corresponding to the line of origin of the ventral roots, is a broad, shallow, almost invisible groove, the *anterolateral sulcus* (sulcus lateralis anterior). And again on either side, corresponding to the line of origin of the dorsal roots, is the narrower but deeper *posterolateral sulcus* (sulcus lateralis posterior). These six furrows extend the entire length of the spinal cord. In the cervical region, an additional longitudinal groove may be seen on the dorsal surface between the posterior median and posterolateral sulci, but somewhat nearer the former. It is known as the *posterior intermediate sulcus* and extends into the thoracic cord, where it gradually disappears.

Funiculi.   By means of these furrows and the subjacent gray matter, each lateral half of the cord is subdivided into columns of longitudinally coursing nerve-fibers known as the anterior, lateral, and posterior funiculi (funiculus anterior, funiculus lateralis and funiculus posterior). In the cervical and upper thoracic regions, the posterior intermediate sulcus divides the posterior funiculus into a medial portion, the fasciculus gracilis, and a lateral portion, the fasciculus cuneatus.

Nerve Roots. From the lateral funiculus in the upper four to six cervical segments there emerge, a little in front of the dorsal roots of the spinal nerves, a series of root filaments which unite to form the spinal root of the *accessory nerve* (Fig. 178). This small nerve trunk ascends along the side of the cord,

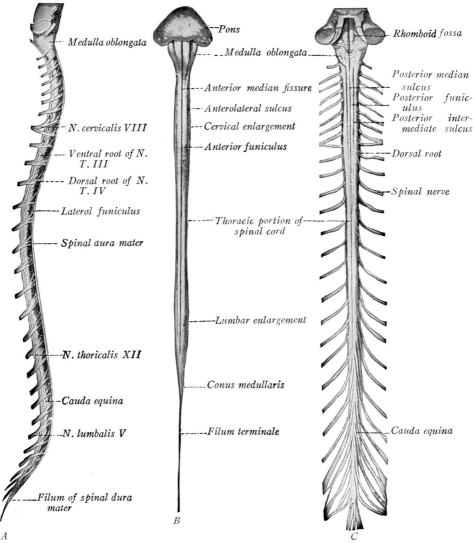

A

Medulla oblongata

N. cervicalis VIII

Ventral root of N. T. III

Dorsal root of N. T. IV

Lateral funiculus

Spinal dura mater

N. thoricalis XII

Cauda equina

N. lumbalis V

Filum of spinal dura mater

B

Pons

Medulla oblongata

Anterior median fissure

Anterolateral sulcus

Cervical enlargement

Anterior funiculus

Thoracic portion of spinal cord

Lumbar enlargement

Conus medullaris

Filum terminale

C

Rhomboid fossa

Posterior median sulcus

Posterior funiculus

Posterior intermediate sulcus

Dorsal root

Spinal nerve

Cauda equina

FIGURE 23. Three views of the spinal cord and rhombencephalon: *A*, Lateral view with spinal nerves attached; *B*, ventral view with spinal nerves removed; *C*, dorsal view with spinal nerves attached. (Modified from Spalteholz.)

enters the cranial cavity through the foramen magnum, and carries to the accessory nerve the fibers for the innervation of the sternocleidomastoid and trapezius muscles.

From the posterolateral sulcus throughout the entire length of the spinal cord emerges an almost uninterrupted series of root filaments (fila radicularia). Those from a given segment of the cord unite to form the *dorsal root* of the corresponding spinal nerve. The filaments of the *ventral roots* emerge from the broad, indistinct anterolateral sulcus in groups, several appearing side by side,

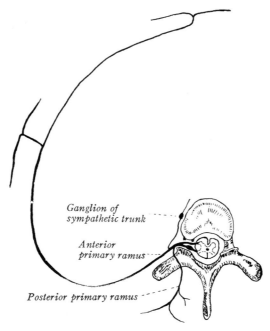

Ganglion of sympathetic trunk

Anterior primary ramus

Posterior primary ramus

FIGURE 24.   Diagram of a typical spinal nerve showing its general pattern of roots and rami.

rather than in the accurate linear order characteristic of the dorsal roots. Those from a given segment unite with each other to form a ventral root; and that in turn joins with the corresponding dorsal root just beyond the spinal ganglion to form the mixed nerve (Figs. 23, 24). The muscles supplied by various spinal segments are indicated in Fig. 26.

Relation of the Spinal Cord and Nerve Roots to the Vertebral Column. At an early fetal stage the spinal cord occupies the entire length of the vertebral canal and the spinal nerves pass horizontally lateralward to their exit through the intervertebral foramina. As development progresses, the vertebral column increases in length more rapidly than the spinal cord, which, being firmly anchored above by its attachment to the brain, is drawn upward along the canal, until in the adult it ends at about the *lower border of the first lumbar vertebra* (Fig. 25). At the same time the roots of the lumbar and sacral nerves become greatly elongated. They run in a caudal direction from their origin to the same intervertebral foramina through which they made their exit before the shift in the relative position of the cord occurred. Since the thoracic portion of the cord has changed its relative position but little, and the cervical part even less, most of the cervical roots run almost directly lateralward, while those of the thoracic nerves incline but little in a caudal direction.

Since the spinal cord ends opposite the first or second lumbar vertebra, the roots of the lumbar, sacral, and coccygeal nerves, in order to reach their proper intervertebral foramina, descend vertically in the canal around the conus medul-

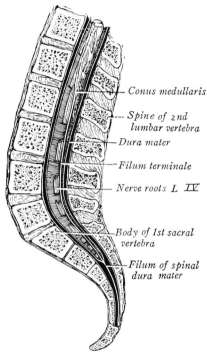

Conus medullaris

Spine of 2nd
lumbar vertebra

Dura mater

Filum terminale

Nerve roots L IV

Body of 1st sacral
vertebra

Filum of spinal
dura mater

FIGURE 25. Sagittal section of the caudal portion of the vertebral column showing spinal cord and filum terminale, and ends of the lower nerve roots making exit from the vertical canal.

laris and filum terminale. In this way there is formed a large bundle, which is composed of the roots of all the spinal nerves below the first lumbar and has been given the descriptive name *cauda equina* (Fig. 23).

The amount of relative shortening of the various segments of the cord differs in different individuals. In Fig. 26, where the quadrilateral areas represent bodies of the vertebrae, the average position of each segment of the spinal cord is indicated. It is obvious that the segments are longer in the thoracic than in the cervical and lumbar portions of the cord, while the sacral segments are the shortest (see also Fig. 130).

The position of a particular point on the spinal cord is subject to slight variation with changes in posture. In body flexion in the monkey, there is downward movement of points above the fourth cervical segment and upward movement of points below this amounting to as much as half a centimeter; this fact implies stretching of the cord (Smith, 1956).

The development of the cauda equina and the vertebral level of the various segments of the spinal cord are of practical importance. In spinal puncture the needle is made to enter the subarachnoid space caudal to the termination of the

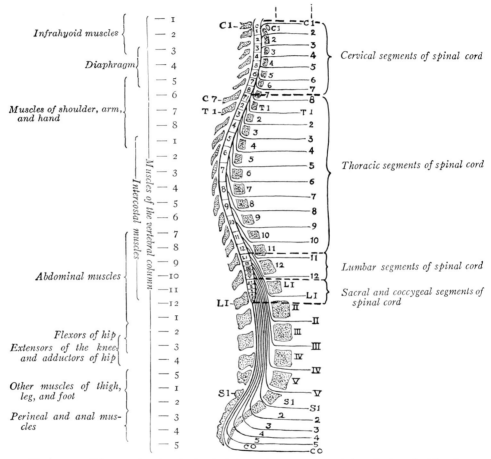

Figure 26. Diagram showing the level of the various segments of the spinal cord with reference to the vertebrae, with a table showing the distribution of the fibers of the several ventral roots; C, cervical; T, thoracic; L, lumbar; S, sacral; co, coccygeal.

cord. In locating lesions of the spinal cord it is necessary to take into consideration the position of its various segments with reference to the vertebrae. It is particularly important to be able to distinguish between an injury to the lower part of the spinal cord and one which involves only the nerve roots in the cauda equina, for though the symptoms in the two cases may be nearly identical, damage to the spinal cord is irreparable, while the motor nerve roots can regenerate.

THE GENERAL TOPOGRAPHY OF THE BRAIN

The topography of the brain as projected to the surface of the skull in the living person is often significant. Figure 27 illustrates the relationship of the main landmarks which are not always exactly comparable in different individuals. The *pterion*, where frontal, temporal, sphenoid, and parietal bones come close together in the temporal fossa, lies approximately over the anterior end of the lateral fissure of the cerebrum, and so between the frontal and temporal lobes. The anterior branch of the middle meningeal artery courses upward be-

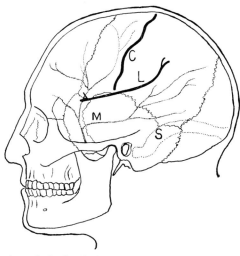

FIGURE 27. Lateral view of the head showing bony landmarks of the skull and the position relative to these of the central sulcus (*C*) and lateral fissure (*L*) of the cerebrum; the middle meningeal artery (*M*) and the sigmoid sinus (*S*).

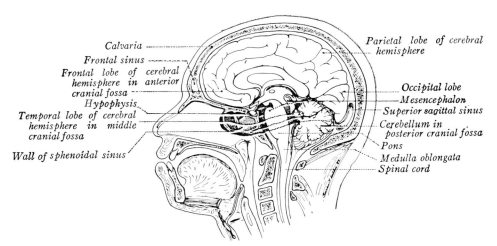

FIGURE 28. Median sagittal section of the head showing the relation of the brain to the cranium. The sphenoid bone is shown in transparency, and through it the temporal lobe may be seen.

neath the pterion. The external occipital protuberance is approximately superficial to the internal occipital protuberance; this is where the occipital poles of
the cerebral hemispheres are separated from the cerebellum by the tentorium
cerebelli, and further marks the location of the sinus confluens.

The brain rests upon the floor of the cranial cavity, which presents three
well marked fossae. In the posterior cranial fossa are lodged the medulla oblon-

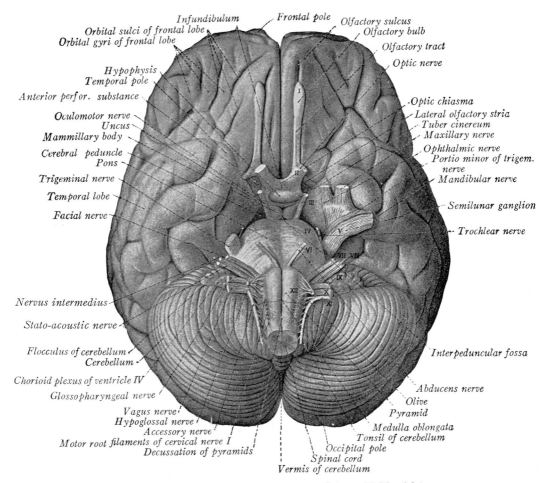

FIGURE 29.   Base of the human brain. (Sobotta-McMurrich.)

gata, pons, and cerebellum, which together constitute the rhombencephalon.
This fossa is roofed over by a partition of dura mater, called the *tentorium
cerebelli*, that separates the cerebellum from the cerebral hemispheres (Fig. 60).
Through the notch in the ventral border of the tentorium projects the mesencephalon, connecting the rhombencephalon below with the prosencephalon
above that partition. The cerebral hemispheres form the largest part of the

prosencephalon, occupy the anterior and middle cranial fossae, and extend to the occiput on the upper surface of the tentorium.

The **dorsal** or **convex aspect** of the human brain presents an ovoid figure. The large *cerebral hemispheres* cover the other parts from view. The cerebral hemispheres, which are separated by a deep cleft called the *longitudinal fissure of the cerebrum*, together present a broad convex surface which lies in close relation to the internal aspect of the calvaria. From the latter it is separated

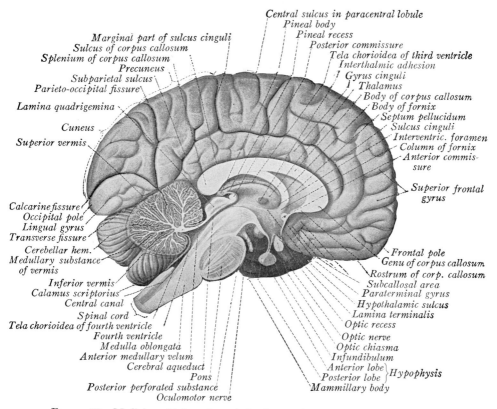

FIGURE 30. Medial sagittal section of the human brain. (Sobotta-McMurrich.)

only by the investing membranes or meninges of the brain. The thin convoluted layer of gray matter upon the surface of the hemispheres is known as the *cerebral cortex* and that on the surface of the cerebellum is known as the *cerebellar cortex*. So great is the folding of the surface that less than a third of the cerebral cortex is exposed, and only about one-sixth of the cerebellar cortex.

The **ventral aspect** or **base** of the brain presents an irregular surface adapted to the uneven floor of the cranial cavity (Figs. 29, 31). The *medulla oblongata*, which is continuous through the foramen magnum with the spinal cord, lies on the ventral aspect of the cerebellum in the vallecula between the two cerebellar hemispheres. Rostral to the medulla oblongata and separated from it only by a transverse groove is a broad elevated band of fibers, which plunges into the cerebellum on either side and is known as the *pons*. The *cerebellum* can be seen occupying a position dorsal to the pons and medulla oblongata, and can easily be recognized by its grayish color and many parallel fissures. A pair of large rope-like strands are seen to emerge from the rostral border of the pons

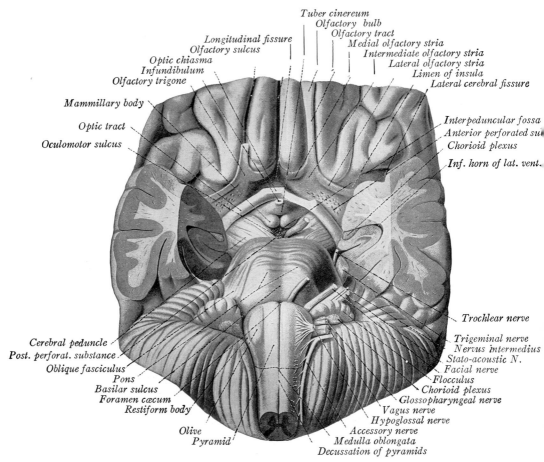

FIGURE 31. Ventral view of the human brain. The temporal lobes have been partly cut away. (Sobotta-McMurrich.)

and to diverge from each other as they run toward the under surface of the cerebral hemispheres. These are the *cerebral peduncles* and they form the ventral part of the mesencephalon. At its rostral extremity each peduncle is partially encircled by a flattened band, known as the *optic tract*, which is continuous through the *optic chiasma* with the optic nerves. A depression, known as the *interpeduncular fossa*, is outlined by the diverging cerebral peduncles and by the optic chiasma and tracts (Fig. 31). Within the area thus outlined and beginning at its caudal angle may be distinguished the following parts: the *posterior perforated substance,* the *mammillary bodies,* the *tuber cinereum,* and the *infundibulum.* Rostral to the optic tract there is on either side a triangular field of gray matter, studded with minute pit-like depressions and known as the *anterior perforated substance.* The perforations here and posteriorly are due to the penetration of small arteries reaching the interior of the cerebrum (p. 80). The olfactory bulb and tract belong to the rhinencephalon but lie in contact with the underside of the frontal part of the cerebral hemispheres. The tract is continuous with lateral and medial olfactory striae bordering the olfactory trigone adjacent to the anterior perforated substance.

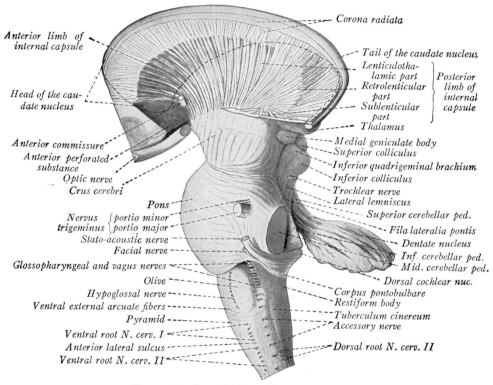

FIGURE 32. Lateral view of human brain stem.

Interrelation of the Various Parts of the Brain. An examination of a medial sagittal section of the brain will make clearer the relation which the various parts bear to each other (Fig. 30). The *medulla oblongata, pons,* and *cerebellum* are seen surrounding the fourth ventricle, and are intimately connected with one another. The medulla oblongata is directly continuous with the pons, and on either side a large bundle of fibers from the dorsal aspect of the former runs into the cerebellum. These two strands, which are known as the *restiform bodies* or *inferior cerebellar peduncles,* constitute the chief avenues of communication between the spinal cord and medulla oblongata on the one hand and the cerebellum on the other (Fig. 32). The ventral prominence of the pons is produced in large part by transverse bundles of fibers, which when traced lateralward are seen to form a large strand, the *brachium pontis* or *middle cerebellar peduncle*, that enters the corresponding cerebellar hemisphere (Figs. 29, 33). The *superior cerebellar peduncle* can be traced rostrally from the cerebellum to the mesencephalon. The three peduncles are paired structures, symmetrically placed on the two sides of the brain (Figs. 32, 33).

The *mesencephalon* surrounds the cerebral aqueduct and consists of the ventrally placed *cerebral peduncles,* and a dorsal plate with four rounded elevations, the *lamina* and *corpora quadrigemina* (superior and inferior colliculi).

The cerebral hemispheres form the most prominent part of the cerebrum and are separated from each other by the longitudinal fissure, at the bottom of which is a broad commissural band, the *corpus callosum,* which joins the two hemispheres together (Fig. 30). Under cover of the cerebral hemispheres and concealed by them, except on the ventral aspect of the brain, is the *diencephalon.* This includes most of the parts which help to form the walls of the third ventricle. These are from above downward, the *epithalamus,* including the habenular trigone and pineal body near the roof of the ventricle; the *thalamus,* which forms most of the lateral wall of the ventricle, and is commonly united with its fellow across the cavity by a short bar of gray substance, the interthalamic adhesion; and the *hypothalamus,* including the mammillary bodies, infundibulum, and part of the hypophysis (Fig. 30).

The Brain Ventricles. The *central canal* of the spinal cord is prolonged through the caudal portion of the medulla oblongata and finally opens out into the broad rhomboidal *fourth ventricle* of the rhombencephalon. At its pointed rostral extremity this ventricle is continuous with the *cerebral aqueduct,* the elongated slender cavity of the mesencephalon. This, in turn, opens into the *third ventricle,* which is a narrow vertical cleft between the two laterally symmetric halves of the diencephalon. It is bridged by the massa intermedia and communicates through a small opening in each lateral wall, the *interventricular foramen,* with the cavity of the cerebral hemisphere or *lateral ventricle.* The ventricles in life are filled with cerebrospinal fluid which also fills the subarachnoid space. Communication between this space and the cavity of the brain ventricles exists at the lateral apertures and the median aperture, in the walls and roof of the fourth ventricle. (Figs. 53, 55).

The **weight of the brain** varies with the sex, age, and size of the individual. The average weight of the brain in young adult men of medium stature is 1360 grams. It is less in women and in persons of small size or advanced age. It is doubtful if there is any close correlation between the brain weight and intelligence or between the latter and the size and arrangement of the cerebral convolutions. The accomplishments of man's nervous system as demonstrated in an elaborate civilization and its artifacts must depend not so much on the volume of the brain as on the facility of its action. The cranial capacity of primitive man is not appreciably different from that of civilized man.

THE ANATOMY OF THE MEDULLA OBLONGATA

At its rostral end the spinal cord increases in size and goes over without sharp line of demarcation into the medulla oblongata, or myelencephalon, which, as was stated earlier, is derived from the posterior part of the third brain vesicle. The medulla oblongata may be said to begin just rostral to the highest rootlet of the first cervical nerve at about the level of the foramen magnum; and at the opposite extremity it is separated from the pons by a horizontal groove (Figs. 28, 30). Its ventral surface rests upon the basilar portion of the occipital bone, while its dorsal surface is in large part covered by the cerebellum. The shape of the medulla oblongata is roughly that of a truncated cone, the smaller end of which is directed caudally and is continuous with the spinal cord. In man it measures about 3 cm., or a little more than 1 inch, in length (Fig. 29). Within this small mass are located central connections concerned with respiration, heart rate, etc., so essential to the life of the owner that a small lesion of any type in this area may be fatal.

Like the spinal cord, the medulla oblongata presents a number of more or less parallel longitudinal grooves. These are *the anterior and posterior median fissures,* and a pair each of *anterior lateral* and *posterior lateral sulci* (Figs. 29, 33). By means of the fissures it is divided symmetrically into right and left halves; these, in turn, are marked off by the sulci into *ventral, lateral,* and *dorsal areas,* which, as seen from the surface, appear to be the direct upward continuation of the anterior, lateral and posterior funiculi of the spinal cord. But this continuity is not as perfect as it appears from the surface; the tracts of the cord undergo a rearrangement as they enter the medulla oblongata. The posterior median fissure does not extend beyond the middle of the medulla, at which point its lips separate to help form the lateral boundaries of the fourth ventricle. The caudal half or *closed portion of the medulla oblongata* contains a canal, the direct continuation of the central canal of the spinal cord (Fig. 30). This canal opens into the fourth ventricle whose floor is formed in part by the rostral half or *open part of the medulla oblongata.*

Fissures and Sulci. The *posterior median fissure* represents the continuation of the posterior median sulcus of the spinal cord and, as noted above, ends near the middle of the medulla oblongata. The *anterior median fissure* is continued from the spinal cord to the border of the pons, where it ends abruptly in a pit known as the *foramen caecum.* Near the caudal extremity of the medulla oblongata this fissure is interrupted by interdigitating bundles of fibers which pass obliquely across the median plane. These are the fibers of the lateral corticospinal tract, which undergo a decussation on passing from the medulla oblongata into the spinal cord, known as the *decussation of the pyramids.* The *anterior lateral sulcus* also extends throughout the length of the medulla oblongata and represents the upward continuation of a much more indefinite groove bearing the same name in the spinal cord. From it emerge the root filaments of the hypoglossal nerve. From the *posterior lateral sulcus* emerge the rootlets of the glossopharyngeal, vagus, and accessory nerves (Figs. 31, 32).

The **ventral area of the medulla oblongata** is included between the anterior median fissure and the anterior lateral sulcus, and has the false appearance of being a direct continuation of the anterior funiculus of the spinal cord. On either side of the anterior median fissure there is an elongated eminence, tapering toward the spinal cord, and known as the *pyramid* (Fig. 29). It is formed by the fibers of the corticospinal or pyramidal tract. Just before the fibers of this tract enter the spinal cord, they undergo a more or less complete decussation, crossing the median plane in large obliquely interdigitating bundles, which fill up and almost obliterate the anterior median fissure in the caudal part of the medulla oblongata. This is known as the *decussation of the pyramids* (decussatio pyramidum). In the sheep these fibers pass into the opposite posterior funiculus of the spinal cord. In man the crossing is incomplete, a majority of the fibers descending into the lateral funiculus of the opposite side, a minority into the anterior funiculus of the same side (Fig. 271, 272). Being covered by other tracts in the spinal cord, they do not show on the surface but will be encountered as the *ventral* and *lateral corticospinal tracts* (direct and crossed pyramidal tracts).

The **lateral area of the medulla oblongata,** included between the anterolateral and posterolateral sulci, appears as a direct continuation of the lateral funiculus of the spinal cord; but, as a matter of fact, many of the fibers of that funiculus find their way into the anterior area (as, for example, the lateral corticospinal tract) or into the posterior area (dorsal spinocerebellar tract). In the rostral part of the lateral area, between the root filaments of the glossopharyngeal and vagus nerves, on the one hand, and those of the hypoglossal, on the other, is an oval eminence, the *olive* (oliva, olivary body), which is produced by a large irregular mass of gray substance, the inferior olivary nucleus, located just beneath the surface (Fig. 32). By a careful inspection of the surface of the medulla oblongata, it is possible to distinguish numerous fine bundles of fibers, which emerge from the anterior median fissure or from the groove between the pyramid and the olive and run dorsally upon the surface of the medulla to enter the restiform bodies. These are the *ventral external arcuate fibers* and are most conspicuous on the surface of the olive (Fig. 32).

The **dorsal area of the medulla oblongata** is bounded ventrally by the posterolateral sulcus and emergent root filaments of the glossopharyngeal, vagus, and accessory nerves. In the closed part of the medulla it extends to the posterior median fissure, while in the open part its dorsal boundary is formed by the lateral margin of the floor of the fourth ventricle. The caudal portion of this area is, in reality, as it appears, the direct continuation of the posterior funiculus of the spinal cord. On the dorsal aspect of the medulla oblongata the fasciculus cuneatus and fasciculus gracilis of the cord are continued as the *funiculus cuneatus* and *funiculus gracilis,* which soon enlarge into elongated eminences, known respectively as the *cuneate tubercle* and the *clava* (Fig. 33). These enlargements are produced by gray masses, the *nucleus gracilis* and *nucleus cuneatus,* within which end the fibers of the corresponding fasciculi of the spinal cord. The clava and cuneate tubercle are displaced laterally by the caudal angle of the fourth ventricle. Somewhat rostral to the middle of the medulla oblongata they gradually give place to the *restiform body.*

More laterally, between the cuneate funiculus and tubercle on the one hand and the roots of the glossopharyngeal, vagus, and accessory nerves on the other, is a third longitudinal club-shaped elevation called the *tuberculum cinereum.* It is produced by a tract of descending fibers, derived from the sensory root of the trigeminal nerve, and by an elongated mass of substantia gelatinosa which forms one of the nuclei of this nerve. This bundle of fibers and the associated mass of gray matter are known as the *spinal tract* and *nucleus of the spinal tract of the trigeminal nerve* (Fig. 304–312).

The **inferior cerebellar peduncle** lies between the lateral border of the fourth ventricle and the roots of the vagus and glossopharyngeal nerves in the rostral part of the medulla oblongata (Fig. 32, 33). There is no sharp line of demarcation between it and the more caudally placed clava and cuneate tubercle. It is produced by a large strand of nerve fibers, which runs along the lateral border of the fourth ventricle and then turns dorsally into the cerebellum. These fibers serve to connect the medulla oblongata and spinal cord on the one hand with the cerebellum on the other. By a careful inspection of the surface of the medulla it is possible to recognize the source of some of the fibers entering into the composition of the restiform body. The *ventral external arcuate fibers* can be seen entering it after crossing over the surface of the lateral area; and the *dorsal spinocerebellar* tract can also be traced into it from a position dorsal to the caudal extremity of the olive.

At the point where the restiform body begins to turn dorsally toward the cerebellum, it is partly encircled by an elongated transversely placed elevation formed by the *ventral and dorsal cochlear nuclei* (Fig. 32). This ridge is continuous with the cochlear nerve. Just caudal to this ridge there is sometimes seen another, running more obliquely across the restiform body, which is an outlying portion of the pons and has been described under the name *corpus pontobulbare* (Fig. 32).

Nerve Roots.   From the surface of the medulla oblongata there emerges in roughly linear order along the posterior lateral sulcus a series of root filaments, which continues the line of the dorsal roots of the spinal nerves. These are the rootlets of the *glossopharyngeal, vagus,* and *accessory nerves.* Unlike the dorsal roots, which are made up of afferent fibers, the spinal accessory nerve contains efferent fibers, while the vagus and glossopharyngeal are mixed nerves. The line of the ventral or motor roots of the spinal nerves is continued in the medulla oblongata by the root filaments of the *hypoglossal nerve,* which is also composed of motor fibers. The *abducens, facial,* and *stato-acoustic nerves* make their exit along the caudal border of the pons in the order named from within outward. The abducens emerges between the pons and the pyramid, the acoustic far lateralward in line with the restiform body, and the facial with its sensory root, the *nervus intermedius,* near the stato-acoustic nerve (Figs. 31, 32).

THE ANATOMY OF THE PONS

The pons, which forms the ventral part of the metencephalon, is interposed between the medulla oblongata and the cerebral peduncles and lies ventral to the cerebellum. As seen from the ventral surface, it is formed by a broad transverse band of nerve fibers, which on either side become aggregated into a large rounded strand, the *middle cerebellar peduncle,* and finally enter the corresponding hemisphere of the cerebellum (Figs. 31, 32). This transverse band of fibers, which gives the bridge-like form from which this part derives its name, belongs to the *basilar portion of the pons* and is superimposed upon a deeper *dorsal portion* that may be regarded as a direct upward continuation of the medulla oblongata. The transverse fibers form a part of the pathway connecting the cerebral hemispheres with the opposite cerebellar hemispheres; and the size of the pons, therefore, varies with the size of these other structures. It is instructive to compare the brains of the shark, sheep, and man with this point in mind (Figs. 10, 30, 419).

The **ventral surface of the pons** is convex from above downward and from side to side and rests upon the basilar portion of the occipital bone and upon the dorsum sellae (Fig. 28). A groove along the median line, the *basilar sulcus*, lodges the basilar artery (Figs. 29, 65).

The *trigeminal nerve* emerges from the ventral surface of the pons far lateralward at the point where its constituent transverse fibers are converging to form the brachium pontis. In fact, it is customary to take the exit of this nerve as marking the point of junction of the pons with its brachium. The nerve has two roots which lie close together: the larger is the *sensory root*, or portio major; the smaller is the *motor root*, or portio minor (Fig. 32).

The **posterior surface of the pons** forms the rostral part of the floor of the fourth ventricle, along the lateral borders of which there are two prominent and rather large strands of nerve fibers, the superior cerebellar peduncle (Figs. 32, 33).

The **superior cerebellar peduncles** lie under cover of the cerebellum. As they emerge from the white centers of the cerebellar hemispheres, they curve rostrally and take up positions along the lateral borders of the fourth ventricle. They converge as they ascend and disappear from view by sinking into the substance of the mesencephalon under cover of the inferior quadrigeminal bodies. Each consists of fibers which connect the cerebellum with the *red nucleus,* a large gray mass situated within the midbrain ventral to the cerebral aqueduct at the level of the superior colliculus of the corpora quadrigemina. The interval between the two superior cerebellar peduncles, where these form the lateral boundaries of the fourth ventricle, is bridged by a thin lamina of white matter, the *anterior medullary velum* (Figs. 30, 33). This is stretched between the free dorsomedial borders of the two peduncles and forms the roof of the rostral portion of the ventricle. Caudally it is continuous with the white center of the cerebellum. The fibers of the *trochlear nerves* decussate in the anterior medullary velum and emerge from its dorsal surface (Fig. 33). As they run through the velum they produce a raised white line which extends transversely from one peduncle to the other.

THE FOURTH VENTRICLE

The diamond-shaped cavity of the rhombencephalon is known as the fourth ventricle. It lies between the pons and medulla oblongata ventrally, and the cerebellum dorsally, and is continuous with the central canal of the closed portion of the medulla, on the one hand, and with the cerebral aqueduct on the other (Fig. 30). On each side a narrow curved prolongation of the cavity extends laterally on the dorsal surface of the restiform body. This is known as the *lateral recess* (Fig. 33). It opens into the subarachnoid space near the flocculus of the cerebellum; and through this *lateral aperture* of the fourth ventricle (foramen of Luschka) protrudes a small portion of the chorioid plexus (Figs. 31, 34). There is also a median aperture (foramen of Magendie) through the roof of the ventricle near the caudal extremity. By means of these three openings, one medial and two lateral, the cavity of the ventricle is in communication with the subarachnoid space, and cerebrospinal fluid may escape from the former into the latter.

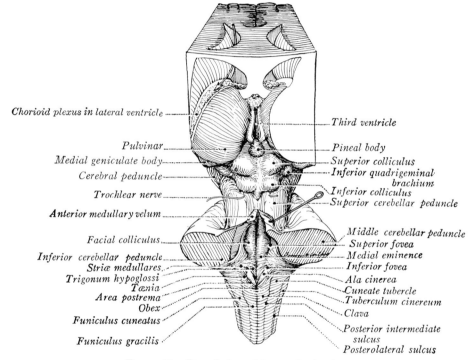

Chorioid plexus in lateral ventricle

Pulvinar
Medial geniculate body
Cerebral peduncle
Trochlear nerve
Anterior medullary velum

Facial colliculus
Inferior cerebellar peduncle
Striæ medullares
Trigonum hypoglossi
Tænia
Area postrema
Obex
Funiculus cuneatus
Funiculus gracilis

Third ventricle

Pineal body
Superior colliculus
Inferior quadrigeminal brachium
Inferior colliculus
Superior cerebellar peduncle

Middle cerebellar peduncle
Superior fovea
Medial eminence
Inferior fovea
Ala cinerea
Cuneate tubercle
Tuberculum cinereum
Clava
Posterior intermediate sulcus
Posterolateral sulcus

FIGURE 33. Dorsal view of human brain stem.

The **floor of the fourth ventricle** is known as the *rhomboid fossa* and is formed by the dorsal surfaces of the pons and open part of the medulla oblongata, which are continuous with each other without any line of demarcation and are irregularly concave from side to side (Fig. 34). The small markings on the floor of the fourth ventricle are valuable aids in the localization of several cranial nerve nuclei which lie beneath them. The fossa is widest opposite the points where the restiform bodies turn dorsally into the cerebellum; and it gradually narrows toward its rostral and caudal angles. The *lateral boundaries* of the fossa, which are raised some distance above the level of the floor, are formed by the following structures: the *brachia conjunctiva, restiform bodies, cuneate tubercles,* and *clavae.* Of the four angles to the rhomboid fossa, two are laterally placed and correspond to the lateral recesses. At its caudal angle the ventricle is continuous with the central canal of the closed part of the medulla oblongata, and at its rostral angle with the cerebral aqueduct. Joining the two last named angles there is a median sulcus which divides the fossa into two symmetric lateral halves.

Lateral to the median sulcus is a shallower groove, the *sulcus limitans,* which is not as straight and which possesses two deeper portions called the superior and inferior foveae.

The rhomboid fossa is arbitrarily divided into three parts. The *superior part* is triangular, with its apex directed rostrally and its base along an imaginary line through the superior fovea. The *inferior part* is also triangular, but with its apex directed caudally and its base at the level of the horizontal portions of the taeniae of the ventricle. Between these two triangular portions is the *intermediate part* of the fossa, which is prolonged outward into the lateral recesses. The floor is covered with a thin lamina of gray matter continuous with that which lines the central canal and cerebral aqueduct. Crossing the fossa transversely in its intermediate portion are several strands of fibers known as the *striae medullares.* These are subject to considerable variation in different specimens. It is said that they run to the cerebellum (Alphin and Barnes, 1944).

The *inferior portion* of the fossa bears some resemblance to the point of a pen and was called the *calamus scriptorius* by ancient anatomists. In this part of the fossa there is on either side a small depression, the *inferior fovea.* From this point run two diverging sulci; a medial groove toward the opening of the central canal and a lateral groove more nearly parallel to the median sulcus. By these sulci the inferior portion of the fossa is divided into three triangular areas. Of these the most medial is called the *trigone of the hypoglossal nerve* or *trigonum nervi hypoglossi.* Beneath the medial part of this slightly elevated area is located the nucleus of the hypoglossal nerve. The area between the two sulci, which diverge from the fovea inferior, is the *ala cinerea* or triangle of the vagus nerve. The third triangular field, placed more laterally, forms a part of the *vestibular area.*

The vestibular area is, however, not restricted to the inferior portion of the fossa, but extends into the *intermediate part* as well. Here it forms a prominent elevation over which the striae medullares run. Subjacent to this area lie the nuclei of the vestibular nerve. A part of the acoustic area and all of the ventricular floor rostral to it belong to the pons.

Rostral to the striae medullares there may be seen a shallow depression in the sulcus limitans, the *fovea superior,* medial to which there is a rounded elevation, the *facial colliculus.* Under cover of this eminence the fibers of the facial nerve bend around the abducens nucleus. Extending from the fovea superior to the cerebral aqueduct is a shallow groove, usually faint blue in color, the *locus caeruleus,* beneath which lies a nucleus, composed of pigmented nerve cells.

Beginning at the cerebral aqueduct and extending through both the superior and inferior foveae is the *sulcus limitans,* which represents the line of separation between the parts derived from the alar plate and those which originate from the basal plate of the embryonic rhombencephalon. Lateral to this sulcus lie the sensory areas of the ventricular floor, including the area acustica, all of which are derived from the alar plate. Medial to this sulcus there is a prominent longitudinal elevation, known as the *medial eminence* which includes two structures already described, namely, the facial colliculus and the trigone of the hypoglossal nerve. Beneath the medial part of this trigone lies the *nucleus of the hypoglossal nerve* and beneath the lateral part is a group of cells designated as the *nucleus intercalatus.*

One or two features remain to be mentioned. At the caudal end of the ala cinerea is a narrow translucent obliquely placed ridge of thickened ependyma,

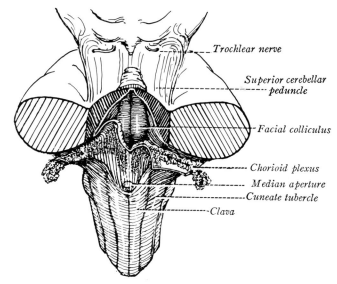

FIGURE 34. Dorsal view of human rhombencephalon showing tela chorioidea and chorioid plexus of the fourth ventricle.

known as the *funiculus separans.* Between this ridge and the clava is a small strip, called the *area postrema,* which on microscopic examination is found to be rich in blood vessels, neuroglial tissue, and nerve fibers. It has been considered to be a kind of neurovegetative nucleus, but whether it has a nervous or an endocrine function is not known (Cammermeyer, 1947).

The **roof of the fourth ventricle** is formed by the *anterior medullary velum,* a small part of the *white substance of the cerebellum,* and by the *tela chorioidea* lined internally by *ependymal epithelium* (Fig. 30). Caudal to the cerebellum the true roof of the cavity is very thin and consists only of a layer of ependymal epithelium, which is continuous with that lining the other walls of the ventricle. This is supported on its outer surface by a layer of pia mater, the *tela chorioidea,* rich in blood vessels. From this layer vascular tufts, covered by epithelium, are invaginated into the cavity and form the *chorioid plexus* of the fourth ventricle (Fig. 34). The plexus is invaginated along two vertical lines close to the median plane and along two horizontal lines, which diverge at right angles from the vertical ones and run toward the lateral recesses. These right and left halves are joined together at the angles so that the entire plexus has the shape of the letter T, the vertical limb of which, however, is double.

After the tela chorioidea with its epithelial lining has been torn away to expose the floor of the ventricle, there remains attached to the lateral boundaries of the caudal part of the cavity the torn edges of this portion of the roof. These appear as lines, the *taeniae of the fourth ventricle,* which meet over the caudal angle of the cavity in a thin triangular lamina, the *obex* (Fig. 33). Rostrally each taenia turns lateralward over the restiform body and forms the caudal boundary of the corresponding lateral recess.

The *anterior medullary velum* is stretched between the dorsomedial borders of the two superior cerebellar peduncles (brachia conjunctiva) and extends from the white center of the cerebellum to the lamina quadrigemina (Figs. 30, 33). Adherent to its dorsal surface is a thin tongue-shaped lobule of the cerebellum, gray in color, known as the *lingula* (Fig. 348).

THE MESENCEPHALON

The *midbrain* or mesencephalon occupies the notch in the tentorium and connects the rhombencephalon, on the one side of that shelf-like process of dura, with the prosencephalon on the other (Fig. 30). It consists of a dorsal part, the *lamina* and *corpora quadrigemina,* and a larger ventral portion, the cerebral *peduncles.* It is tunneled by a canal of relatively small caliber, called the cerebral aqueduct, which connects the third and fourth ventricles and is placed nearer the dorsal than the ventral aspect of the midbrain (Figs. 30, 168).

The **cerebral peduncles** (pedunculi cerebri, crura cerebri), as seen on the ventral aspect of the brain, diverge like a pair of legs from the rostral border of the pons (Fig. 31). Just before they disappear from view by entering the ventral surface of the prosencephalon they enclose between them parts of the hypothalamus, and are encircled by the optic tracts (Fig. 31). On section, each peduncle is seen to be composed of a dorsal part, the *tegmentum,* and a ventral part, the *basis pedunculi.* Between the basis pedunculi and the tegmentum there intervenes a strip of darker color, the *substantia nigra* (Fig. 168). By dissection it is easy to show that the basis pedunculi is composed of longitudinally coursing fibers which can be traced rostrally to the internal capsule (Fig. 32). In the other direction some of these fibers can be followed into the corresponding pyramid of the medulla oblongata. On the surface two longitudinal sulci mark the plane of separation between the tegmentum and the basis pedunculi. The groove on the medial aspect of the peduncle, through which emerge the fibers of the third nerve, is known as the *sulcus of the oculomotor nerve,* while that on the lateral aspect is called the *lateral sulcus* of the mesencephalon. Dorsal to this latter groove the tegmentum comes to the surface and is faintly marked by fine bundles of fibers which curve dorsally toward the inferior colliculus of the corpora quadrigemina (Fig. 32). These fibers belong to the lateral lemniscus, the central tract associated with the cochlear nerve.

The **corpora quadrigemina** form the dorsal portion of the mesencephalon, and consist of four rounded eminences, the quadrigeminal bodies or *colliculi,* which arise from the dorsal aspect of a plate of mingled gray and white matter known as the *quadrigeminal lamina* (Fig. 33). A median longitudinal groove separates the right and left colliculi. In the rostral end of this groove rests the *pineal body,* while attached to its caudal end is a band which runs to the anterior medullary velum, and is known as the *frenulum veli.* A transverse groove runs between the superior and inferior colliculi and extends onto the lateral aspect of the mesencephalon, where it intervenes between the superior colliculus and the inferior quadrigeminal brachium (Fig. 33).

From each colliculus there runs laterally an arm or brachium (Fig. 41). The *inferior quadrigeminal brachium* is the more conspicuous. It runs from the inferior colliculus to the *medial geniculate body,* an oval eminence belonging to the diencephalon, which has been displaced caudally so as to lie on the lateral aspect of the mesencephalon. The *superior quadrigeminal brachium* runs from the superior colliculus toward the *lateral geniculate body,* passing between the pulvinar of the thalamus and the medial geniculate body. The bundle can be shown to connect with the optic tract beyond the lateral geniculate body.

THE CEREBELLUM

The Anatomy of the Cerebellum. The cerebellum is developed from the dorsal aspect of the metencephalon and lies as one of the three major supra-segmental structures above the main axis of the central nervous system, a little out of the direct line, but well connected. Its size and appearance in different animal species can be matched roughly by stages in the development of the human cerebellum (Fig. 35). In animals with simple movements, such as the lamprey which only wiggles or the frog which hops, and in which the center of gravity of the individual is never far from its base of support, the cerebellum is small. In higher animals with more elaborate movements of trunk and limbs and a center of gravity not so close to the base of support, the cerebellum is appropriately more elaborate. Knowledge of the relation of separate parts of the cerebellum to the muscular activity of separate bodily parts has been gained largely through a study of comparative series. Midline portions of the cerebellum developed in those animals with movements that are largely bilaterally symmetrical, as in birds in flight. In animals in which individual movements of limbs become elaborate, the lateral portions of the cerebellum become more prominent. Phylogenetically older parts of the cerebellum are termed paleocerebellum, and the more recent developments neocerebellum. It is customary to consider the cerebellum as composed of three parts: a small unpaired median portion, called the *vermis,* because superficially it resembles a worm bent on itself to form almost a complete circle; and two large lateral masses, the *cerebellar hemispheres.* On the dorsal surface of the cerebellum the vermis (Fig. 36) forms a median ridge, not sharply marked off laterally from the hemispheres. This part has been called the *superior vermis,* and in contradistinction the remainder is known as the *inferior vermis.* The latter forms a prominent ridge and lies in a deep groove between the hemispheres on the ventral surface of the cerebellum (Figs. 37–39). The cerebellar cortex is folded to form long slender convolutions or *folia* separated by parallel sulci.

As in other portions of the nervous system, names have been applied to parts of the cerebellum because of their external appearance rather than from an understanding of function. More recent terminology has been applied to comparable parts of the cerebella of different species of animals in the hope of simplification.

A fundamental plan of the mammalian cerebellum is recognizable from comparative studies and especially from the viewpoint of the embryology, where similar patterns can be seen at early stages (Larsell, 1952, 1953, 1954), when the folding is simpler. Of the various fissures that subdivide the cerebellum, some

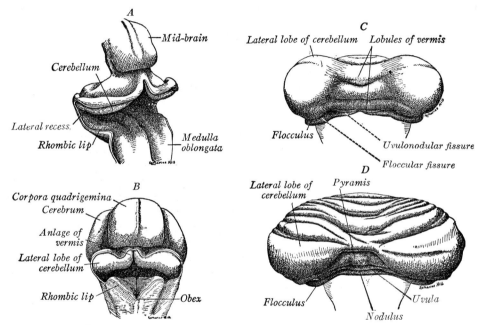

FIGURE 35. Dorsal view of four stages in the development of the cerebellum: *A*, of a 13.6 mm. embryo (His); *B*, of a 24 mm. embryo; *C*, of a 110 mm. fetus; *D*, of a 150 mm. fetus. (Prentiss and Arey.)

are especially significant. The *posterolateral fissure* separates the more caudal *flocculonodular* lobe, having heavy vestibular connections, from the *corpus cerebelli*, which constitutes the main bulk of the cerebellum. The flocculonodular lobe belongs to paleocerebellum, while the corpus cerebelli has both paleo- and neocerebellar origin.

As its name implies, the flocculonodular lobe includes the two flocculi laterally connected by a peduncle with the nodulus medially. In man the flocculi are small irregular lobules situated on the inferior surface of the hemisphere close to the brachia pontis (Fig. 37).

The corpus cerebelli is divided by the *primary fissure* into an anterior and a posterior lobe. The *anterior lobe* includes all that part of the cerebellum that lies on the rostral side of the primary fissure (Fig. 36). In this lobe the folia have a transverse direction and extend without interruption across the vermis into both hemispheres. It includes the three most rostral lobules of the superior vermis, which are designated in order from before backward, the *lingula, lobulus centralis* and *culmen*. In man it also includes a large wing-shaped portion of each hemisphere.

The *posterior lobe* includes that part of the cerebellum between the primary fissure and the posterolateral fissure, and it shows certain subdivisions. The most rostral portion is the *lobulus simplex* or simple lobule, which is separated from the anterior lobe by the primary fissure, and like that lobe it consists of transverse folia which extend across the superior vermis into both hemispheres (Figs. 36, 39). In man the simple lobule and its neighbor across the primary fissure

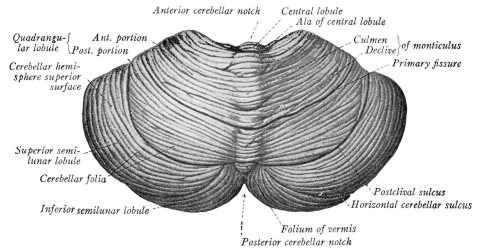

FIGURE 36. Superior view of the human cerebellum. (Modified from Sobotta-McMurrich.)

have in the past been called together the *quadrangular lobule*, but from a comparative anatomical view it seems more reasonable to refer to these divisions as *anterior* and *posterior semilunar lobules*. The remainder of the neocerebellar part of the posterior lobe is subdivided into median and paired lateral portions. The median part from before backwards includes *folium* and *tuber* of the neocerebellum, and *pyramis* and *uvula* of the paleocerebellum. Paired lateral parts associated with the folium and tuber are the neocerebellar *ansiform* and *paramedian* lobules, of which the ansiform contributes the greatest bulk to the cerebellar hemispheres. Associated with the pyramis and uvula laterally are the *parafloculi* which are also paleocerebellar, and incidentally are rudimentary in man, though they are highly developed in aquatic mammals.

The folium and tuber vermis may be identified in man at the occipital extremity of the inferior vermis. The ansiform lobule in man is continuous around the posterior border from the superior surface of the hemisphere (where it is known as the *superior semilunar lobule*) to the inferior surface (*inferior*

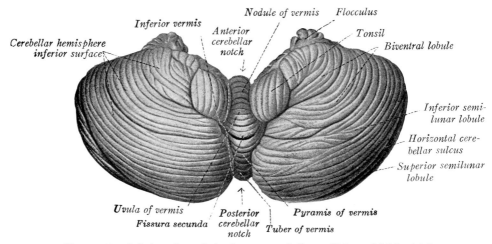

FIGURE 37. Inferior view of the human cerebellum. (Sobotta-McMurrich.)

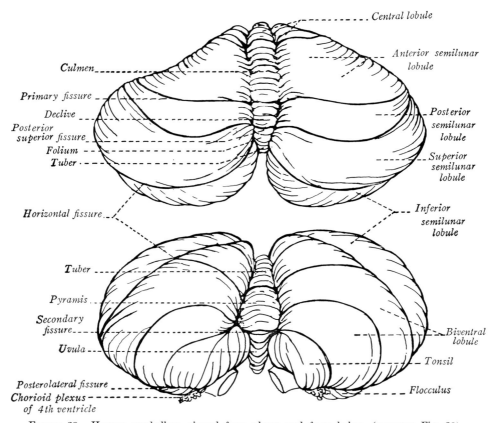

FIGURE 38. Human cerebellum viewed from above and from below (compare Fig. 39).

semilunar lobule, Figs. 36 to 39). These are referred to in comparative anatomy as *Crus I* and *Crus II* of the ansiform lobule.

The paramedian lobule, for which homology with that of lower forms is not entirely clear though it apparently includes the tonsil and at least part of the biventral lobule of old terminology, is found in the caudal surface in man, behind the greatly expanded lobulus ansiformis.

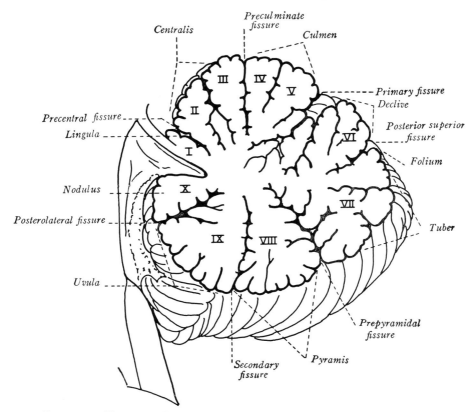

FIGURE 39. Human cerebellum, sagittal view. Numbering follows Larsell's plan.

It has long been known that the *degree of development of the cerebellar hemispheres* in the different classes of vertebrates is closely correlated with that of the pons and cerebral cortex. This is particularly true of the ansiform and paramedian lobules, which, like the neopallium, are recent phyletic developments, i.e., belong to the neocerebellum.

THE DIENCEPHALON

Development. In an earlier chapter we traced briefly the development of the prosencephalon and showed that the cerebral hemispheres were developed through the evagination of the lateral walls of the telencephalon (Fig. 16). It is, however, only the alar lamina which is involved in this evagination. It has been shown that the basal lamina and sulcus limitans do not extend into the prosencephalon, which is formed entirely from the alar plates (Schulte and Tilney, 1915; Kingsbury, 1922). The floor of the neural tube in this region is formed by the union of these plates across the median plane. Through the excessive growth of the hemisphere the diencephalon becomes covered from view (Fig. 17), and appears to occupy a central position in the adult human brain. It is separated from the hemisphere by the *transverse cerebral fissure*, which is formed by the folding back of the hemisphere over the diencephalon. The roof of the prosencephalon remains thin and constitutes the epithelial roof of the third ventricle, which along the median plane becomes invaginated into the ventricle as the covering of a vascular network to form the chorioid plexus.

There is but one pair of nerves associated with the diencephalon, and these, the optic nerves, are not true nerves, but fiber tracts joining the retinae with the brain. It will be remembered that the retina develops as an evagination of the lateral wall of the prosencephalon in the form of a vesicle whose cavity is continuous with that of the forebrain. By a folding of its walls in the reverse direction, i.e., by invagination, the *optic vesicle* becomes transformed into the *optic cup* (Fig. 13); and the cavity of the vesicle becomes reduced to a mere slit between the two layers forming the wall of the cup. The inner of these two layers develops into the nervous portion of the retina, and nerve fibers arising in it grow back to the brain along the course of the *optic stalk*, which still connects the optic cup with the forebrain. This mode of development serves to explain why the structure of the retina resembles that of the brain more than it does that of other sense organs, and why the optic nerve fibers, like those of the fiber tracts of the central nervous system, are devoid of neurilemma sheaths.

The *diencephalon* which encloses the third ventricle is composed of the following parts: (1) epithalamus, (2) thalamus, including the geniculate bodies, termed metathalamus, (3) subthalamus or ventral thalamus, and (4) hypothalamus.

THE THIRD VENTRICLE

Since the third ventricle is chiefly surrounded by structures belonging to the diencephalon, it will be convenient to consider it at this point and to give at the same time an account of the *parts of the telencephalon* which help to form its walls. These include the lamina terminalis and anterior commissure (Fig. 40). The *lamina terminalis* is a thin plate joining the two hemispheres, which stretches from the optic chiasma in a dorsal direction to the anterior commissure. Here it becomes continuous with the thin edge of the rostrum of the corpus callosum, known as the *rostral lamina*. The *anterior commissure* is a bundle of fibers which crosses the median plane in the lamina terminalis and serves to connect certain parts of the two cerebral hemispheres, which are associated with the olfactory nerves. The anterior commissure and the lamina terminalis form the *rostral boundary* of the third ventricle, and between the latter and the optic chiasma is a diverticulum, known as the optic recess.

The *third ventricle* is a narrow vertical cleft. The *lateral walls* are formed

for the greater part by the medial surfaces of the two thalami which are usually
fused across the middle portion forming the interthalamic adhesion (massa
intermedia). Ventral to the interthalamic adhesion is seen a groove known as the
hypothalamic sulcus, which if followed rostrally leads to the interventricular
foramen, while in the other direction it can be traced to the cerebral aqueduct.
Below this groove the lateral wall and floor of the ventricle are formed by the
subthalamus and hypothalamus.

In the *floor* of the ventricle there may be enumerated the following structures, beginning at the rostral end: the optic chiasma, infundibulum, tuber
cinereum, mammillary bodies, and the subthalamus.

The *roof* of the third ventricle is formed by the thin layer of *ependyma,*
which is stretched between the striae medullares thalami of the two sides (Figs.
40, 42). Upon the outer surface of this ependymal roof is a fold of pia mater
in the transverse fissure. This is known as the *tela chorioidea;* and from it delicate vascular folds are invaginated into the ventricle, carrying a layer of
ependyma before them by which they are, in reality, excluded from the cavity.
These folds are the *chorioid plexuses* (Figs. 41, 42). There are two of them
extending side by side from the interventricular foramina to the caudal extremity
of the roof. Here they extend into an evagination of the roof above the pineal
body, known as the suprapineal recess.

There are three openings into the third ventricle. The aqueduct of the cerebrum opens into it at the caudal end; while at the opposite extremity it communicates with the lateral ventricles through the two interventricular foramina.

THE THALAMUS

The thalamus is a large ovoid mass, consisting chiefly of gray matter,
placed obliquely across the rostral end of the cerebral peduncle (Figs. 40, 42).
Between the two thalami a deep median cleft is formed by the third ventricle.
The *rostral or anterior end* is small and lies close to the median plane. It projects
slightly above the rest of the dorsal surface, forming the *anterior tubercle* of
the thalamus, and helps to bound the interventricular foramen (Fig. 40). The
caudal or posterior extremity is larger and is separated from its fellow by a
wide interval, in which the corpora quadrigemina appear. It forms a marked
projection, the *pulvinar,* which overhangs the medial geniculate body and the
brachia of the corpora quadrigemina. For purposes of description it is convenient to recognize four thalamic surfaces, namely, dorsal, ventral, medial, and
lateral.

The **dorsal surface** of the thalamus is free and directed upward (Fig. 41).
It forms the floor of the transverse fissure of the cerebrum and is separated by
this fissure from the parts of the cerebral hemisphere which overlie it, that is,
from the fornix and corpus callosum. *Laterally* it is bounded by a groove which
separates it from the caudate nucleus and which contains a strand of longitudinal fibers, the *stria terminalis* and a vein, the *vena terminalis* (Figs. 41,
42). The dorsal surface is separated from the medial by a sharp ridge, the *taenia
thalami,* which represents the torn edge of the ependymal roof of the third
ventricle. The taeniae of the two sides meet on the stalk of the pineal body.

The prominence of this torn edge of the roof is increased by a longitudinal bundle of fibers, the *stria medullaris thalami*. This fascicle, together with the closely related habenular trigone and the pineal body, belongs to the epithalamus and will be described later.

The *dorsal surface* of the thalamus is slightly convex and is divided by a faint groove into two parts: a lateral area, covered by the *lamina affixa* and forming a part of the floor of the lateral ventricle; and a larger medial area, which forms the floor of the transverse fissure of the cerebrum. The oblique groove separating these two areas corresponds to the lateral border of the fornix

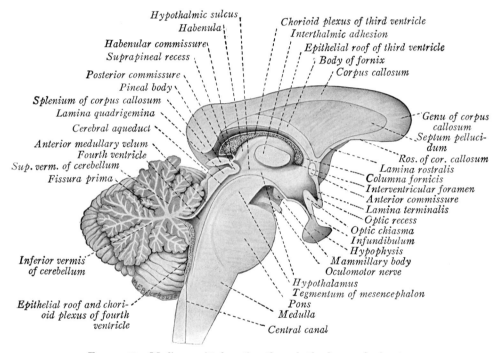

FIGURE 40.   Median sagittal section through the human brain stem.

(Figs. 41, 42). The lamina affixa is part of the ependymal lining of the lateral ventricle superimposed upon this part of the thalamus. Along its medial edge is the *taenia chorioidea*, where the epithelium of the chorioid plexus is continuous with the ventricular ependymal lining. The transverse fissure intervenes between the thalamus and the cerebral hemisphere. It contains a fold of pia mater, known as the *tela chorioidea*, bearing as it does the chorioid plexus of the third ventricle in the midline and the chorioid plexuses of the lateral ventricles along its edges (Figs. 40, 42, 58).

The **medial surface** of the thalamus is covered by the ependyma and forms the lateral wall of the third ventricle (Fig. 40). As the ventricle is a narrow cleft, the medial surfaces of the two thalami are closely approximated, and are united across the median plane by a short bar of gray substance, the interthalamic adhesion, which represents a secondary fusion during growth and is absent in about 20 per cent of cases.

Occasionally, but not very often, an additional small band of gray matter stretches across the third ventricle from one wall to the other (Vonderahe, 1937).

The **lateral surface** of the thalamus is hidden from view. It lies against the broad band of fibers, known as the internal capsule, which connects the cerebral

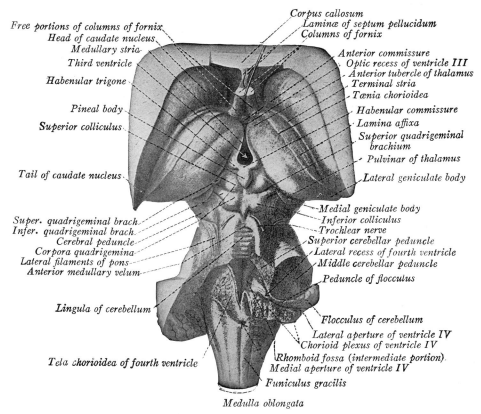

FIGURE 41.   Dorsal view of the human brain stem.   (Sobotta-McMurrich.)

hemispheres with the lower levels of the central nervous system. This surface is best examined in sections through the entire cerebrum (Figs. 42, 206, 207, 226). Many fibers stream out of the thalamus through its lateral surface and enter the internal capsule, through which they reach the cerebral cortex. To this important stream of fibers the name *thalamic radiation* is applied.

The **ventral surface** of the thalamus is directed downward and lies on the subthalamus and the tegmentum of the mesencephalon (Figs. 42, 206, 207, 217, 218, 222, 223). Many fibers, representing such ascending tegmental paths as the medial lemniscus, spinothalamic tract, and brachium conjunctivum, enter the thalamus through this surface. A part of this ventral surface is formed by the

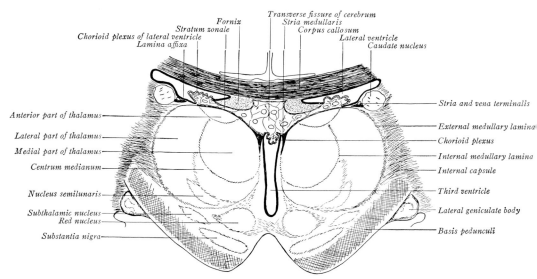

FIGURE 42. Diagrammatic frontal section through the human thalamus and the structures which immediately surround it.

medial and lateral geniculate bodies. They lie lateral to the rostral end of the mesencephalon (Fig. 400).

THE EXTERNAL CONFIGURATION OF THE CEREBRAL HEMISPHERES

Development. The *cerebral hemispheres* are formed by the evagination of the lateral walls of the telencephalon, the rest of which remains as the boundary of the rostral part of the third ventricle, and is known as the *telencephalon medium.* The cavities of the evaginated portions are known as the *lateral ventricles* and communicate with the third ventricle by way of the interventricular foramina (Figs. 13, 16, 17). Each of the cerebral hemispheres consists of two ventrally placed portions, the *rhinencephalon* or olfactory lobe and the *corpus striatum,* and a third part, more extensive than the others, the *pallium* or primitive cerebral cortex. The pallium expands more rapidly than the other parts, both rostrally and caudally, and comes to overlie the diencephalon, from which it is separated by the transverse fissure (Fig. 17). The fold of pia mater which is inclosed within this fissure is known as the *tela chorioidea;* from it a vascular plexus grows into the lateral ventricle through the thin portion of the medial wall of the hemisphere, where this is attached to the diencephalon. This forms the *chorioid plexus* of the lateral ventricle and carries before it an epithelial covering from the ependymal lining, by which it is, in reality, excluded from the ventricular cavity. This invagination of the medial wall of the hemisphere produces the *chorioid fissure.* Ventrally the thickened part of the hemisphere, known as the *corpus striatum,* remains in uninterrupted continuity with the thalamus.

At first the *cerebral hemisphere* has a relatively large cavity and thin walls. As the pallium and ventricle enlarge they become bent around the thalamus and corpus striatum (Fig. 17). The hemisphere becomes bean-shaped and expands rostrally to form the *frontal lobe,* caudally to form the *occipital lobe,* and ventrolaterally to form the *temporal lobe* (Fig. 43). Into each of these there is carried a prolongation of the lateral ventricle forming respectively the *anterior, posterior,* and *inferior horns.* Between the temporal and frontal lobes a deep fossa appears, which is the forerunner of the lateral fissure. At the bottom of this fossa is the *insula,* a portion of the cortex which overlies the corpus striatum and develops more slowly than the surrounding areas (labeled lateral fissure, Fig. 43). Folds from the surrounding cortex close in over the insula, burying it from sight in the adult brain. These folds are known as the *opercula,* and the deep cleft which separates them as the *lateral fissure.*

Development of the Cerebral Cortex. At first the pallium, like other parts of the neural tube, consists of three primitive zones: the ependymal, mantle, and marginal layers. But during the third month neuroblasts migrate outward from the ependymal and mantle layers into the marginal zone and there give rise to a superficial layer of gray matter—the cerebral cortex. Nerve fibers from these neuroblasts and others growing into the hemisphere from the thalamus accumulate on the deep surface of the developing cortex and form the white medullary substance of the hemisphere. As the brain increases in size the area of the cortex expands out of proportion to the increase in volume of the white medullary layer upon which it rests, and is thrown into folds or gyri separated by fissures or sulci. All the larger mammalian brains present well developed gyri, while the smaller brains are smooth; it would thus appear that the size of the brain is an important factor in determining the amount of folding that occurs in the cortex.

The cortex does not differentiate in exactly the same manner throughout, but may be subdivided into structurally and functionally distinct areas. The sulci develop in more or less definite relation to these areas, some making their appearance along the boundary lines between them. These are known as *terminal sulci,* of which the rhinal fissure and central sulcus are examples. Sometimes the folding occurs entirely within such an area, i.e., along its axis. There are still others in which the relation to these functional areas is not so evident. The arrangement of the fissures and sulci in a seven months' fetus is shown in Fig. 43.

Development of the Septum and Commissures. The two hemispheres are connected by the *lamina terminalis,* which serves as a bridge for fibers which cross from one hemisphere to the other. These form three important bundles: the *anterior commissure,* the *commissure of the fornix,* and the *corpus callosum.* The two former connect the olfactory portions of the hemispheres, while the latter is the great commissure of the non-olfactory cortex or neopallium.

Everyone admits that the anterior commissure develops in the lamina terminalis (Fig. 44); and the corpus callosum and commissure of the fornix (hippocampal commissures) are said to form in its dorsal part (Streeter, 1912). According to this account the lamina terminalis becomes stretched by the great development of the corpus callosum and appropriates part of the paraterminal body. This is the portion of the rhinencephalon that lies immediately rostral to the lamina terminalis in the medial wall of each hemisphere. Eventually the lamina terminalis presents a large cut surface in the median sagittal section and includes the commissures as well as the septum pellucidum. The portion of the lamina terminalis which enters into the formation of the septum becomes hollow as a result of the stretching to which it is subjected, and the resulting cavity is known as the *cavum septi pellucidi.*

The **cerebral hemispheres** are incompletely separated from each other by the *longitudinal fissure* of the cerebrum, at the bottom of which lies a broad band of commissural fibers, the *corpus callosum,* which forms the chief bond of union

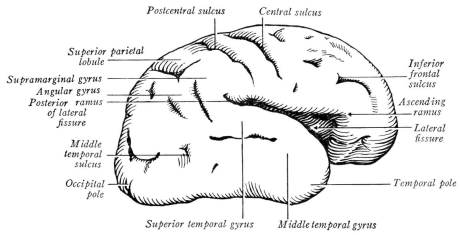

FIGURE 43.   Lateral view of the right cerebral hemisphere from a seven months' fetus. (Kollmann.)

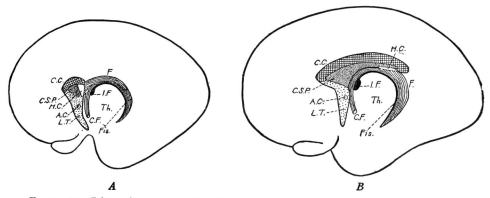

A   *B*

FIGURE 44.   Schematic representation of the development of the septum pellucidum and telencephalic commissures: *A. C.,* Anterior commissure; *C. C.,* corpus callosum; *C. F.,* columna fornicis; *C. S. P.,* cavum septi pellucidi; *F.,* fornix; *H. C.,* commissure of the fornix (hippocampal commissure); *I. F.,* interventricular foramen; *Fis.,* chorioid fissure; *L. T.,* lamina terminalis. (Based on drawings of models of the telencephalon of a four months' fetus (*A*) and of a five months' fetus (*B*) by Streeter.)

between them. Each hemisphere has three surfaces: a convex *dorsolateral surface* (Fig. 45), a *median surface* flattened against the opposite hemisphere (Fig. 49), and a very irregular ventral or *basal surface.* A *dorsal border* separates the dorsolateral from the medial surface, and a *lateral border* marks the transition between the dorsolateral and basal surfaces. One may recognize also *frontal, occipital,* and *temporal poles* (Fig. 45). The long axis of the hemisphere extends between the frontal and occipital poles, and in man is placed almost at right angles to the long axis of the body (Fig. 20), while in other mammals it corresponds more nearly to the body axis. On this account it will be convenient in the description of the human cerebral hemisphere to take the occiput as a point of reference and use the term "posterior" in place of "caudal." Otherwise our directive terms remain the same as in the diencephalon—rostral or anterior, dorsal or superior, and ventral or inferior— except that for the term "ventral" we shall often use the word "basal."

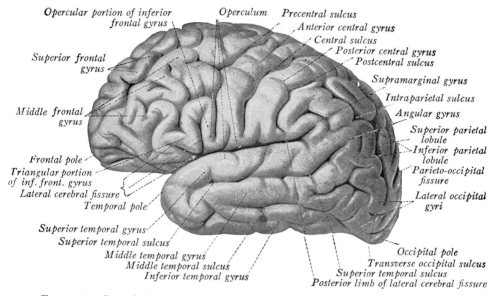

FIGURE 45. Lateral view of the human cerebral hemisphere. (Sobotta-McMurrich.)

The **cerebral cortex** is a layer of gray matter spread over the surface of the hemisphere; its area is greatly increased by the occurrence of folds or gyri separated by deep sulci. That part of the cortex which belongs to the rhinencephalon and is phylogenetically the oldest is designated as the archipallium. It is separated from the newer and in mammals much larger neopallium or non-olfactory cortex by the *rhinal fissure* (Fig. 50), which is less obscured in sheep than in man (Fig. 420).

THE DORSOLATERAL SURFACE OF THE HEMISPHERE

By means of some of the more important sulci and a few arbitrary lines the cortex is marked off into well defined areas, known as the *frontal, parietal, temporal,* and *occipital lobes* (Fig. 46). To these should be added a lobe buried at the bottom of the lateral fissure and known as the *insula* (Fig. 48). In the delimitation of these lobes the *lateral fissure* and the *central sulcus* play a prominent part. Some of the more important sulci are designated as fissures.

This usage is regulated by custom but it may be said that some of the fissures are invaginations of the entire thickness of the wall of the hemisphere and produce corresponding elevations projecting into the lateral ventricle.

The **lateral cerebral fissure** or fissure of Sylvius begins on the basal surface of the brain as a deep cleft lateral to the anterior perforated substance (Fig. 51). From this point it extends lateralward between the temporal and frontal lobes to the lateral aspect of the brain, where it divides into three branches (Figs. 45, 46). The *anterior horizontal ramus* of the lateral fissure runs rostrally, and the *anterior ascending ramus* dorsally into the frontal lobe. The *posterior ramus* of the lateral fissure is much longer, and runs obliquely toward the occiput and at

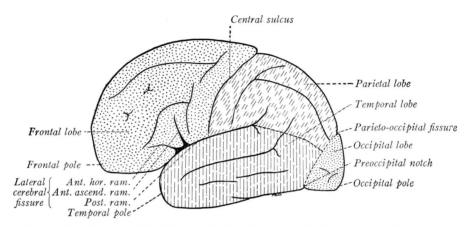

FIGURE 46.   Diagram of the lobes on the lateral aspect of the human cerebral hemisphere.

the same time somewhat dorsally. The terminal part turns dorsally into the parietal lobe. This fissure is, in reality, a deep fossa, at the bottom of which lies the *insula*. It separates the frontal and parietal lobes, which lie dorsal to it, from the temporal lobe.

The **central sulcus** or fissure of Rolando runs obliquely across the dorsolateral surface of the hemisphere, separating the frontal from the parietal lobe (Figs. 27, 45, 46). It begins on the medial surface of the hemisphere a little behind the middle of the dorsal border and extends in a sinuous course rostrally and toward the base, nearly reaching the posterior ramus of the lateral fissure. It makes an angle of about 70 degrees with the dorsal border. It is customary to recognize two knee-like bends in this sulcus; one located at the junction of the dorsal and middle thirds with concavity forward, and the other at the junction of the middle and basal thirds with concavity backward, but these are not always conspicuous. If the margins of the sulcus are pressed apart, a deep annectent gyrus may often be seen extending across it, by which the continuity of the sulcus is to some extent interrupted. This is explained by the fact that the sulcus usually develops in two pieces, which become united as the depth of the sulcus increases.

Lobes.   The *frontal lobe* lies dorsal to the lateral cerebral fissure and rostral to the central sulcus (Fig. 46). The remainder of the dorsolateral surface is sub-divided rather arbitrarily into the parietal, occipital, and temporal lobes. The rostral border of the *occipital lobe* is usually placed at a line joining the end of the parieto-occipital fissure with the preoccipital notch. The latter is a slight indentation on the lateral border of the hemisphere about 4 cm. rostral to the occipital pole, while the parieto-occipital fissure is a deep cleft on the median surface (Fig. 49), which cuts through the dorsal border about midway between the occipital pole and the central sulcus, but a little nearer the former. The *parietal lobe* is situated between the central sulcus and the imaginary line join-ing the parieto-occipital fissure with the preoccipital notch. It lies dorsal to the lateral fissure and to an imaginary line connecting that fissure with the middle of the preceding line. The remainder of the dorsolateral surface belongs to the *temporal lobe.*

The Frontal Lobe. The rostral part of the hemisphere is formed by the frontal lobe. Within it one may identify three chief sulci, which are, however, subject to considerable variation. The *precentral sulcus* is more or less parallel with the central sulcus and is often subdivided into two parts, the superior and inferior precentral sulci (Fig. 47). The *superior frontal sulcus* usually begins in the superior precentral sulcus and runs rostrally, following in a general way the curvature of the dorsal border of the hemisphere which it gradually ap-proaches. The *inferior frontal sulcus* usually begins in the inferior precentral sulcus and extends rostrally, arching at the same time toward the base of the hemisphere. For minor variations compare Figs. 45 and 46.

Between the precentral and central sulci lies the *anterior central gyrus* in which is found the motor area of the cerebral cortex. The remainder of this surface of the frontal lobe is composed of three convolutions, the *superior, middle* and *inferior frontal gyri,* separated from each other by the *superior* and *inferior frontal sulci.* The inferior frontal gyrus, which in the left hemisphere is also known as Broca's convolution, is subdivided by the two anterior rami of the lateral sulcus into three parts, known as the orbital, triangular, and opercular portions. The *orbital part of the inferior frontal gyrus* lies rostral to the anterior horizontal ramus of the lateral sulcus; the *triangular* part is a wedge-shaped convolution between the two anterior rami of that fissure; while the *opercular portion* lies in the frontal operculum between the precentral sulcus and the anterior ascending ramus of the lateral fissure.

The Temporal Lobe. Ventral to the lateral fissure is the long tongue-shaped temporal lobe which terminates rostrally in the temporal pole. The *superior temporal sulcus* is a very constant fissure, which begins near the temporal pole and runs nearly parallel with the lateral cerebral fissure. Its terminal part turns dorsally into the parietal lobe. The *middle temporal sulcus,* ventral to the pre-ceding and in general parallel with it, is usually composed of two or more dis-connected parts. The *inferior temporal sulcus* is located for the most part on the basal surface of the temporal lobe. Dorsal to each of these fissures is a gyrus which bears a similar name: the *superior temporal gyrus,* between the lateral fissure and the superior temporal sulcus; the *middle temporal gyrus,* between the superior and middle temporal sulci; and the *inferior temporal gyrus,* between the middle and inferior temporal sulci. The lateral fissure is very deep; and the surface of the superior temporal gyrus that bounds it is broad and marked near its posterior extremity by horizontal convolutions, known as the transverse temporal gyri. One of these, more marked than the others, has been called the *anterior transverse temporal gyrus* or Heschl's convolution and represents the cortical center for hearing (Fig. 52).

The Parietal Lobe.   *The postcentral sulcus* runs nearly parallel with the central sulcus and consists of two parts, the *superior* and *inferior postcentral sulci,* which may unite with each other or with the *intraparietal sulcus.* Often all three are continuous, forming a complicated fissure, as shown in Fig. 47. The intraparietal sulcus extends in an arched course toward the occiput and may end

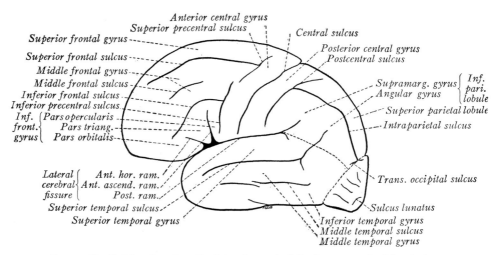

FIGURE 47.   Sulci and gyri on the lateral aspect of the human cerebral hemisphere.

in th*e transverse occipital sulcus.* These four sulci are often included under the term "intraparietal sulcus." The intraparietal sulcus proper is then designated as the horizontal ramus.

The *posterior central gyrus* lies between the central and postcentral sulci. The intraparietal sulcus separates the *superior parietal lobule* from the *inferior parietal lobule.* Within the latter there are to be seen two convolutions: the *supramarginal gyrus,* which curves around the upturned end of the lateral fissure; and the *angular gyrus,* similarly related to the terminal ascending portion of the superior temporal fissure.

The Occipital Lobe.   Only a small part of the dorsolateral surface of the hemisphere is formed by the occipital lobe. This is a triangular area at the occipital extremity, bounded rostrally by a line joining the parieto-occipital fissure and the preoccipital notch (Figs. 46, 48). The transverse occipital sulcus may help to bound this area or may lie within it. Other inconstant sulci help to divide it into irregular convolutions. Sometimes the visual area which lies on the mesial aspect of this lobe is prolonged over the occipital pole to the lateral aspect. In this case a small semilunar furrow develops around it on the lateral surface and is known as the *sulcus lunatus* (Fig. 47).

The Insula. The part of the cortex which overlies the corpus striatum lags behind in its development and becomes overlapped by the surrounding pallium. The cortex, which thus becomes hidden from view at the bottom of the lateral fissure, forms in the adult a somewhat conical mass called the insula or island of Reil (Fig. 48). Its base is surrounded by a limiting furrow, the *circular sulcus,* which is, however, more triangular than circular, and in which we may recognize three portions: superior, inferior and anterior. The apex of this conical lobe is known as the *limen insulae;* and the remainder is subdivided by an oblique groove

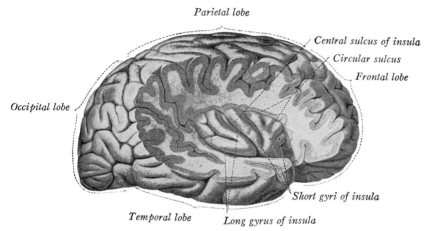

FIGURE 48. Lateral view of the human cerebral hemisphere with the insula exposed by removal of the opercula. (Sobotta-McMurrich.)

(sulcus centralis insulae) into the long gyrus of the insula and a more rostral portion, which is again subdivided into short gyri.

The Opercula. As the adjacent portions of the pallium close over the insula (Fig. 43) they form by the approximation of their margins the three rami of the lateral fissure. These folds constitute the opercula of the insula. Each of the three surrounding lobes takes part in this process; and we may accordingly recognize a *frontal,* a *temporal,* and a *parietal operculum* (Fig. 45).

THE MEDIAN AND BASAL SURFACES

The **occipital lobe** comes more nearly being a structural and functional entity than any of the other lobes. It corresponds in a general way to the "regio occipitalis" as outlined by Brodman (Fig. 255), and it is probably all concerned directly or indirectly with visual processes. We have seen that it forms a small convex area on the lateral surface near the occipital pole; and we now note that it is continued on to the medial surface of the hemisphere, where it forms a somewhat larger triangular field between the parieto-occipital and the anterior portion of the calcarine fissure dorsorostrally and the collateral fissure ventrally. On this aspect of the brain it includes two constant and well defined convolutions: the *cuneus* and the *lingual gyrus* (Figs. 49, 50).

The *calcarine fissure* begins ventrally to the splenium of the corpus callosum and extends toward the occipital pole, arching at the same time somewhat dorsally. It consists of two portions. The rostral part, the calcarine fissure proper, is deeper, more constant in form and position, and phylogenetically much older than the rest, and produces the elevation on the wall of the lateral

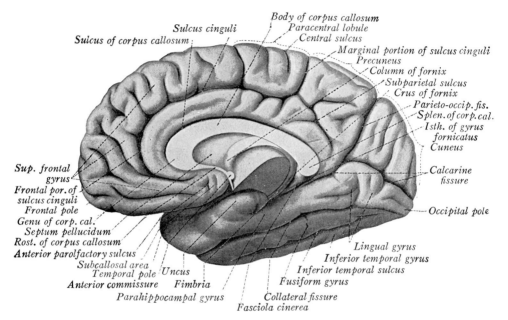

FIGURE 49. Human cerebral hemisphere seen from the medial side. The brain has been divided in the median plane and part of the thalamus has been removed along with the mesencephalon and rhombencephalon. (Sobotta-McMurrich.)

ventricle known as the *calcar avis* (Fig. 57). This part terminates at the point where the calcarine is joined by the parieto-occipital fissure. The other portion, sometimes called the "posterior calcarine sulcus," arches downward and backward from this junction toward the occipital lobe, and occasionally cuts across the border of the hemisphere to its dorsolateral surface. The *parieto-occipital fissure,* which is really a deep fossa with much buried cortex at its depth, appears to be the direct continuation of the rostral part of the calcarine fissure. It cuts through the dorsal border of the hemisphere somewhat nearer to the occipital pole than to the central sulcus. These fissures form a **Y**-shaped figure, whose stem is the calcarine fissure and whose two limbs are the parieto-occipital fissure and the "posterior calcarine sulcus." If the fissures are opened up the stem is seen to be marked off from the two limbs by buried annectent gyri.

The *cuneus* is a triangular convolution with apex directed rostrally, which lies between the diverging parieto-occipital and calcarine fissures. The rest of the medial surface of the occipital lobe belongs to the *lingual gyrus*, which lies between the calcarine and collateral fissures.

The **remaining sulci** and **gyri** on the median and basal surfaces may now be briefly described.

The **sulcus of the corpus callosum** (sulcus corporis callosi) begins ventrally to the rostrum of the corpus callosum, encircles that great commissure on its convex aspect, and finally bends around the splenium to become continuous with the *hippocampal fissure* (Fig. 50). The latter is a shallow groove, which runs from the region of the splenium of the corpus callosum toward the temporal pole near the dorsomedial border of the temporal lobe. It terminates in the bend between the hippocampal gyrus and the uncus.

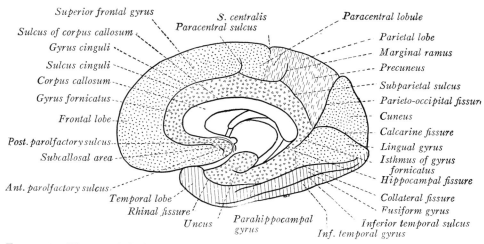

Figure 50.   Diagram of the lobes, sulci, and gyri on the medial aspect of the human cerebral hemisphere.

The **sulcus cinguli** (callosomarginal fissure) begins some distance ventral to the rostrum of the corpus callosum and follows the arched course of the sulcus of the corpus callosum, from which it is separated by the gyrus cinguli. It terminates by dividing into two branches. One of these, the *subparietal sulcus*, continues in the direction of the sulcus cinguli and ends a short distance behind the splenium. The other, known as the *marginal ramus*, turns off at a right angle and is directed toward the dorsal margin of the hemisphere just posterior to the point where the central sulcus turns over the medial border of the hemisphere. A side branch, directed dorsally, is usually given off from the main sulcus some distance rostral to its bifurcation, and is known as the *paracentral sulcus*.

The **collateral fissure** begins near the occipital pole and runs rostrally, separated from the calcarine and hippocampal fissures by the lingual and hippocampal gyri. It is sometimes continuous with the *rhinal fissure*. The latter separates the terminal part of the hippocampal gyrus, which belongs to the archipallium, from the rest of the temporal lobe (Fig. 50).

Convolutions. Dorsal to the corpus callosum is the *gyrus cinguli* between the sulcus of the corpus callosum and the sulcus cinguli. The *superior frontal gyrus* is continued over the dorsal border of the hemisphere from the dorso-lateral surface and reaches the sulcus cinguli. Surrounding the end of the central sulcus is a quadrilateral convolution, known as the *paracentral lobule*. It is bounded by the sulcus cinguli, its marginal ramus, and the paracentral sulcus. Another quadrilateral area, known as the *precuneus,* is bounded by the parieto-occipital fissure, the subparietal sulcus, and the marginal ramus of the sulcus cinguli. The *parahippocampal gyrus* lies between the hippocampal fissure dorsally and the collateral and rhinal fissures ventrally. Its rostral extremity bends around the hippocampal fissure to form the uncus. It is connected with the gyrus cinguli by a narrow convolution, the *isthmus of the gyrus fornicatus.* Under the name *gyrus fornicatus* it has been customary to include the gyrus cinguli, isthmus, hippocampal gyrus, and uncus. Between the collateral fissure and the inferior temporal sulcus is the *fusiform gyrus* which lies on the basal surface of the temporal lobe in contact with the tentorium of the cerebellum (Figs. 49, 51).

It has been customary to apportion parts of the medial and basal surfaces of the cerebral hemisphere to the frontal, parietal, occipital, and temporal lobes, as indicated in Fig. 50. According to this scheme the gyrus fornicatus stands by itself and is sometimes designated as the *limbic lobe.* This plan of subdivision, which was based on the erroneous belief that all portions of the gyrus fornicatus belonged to the rhinencephalon, should be abandoned. A simpler and more logical arrangement assigns the hippocampal gyrus and uncus to the temporal lobe and divides the gyrus cinguli between the frontal and parietal lobes.

The **basal surface** of the hemisphere (Fig. 51) consists of two parts: (1) the ventral surface of the temporal lobe, whose sulci and gyri have been described in a preceding paragraph, and which rests upon the tentorium cerebelli and the floor of the middle cranial fossa; and (2) the orbital surface of the frontal lobe resting upon the floor of the anterior cranial fossa. This orbital surface presents near its medial border the *olfactory sulcus,* a straight, deep furrow, directed rostrally and somewhat medially, that lodges the olfactory tract and bulb. To its medial side is found the *gyrus rectus.* The remainder of the orbital surface of the frontal lobe is subdivided by irregular *orbital sulci* into equally irregular *orbital gyri.*

From the foregoing account it will be apparent that almost the entire surface of the human cerebral hemisphere is formed by *neopallium.* Of the parts already described, only the uncus and adjacent part of the hippocampal gyrus belong to the *archipallium.* Other superficial portions of the rhinencephalon, such as the olfactory bulb, tract and trigone, and the anterior perforated substance, will be described in connection with the hidden parts of the rhinencephalon in Chapter XVII.

THE INTERNAL CONFIGURATION OF THE CEREBRAL HEMISPHERES

When a horizontal section is made through the cerebral hemisphere at the level of the dorsal border of the corpus callosum, the central white substance will be displayed in its maximum extent and will appear as a solid, semioval mass, known as the *centrum semiovale* (Fig. 52). It will also be apparent that lamellae extend from this central white substance to form the medullary centers of the various convolutions, and that over this entire mass the cortex is spread in an uneven layer, thicker over the summit of a convolution than at the bottom of a sulcus. This medullary substance is composed of three kinds of fibers: (1) fibers from the corpus callosum and other commissures joining the cortex of one hemisphere with that of the other; (2) fibers from the internal capsule, uniting

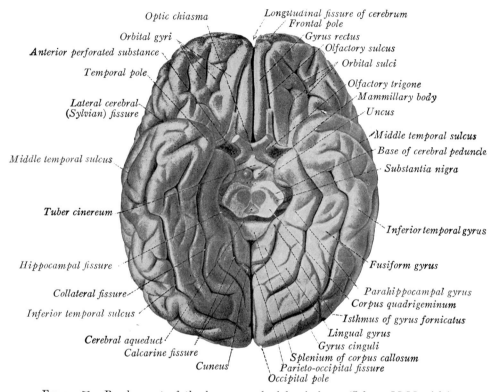

Optic chiasma
Longitudinal fissure of cerebrum
Frontal pole
Orbital gyri
Gyrus rectus
Anterior perforated substance
Olfactory sulcus
Orbital sulci
Temporal pole
Olfactory trigone
Mammillary body
Lateral cerebral (Sylvian) fissure
Uncus
Middle temporal sulcus
Base of cerebral peduncle
Middle temporal sulcus
Substantia nigra
Tuber cinereum
Inferior temporal gyrus
Hippocampal fissure
Fusiform gyrus
Collateral fissure
Parahippocampal gyrus
Corpus quadrigeminum
Inferior temporal sulcus
Isthmus of gyrus fornicatus
Lingual gyrus
Cerebral aqueduct
Gyrus cinguli
Calcarine fissure
Splenium of corpus callosum
Cuneus
Parieto-occipital fissure
Occipital pole

FIGURE 51. Basal aspect of the human cerebral hemisphere. (Sobotta-McMurrich.)

the cortex with the thalamus and lower lying centers; and (3) association fibers running from one part of the cortex to another within the same hemisphere.

The Corpus Callosum. At the bottom of the longitudinal fissure of the cerebrum is a broad white band of commissural fibers, known as the *corpus callosum*, which connects the neopallium of the two hemispheres. While the medial portion of this commissure is exposed in the floor of the longitudinal fissure, its greater part is concealed in the white center of the hemisphere where its fibers radiate to all parts of the neopallium, forming the *radiation of the corpus callosum*. When examined in a median sagittal section of the brain, the corpus callosum is seen to be arched dorsally and to be related on its ventral surface to the fornix and *septum pellucidum* (Figs. 40, 49). The latter consists of two thin membranous plates, stretched between the corpus callosum and the fornix and separated by a narrow cleft-like space, the cavum septi pellucidi (Fig. 56). If the septum has been torn away, it will be possible to look into the lateral ventricle and see that the corpus callosum forms the roof of a large part of that cavity. At its rostral extremity it curves abruptly toward the base of the brain, forming the *genu*, and then tapers rapidly to form the *rostrum*. The latter is triangular in cross-section, with its edge directed toward the anterior commissure to which it is connected by the *rostral lamina*. The body of the corpus

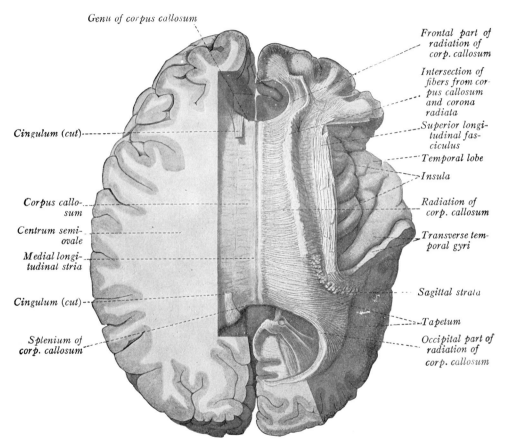

Genu of corpus callosum

Frontal part of radiation of corp. callosum

Intersection of fibers from corpus callosum and corona radiata

Cingulum (cut)

Superior longitudinal fasciculus

Temporal lobe

Insula

Corpus callosum

Centrum semiovale

Medial longitudinal stria

Radiation of corp. callosum

Transverse temporal gyri

Cingulum (cut)

Sagittal strata

Tapetum

Splenium of corp. callosum

Occipital part of radiation of corp. callosum

FIGURE 52. Dissection of the human telencephalon to show the radiation of the corpus callosum. Dorsal view.

callosum (truncus corporis callosi), arching somewhat dorsally, extends toward the occiput and terminates in the *splenium*, a thickened rounded border situated dorsal to the pineal body and corpora quadrigemina. Related to the concave or ventral side of the corpus callosum are the fornix, septum pellucidum, lateral ventricles, tela chorioidea of the third ventricle, and the pineal body (Fig. 40).

Turning again to the dorsal aspect of the corpus callosum, a careful inspection will show that at the bottom of the great longitudinal fissure it is covered by a very thin coating of gray matter, continuous with the cerebral cortex in the depths of the sulcus of the corpus callosum. This is a *rudimentary portion of the hippocampus* and is known as the supracallosal gyrus or *indusium griseum*. In this gray band there are embedded delicate longitudinal strands of nerve fibers. Two of these, placed close together on either side of the median plane, are known as the *medial longitudinal striae* (Fig. 52). Further lateralward on either side, hidden within the sulcus of the corpus callosum, is a less well developed band, the *lateral longitudinal stria*.

The corpus callosum is transversely striated and is composed of fibers that pass from one hemisphere to the other. By dissection these may be followed into the centrum semiovale, where they constitute the *radiation of the corpus cal-*

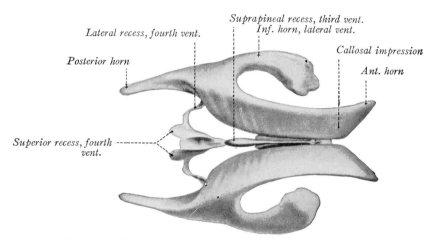

FIGURE 53. Dorsal view of a cast of the brain ventricles of man. (Retzius.)

losum and intersect those from the internal capsule in the corona radiata (Fig. 52). The fibers of the genu sweep forward into the frontal lobe, constituting the frontal part of the radiation or *forceps minor*. Fibers from the splenium bend backward toward the occipital pole, forming the *occipital part of the radiation* or *forceps major*. In the human brain, fibers from the body and splenium of the corpus callosum sweep outward over the lateral ventricle, forming the roof and lateral wall of its posterior horn and the lateral wall of its inferior cornu. Here they constitute a very definite stratum called the *tapetum* (Figs. 52, 399–401).

THE LATERAL VENTRICLE

When the corpus callosum and its radiation are cut away, a cavity, known as the *lateral ventricle*, is uncovered. It is lined by ependyma, continuous with the ependymal lining of the third ventricle by way of the interventricular foramen. This cavity, which contains cerebrospinal fluid, varies in size in different parts, and in some places is reduced to a mere cleft between closely apposed walls. The shape of the ventricle is highly irregular (Figs. 53, 54, 55). As constituent parts we recognize a *central portion* and *anterior, inferior,* and *posterior horns.* The posterior horn develops rather late in the human fetus as a diverticulum from the main cavity.

The **anterior horn,** or cornu anterius, is the part which lies rostral to the interventricular foramen. Its *roof* and *rostral boundary* are formed by the corpus callosum. Its *medial wall* is vertical and is formed by the septum pellucidum, which is stretched between the corpus callosum and the fornix (Fig. 56). The sloping *floor* is at the same time the lateral wall, and is formed by the head of the caudate nucleus, which bulges into the ventricle from the ventrolateral side.

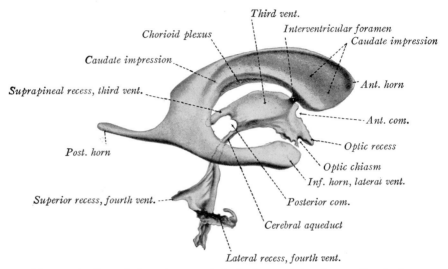

FIGURE 54.   Lateral view of a cast of the brain ventricles of man. (Retzius.)

In frontal section the cavity has a triangular outline; in such a section its walls and the relation which they bear to the rest of the brain can be studied to advantage (Fig. 220).

The **central part** or **body of the lateral ventricle** extends from the interventricular foramen to the splenium of the corpus callosum, where the cavity bifurcates into posterior and inferior horns. The *roof* of the central part is formed by the corpus callosum, and the *medial* wall by the septum pellucidum. The *floor,* which slants to meet the roof at the lateral angle, is composed from within outward of the following structures: the fornix, chorioid plexus, lateral part of the dorsal surface of the thalamus, the stria terminalis, vena terminalis, and the caudate nucleus (Figs. 56, 222). The caudate nucleus tapers rapidly as it is followed from the anterior horn into the body of the ventricle (Fig. 56). The cavity is lined throughout by ependymal epithelium, indicated in Fig. 42. Between the caudate nucleus and the fornix this layer of ependyma constitutes the entire thickness of the wall of the hemisphere. It rests upon the thalamus and becomes adherent to it as the lamina affixa (Fig. 41). At the margin of the fornix, a vascular network from the *tela chorioidea,* i.e., from the pia mater in

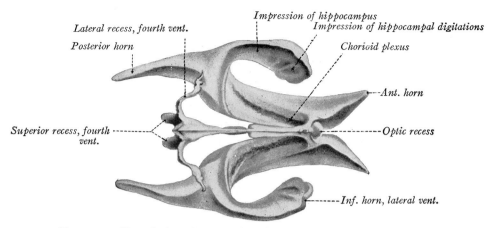

FIGURE 55. Ventral view of a cast of the brain ventricles of man. (Retzius.)

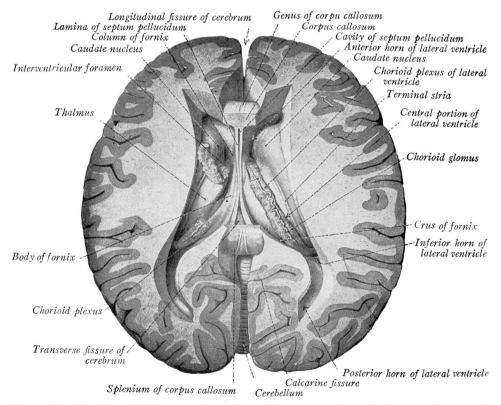

FIGURE 56. Dissection of the human telencephalon. The corpus callosum has been partly removed and the lateral ventricles have been exposed. Dorsal view. (Sobotta-McMurrich.)

the transverse cerebral fissure, is invaginated into the ventricle, pushing this epithelial layer before it and constituting the chorioid plexus (Fig. 56).

The **posterior horn,** or cornu posterius, extends into the occipital lobe, tapering to a point, and describing a gentle curve with concavity directed medially (Figs. 56, 57).

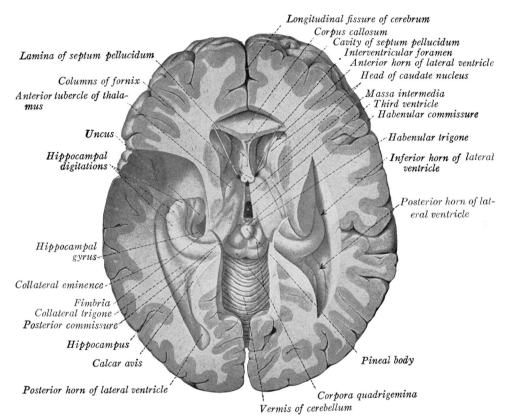

FIGURE 57.   Dissection of the human brain to show the posterior and inferior horns of the lateral ventricle. The body and splenium of the corpus callosum have been removed, as have also the body of the fornix and the tela chorioidea of the third ventricle. A sound has been passed through the interventricular foramina. Dorsal view. (Sobotta-McMurrich.)

The tapetum of the corpus callosum forms a thin but distinct layer in the *roof* and *lateral wall* of the posterior horn, and is covered laterally by a thicker layer of fibers belonging to the sagittal strata (Figs. 224, 390, 399). In the *medial wall* two longitudinal elevations may be seen. Of these, the more dorsal one is known as the *bulb of the posterior horn* (bulbus cornu), and is formed by the occipital portion of the radiation of the corpus callosum or forceps major (Fig. 224). The other elevation, known as the *calcar avis,* is larger and is produced by the rostral part of the calcarine fissure, which here causes a folding of the entire thickness of the pallium.

The **inferior horn,** or cornu inferius, curves ventrally and then rostrally into the temporal lobe (Fig. 57). The angle between the diverging inferior and posterior horns is known as the *collateral trigone*. This horn lies in the medial part of the temporal lobe and does not quite reach the temporal pole. The *roof* is formed by the white substance of the hemisphere, and along its medial border are the *stria terminalis* and *tail of the caudate nucleus*. At the end of the latter

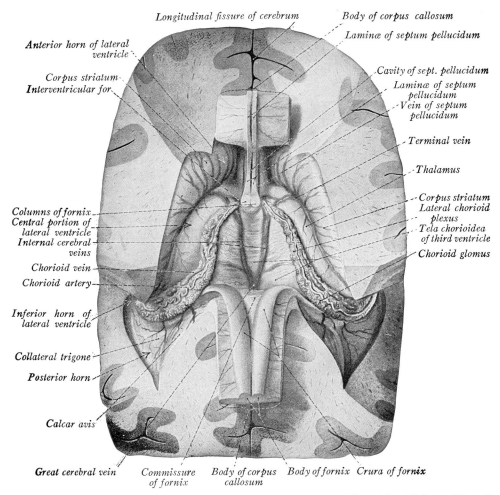

Longitudinal fissure of cerebrum *Body of corpus callosum*

Laminæ of septum pellucidum

Anterior horn of lateral ventricle

Cavity of sept. pellucidum

Corpus striatum
Interventricular for.

Laminæ of septum pellucidum
Vein of septum pellucidum

Terminal vein

Thalamus

Corpus striatum
Lateral chorioid plexus

Columns of fornix
Central portion of lateral ventricle
Internal cerebral veins

Tela chorioidea of third ventricle

Chorioid glomus

Chorioid vein

Chorioid artery

Inferior horn of lateral ventricle

Collateral trigone

Posterior horn

Calcar avis

Great cerebral vein   *Commissure of fornix*   *Body of corpus callosum*   *Body of fornix*   *Crura of fornix*

FIGURE 58. Dissection of the human brain to show the tela chorioidea of the third ventricle and the commissure of the fornix. The body of the corpus callosum and the fornix have been divided and reflected. Dorsal view, except that the ventral surfaces of the reflected corpus callosum and the commissure of the fornix are seen. (Sobotta-McMurrich.)

the *amygdaloid nucleus* bulges into the terminal part of the inferior horn (Figs. 219, 393–395). The *floor* and *medial wall* of the inferior horn are formed in large part by the following structures, named in order from within outward: the fimbria, hippocampus, and collateral eminence (Figs. 57, 223). Upon the fimbria and hippocampus there is superimposed the chorioid plexus. The *hip-*

pocampus is a long, prominent, curved elevation, with whose medial border there is associated a band of fibers, representing a continuation of the fornix and known as the *fimbria*. These parts will be described in connection with the rhinencephalon. The *collateral eminence* is an elevation in the lateral part of the floor produced by the collateral fissure.

The thin epithelial membrane, described above as joining the edge of the fornix with the caudate nucleus (Fig. 42), continues to unite these structures as they both curve downward, the former in the floor, the latter in the roof, of the inferior horn. A vascular plexus from the pia mater is invaginated into the lateral ventricle along this curved line, carrying before it an epithelial cover-

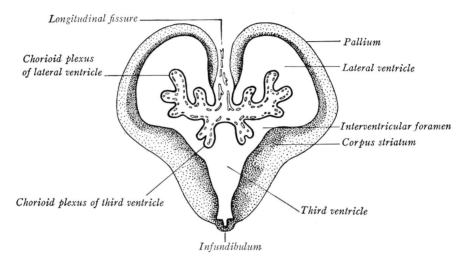

Longitudinal fissure

Chorioid plexus
of lateral ventricle

Pallium

Lateral ventricle

Interventricular foramen

Corpus striatum

Chorioid plexus of third ventricle

Third ventricle

Infundibulum

FIGURE 59. Diagram of a cross-section through the developing forebrain showing relationship of the ependyma covering the chorioid plexuses to the early ventricular spaces (modified from Arey).

ing from this thin membrane. In this way there is formed the *chorioid plexus of the lateral ventricle* (Fig. 58). The line along which this invagination occurs is the chorioid fissure; when the plexus is torn away, the position of the fissure is indicated by an artificial cleft extending into the ventricle, which begins at the interventricular foramen and follows the fornix and fimbria in an arched course into the temporal lobe (Fig. 242). The topography of the lateral ventricle is well illustrated in Figs. 391–402.

The **chorioid plexus** of the lateral ventricle (Figs. 58, 222) is continuous with that of the third ventricle at the interventricular foramen, from which point it can be followed backward through the central part into the inferior horn. It is coextensive with the chorioid fissure and is not found in the anterior or posterior horns. It consists of a vascular network derived from the pia mater, and is covered throughout by a layer of epithelium of ependymal origin, which is adapted to every unevenness of its surface (Fig. 42).

CHAPTER III

Meninges and Blood Vessels of the Central Nervous System

After the closing of the fontanelles and sutures of the skull, the interior of the cranium containing the brain is a closed compartment, and, except for the foramen magnum, the only openings into it from the outside are by way of foramina through which blood vessels and nerves pass. Since the brain case can not be stretched and its contents are incompressible, it is evident that blood enters and leaves in equal quantities constantly. Even a slight increase of the blood pressure is reflected by an increase in the intracranial pressure. Delicate adjustments of this pressure must be maintained (through carotid sinus reflexes and similar mechanisms) so that on the one hand the blood pressure is adequate to give a constant supply of oxygen to the nervous tissue, and on the other it is not too great to interfere with function.

The brain and spinal cord are protected by three membranes or meninges and cushioned by a layer of cerebrospinal fluid, which varies in thickness so as to fill in all the depressions in the brain's uneven surface (Fig. 61).

The **dura mater,** the most superficial of the three membranes covering the brain and spinal cord, is a thick and tough layer of dense collagenous tissue. The spinal dura is separated from the periosteum of the vertebrae by fat and blood vessels, but within the cranium the dura and periosteum are fused. In other words the intracranial dura consists of two layers, the outer of which is periosteum. The inner layer or dura proper separates from the outer at certain points to form folds that project into the cranial cavity: the tentorium cerebelli, falx cerebri, and falx cerebelli (Fig. 60). The *tentorium cerebelli* is stretched like a tent over the posterior cranial fossa and separates the occipital lobes of the cerebral hemispheres from the cerebellum. The *falx cerebri*, a long sickle-shaped fold, projects downward in the midline and separates the two cerebral hemispheres. Beneath its free margin the corpus callosum joins the two hemispheres together. At its posterior end it is attached to the tentorium, drawing this upward in the midline to a tent-like peak. The falx cerebri and tentorium cerebelli are stretched tight and serve mutually to keep each other taut. A

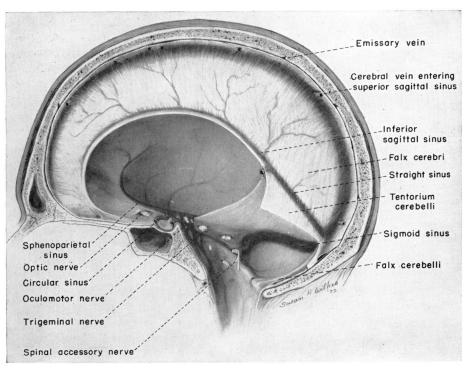

Emissary vein

Cerebral vein entering
superior sagittal sinus

Inferior
sagittal sinus

Falx cerebri

Straight sinus

Tentorium
cerebelli

Sigmoid sinus

Falx cerebelli

Sphenoparietal
sinus
Optic nerve
Circular sinus
Oculomotor nerve

Trigeminal nerve

Spinal accessory nerve

FIGURE 60. Drawing of a parasagittal section of the cranial cavity to show the meninges and dural venous sinuses. The hypophysis is shown just posterior to the lead line for the circular sinus; just beneath it is shown the air sinus of the sphenoid bone. The great cerebral vein (of Galen) is shown joining the straight sinus at an angle at the apex of the tentorium cerebelli. The middle meningeal vein is shown upon the wall of the middle cranial fossa.

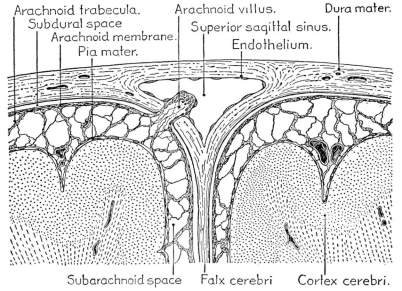

Arachnoid trabecula.   Arachnoid villus.   Dura mater.
Subdural space
Arachnoid membrane.   Superior sagittal sinus.
Pia mater.   Endothelium.

Subarachnoid space   Falx cerebri   Cortex cerebri.

FIGURE 61. Diagrammatic representation of a coronal section through the superior sagittal sinus to illustrate the meninges. (Weed.)

much smaller sickle-shaped fold, the *falx cerebelli*, projects forward in the midline in the posterior cranial fossa. Venous sinuses, to be described in another paragraph are illustrated in Fig. 60, lie within clefts formed by the separation of the inner from the outer layers of dura (superior longitudinal, transverse, and cavernous sinuses, Figs. 61, 194) or by separation of the two layers of the folds forming the falx cerebri and tentorium cerebelli (inferior longitudinal and straight sinuses).

The **arachnoid membrane** is very delicate and lies beneath the dura, from which it is separated by the subdural space. The latter is a mere cleft containing only a little moisture, except when dura and arachnoid are separated by an abnormal accumulation of fluid, such as a subdural hematoma. Between the arachnoid membrane and the pia is the subarachnoid space, containing cerebro-

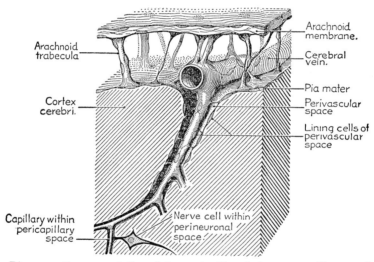

FIGURE 62.   Diagrammatic representation of the arachnoid and pia mater to illustrate the subarachnoid space and perivascular channels. (Weed.)

spinal fluid and bridged by delicate arachnoid trabeculae (Figs. 61, 62). The arachnoid is avascular; the vessels supplying brain and spinal cord run in the pia mater. The binding together of pia and arachnoid by trabeculae results in the use of the term *pia-arachnoid* to describe them both.

The **pia mater** is a delicate membrane which closely invests and is adherent to the brain and spinal cord, extending down to the depths of the fissures and sulci. It is very thin over the cerebral cortex, but thicker over the brain stem. The blood vessels for the brain ramify within it, and as they enter the brain substance they are accompanied for a short distance by a pial sheath (Fig. 62).

The **subarachnoid space** with the cerebrospinal fluid it contains intervenes between the pia and arachnoid. Since the former is closely applied to the brain, following its contour into all the fossae, fissures, and sulci while the latter remains close to the dura, the depth of the subarachnoid space varies, being least over the summits of the cerebral convolutions.

At certain points where the brain does not closely follow the contour of the skull the subarachnoid space is large; these enlargements hold considerable cerebrospinal fluid and have been called cisterns. The largest of these is the *cerebellomedullary cistern* (cisterna magna), which occupies the space between the inferior surface of the cerebellum and the dorsal surface of the medulla (Fig. 63). At its lower end it is continuous with the spinal subarachnoid space, and the cerebrospinal fluid passes freely through the foramen magnum. Other enlargements of the subarachnoid space are designated as follows: the *superior cistern*, between cerebellum and mesencephalon; the *pontine cistern*, ventral to the pons; the *interpeduncular cistern*, in the interpeduncular fossa; the *cistern of the chiasma*, just in front of the optic chiasma; and the *cistern of the lateral fossa of the cerebrum*, associated with the lateral cerebral fissure. When air has been introduced into the subarachnoid spaces, these cisterns show as shadows in x-ray photographs of the head. Changes from normal in their size and shape seen in such photographs give information concerning pathologic changes within the cranium.

The *arachnoid villi* are small tufts of arachnoid which project into the venous sinuses, chiefly into the superior sagittal sinus, and which carry with them a prolongation of the subarachnoid space (Fig. 61). Through these villi cerebrospinal fluid can filter into the venous sinuses and join the blood stream.

Perivascular spaces (Virchow-Robin spaces) surround the blood vessels as they enter the brain substance (Fig. 62). The inner wall of such a space is formed by a prolongation of a membrane like the arachnoid, the outer wall is continuous with the pia, and the intervening channel opens into the subarachnoid space. Along these perivascular spaces tissue fluids can pass slowly to the surface to join the cerebrospinal fluid. Deep within the nervous tissue the perivascular spaces lie within the adventitia of the blood vessels and extend as far as the transition of arterioles and venules to capillaries. It is thought that the pericapillary and perineuronal spaces are artifacts. India ink particles in the cerebrospinal fluid penetrate perivascular spaces to small vessels but do not enter the "perineural space" (Brierley, 1950). Studies with the electron microscope confirm the belief that there is no perineuronal space or perivascuiar space about capillaries, though these structures are nearly surrounded by the perivascular feet of astrocytes which may have given the appearance of spaces (Maynard, Schultz and Pease, 1957). Along the capillaries there is a glial limiting membrane, which with the endothelium forms the hemoencephalic barrier.

The term hemoencephalic barrier refers to a conception rather than a constant anatomical structure, for the separation of the blood from the parenchyma of any organ is primarily and simply endothelium, though additional structures may be applied to this and perhaps modify the diffusion process between blood and the intercellular fluid. This barrier varies widely in histological structure, from the columnar epithelium of the chorioid plexus plus the endothelium of capillaries to the endothelium alone. It is permeable to various substances, but to some of them apparently in only one direction (Rodriguez-Peralta, 1957). It is of interest that in fish, amphibians and reptiles the perivascular spaces communicate directly with the ventricles, but this is not so in birds and mammals.

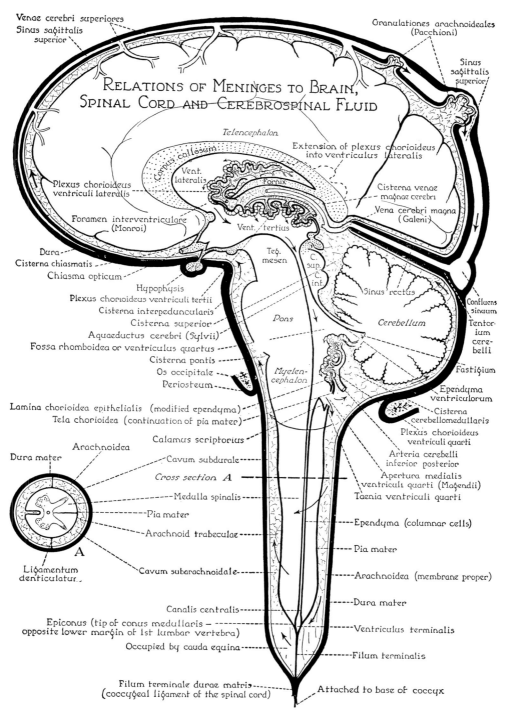

Venae cerebri superiores
Sinus sagittalis superior
Granulationes arachnoideales (Pacchioni)
Sinus sagittalis superior

RELATIONS OF MENINGES TO BRAIN, SPINAL CORD AND CEREBROSPINAL FLUID

Telencephalon

Corpus callosum
Vent. lateralis
Fornix
Extension of plexus chorioideus into ventriculus lateralis
Plexus chorioideus ventriculi lateralis
Cisterna venae magnae cerebri
Vena cerebri magna (Galeni)
Foramen interventriculare (Monroi)
Vent. tertius
Dura
Cisterna chiasmatis
Chiasma opticum
Teg. mesen
C. sup.
C. inf.
Sinus rectus
Confluens sinuum
Hypophysis
Plexus chorioideus ventriculi tertii
Cisterna interpeduncularis
Cisterna superior
Aquaeductus cerebri (Sylvii)
Fossa rhomboidea or ventriculus quartus
Cisterna pontis
Os occipitale
Periosteum
Pons
Cerebellum
Tentorium cerebelli
Myelencephalon
Fastigium
Ependyma ventriculorum
Lamina chorioidea epithelialis (modified ependyma)
Tela chorioidea (continuation of pia mater)
Cisterna cerebellomedullaris
Plexus chorioideus ventriculi quarti
Calamus scriptorius
Arteria cerebelli inferior posterior
Apertura medialis ventriculi quarti (Magendii)
Taenia ventriculi quarti
Arachnoidea
Dura mater
Cavum subdurale
Cross section A
Medulla spinalis
Ependyma (columnar cells)
Pia mater
Pia mater
Arachnoid trabeculae
Arachnoidea (membrane proper)
A
Dura mater
Ligamentum denticulatum
Cavum subarachnoidale
Canalis centralis
Ventriculus terminalis
Epiconus (tip of conus medullaris — opposite lower margin of 1st lumbar vertebra)
Occupied by cauda equina
Filum terminalis
Filum terminale durae matris (coccygeal ligament of the spinal cord)
Attached to base of coccyx

FIGURE 63. Diagram of the meninges, brain ventricles, and subarachnoid spaces. The arrows indicate the direction of the flow of the cerebrospinal fluid. (From Rasmussen, The Principal Nervous Pathways. By permission of The Macmillan Co., Publishers.)

The **chorioid plexuses** and **ventricles** of the brain should be considered along with the meninges because of their close relationship to the cerebrospinal fluid which fills the ventricles and the subarachnoid space. The chorioid plexuses (Fig. 64) are tufts of capillaries covered by a simple columnar epithelium, derived from the ependyma, which are suspended from the roof of the third and fourth ventricles and the walls of the lateral ventricles. The ependymal epithelium represents the total wall of the neural tube at this point. The epithelium, a small amount of connective tissue, and the endothelium of the capillaries constitute a barrier interposed between the blood stream and the cerebrospinal

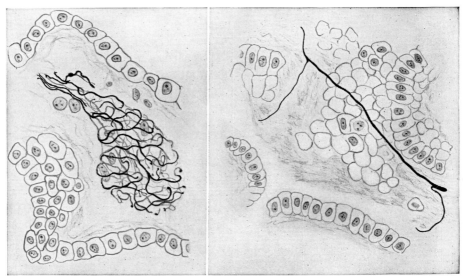

FIGURE 64. Innervation of the chorioid plexus. (Clark.) To the left is a typical tangled skein of knobbed fibers surrounded by connective tissues; to the right is a simply branching fiber which lies close to the base of the epithelium.

fluid. (For the chorioid plexuses of the lateral ventricles, see p. 70, Figs. 42, 58, 221–223; the chorioid plexus of the third ventricle, p. 49, Figs. 40, 42; and that of the fourth ventricle, p. 38, Fig. 34.)

The **cerebrospinal fluid** is a clear watery fluid of low specific gravity. Being separated by a semipermeable membranous barrier from the blood stream, it is in osmotic balance with the blood. The cerebrospinal fluid contains more dissolved electrolytes than the blood, but is low in protein (15–45 mg. per 100 cc.); it has less than 5 cells per cubic millimeter and a pressure of 70–180 mm. of water and 50–100 mg. of glucose per 100 cc. The barrier between the blood and cerebrospinal fluid varies in different regions. Aside from the endothelium of the blood vessels, there is the ependymal simple columnar epithelium covering the chorioid plexuses and the regular ependymal lining of the ventricles of the brain; there is the thin wall of the arachnoidal granulations invaginated into the dural sinuses; and there is the ultimate extension of the perivascular spaces in the substance of the central nervous system.

The source of the cerebrospinal fluid is commonly said to be the chorioid plexuses, and it has been observed to accumulate in drops on exposed plexuses (Cushing, 1914). Furthermore Dandy (1919) was able to show that plugging one interventricular foramen resulted in a unilateral internal hydrocephalus, while the hydrocephalus did not occur if the chorioid plexus of the plugged ventricle had been previously removed.

While these and other facts indicate that cerebrospinal fluid is produced through the chorioid plexuses, there is evidence that it can also accumulate through other regions of the barrier between blood and the fluid. Much discussion has arisen as to whether the fluid is a product of secretion or dialysis. There are no new substances formed by the chorioid plexuses and put into the fluid. Histologic studies of the columnar cells covering the chorioid plexus do not give definite evidence of secretory activity, but experiments with demonstrable diffusible substances show that the cells allow passage of substances from blood stream to ventricular space and in the reverse direction. However, cells of chorioid plexuses grown in tissue culture showed granules in the cytoplasm, and globular swellings along the surface were pinched off in the manner of cells secreting by the apocrine method. There are only slight traces of alkaline phosphatase in the epithelium of the chorioid plexus and relatively little in the endothelium of the capillaries within it. Some acid phosphatase is demonstrable in the chorioidal epithelium and a few basophilic granules which appear to be ribonucleoprotein occur. In the cells of the meninges lining the subarachnoid spaces there is little evidence of the presence of phosphatase (Wislocki and Dempsey, 1948). Nerve endings in the chorioid plexuses are suggestive of a sensory rather than secretory function (Fig. 64).

Though a considerable quantity of cerebrospinal fluid can be drained off from an opening in the subarachnoid space within a day's time, it appears that this is a result of altered pressure relationships. The usual description of a "direction of flow" of the cerebrospinal fluid is not to be taken as evidence of a constant rate of production. As Becht (1920) observed, the changes in pressure and outflow of the fluid are related to the alterations in the venous and arterial pressures within the cranium. Obstruction of the interventricular foramina, cerebral aqueduct, or apertures of the fourth ventricle results in an accumulation of the fluid behind the block and the development of hydrocephalus.

Arteries of the Brain.   The brain receives its blood supply through the vertebral and internal carotid arteries. The two *vertebral arteries* enter the cranial cavity through the foramen magnum, run rostrally and toward the median plane along the ventral surface of the medulla oblongata, and unite at the lower border of the pons to form the basilar artery (Fig. 65). The chief branch of the vertebral artery within the cranium is the *posterior inferior cerebellar artery,* which winds around the medulla oblongata to the inferior surface of the cerebellum. This branch is of clinical importance because it supplies the lateral portion of the medulla oblongata. Thrombosis of this artery gives rise to a well defined symptom complex (see Chapter XXI, Case 8).

The *basilar artery* is formed by the junction of the two vertebral arteries at the lower border of the pons and ends at the upper border of the pons by dividing into the two *posterior cerebral arteries*. In addition to those just named, it gives off the following branches: two *anterior inferior cerebellar arteries*, two *internal auditory arteries*, several *pontile branches*, and two *superior cerebellar arteries*.

The *posterior cerebral arteries* formed by the bifurcation of the basilar artery run dorsalward around the cerebral peduncles close to the upper border of the

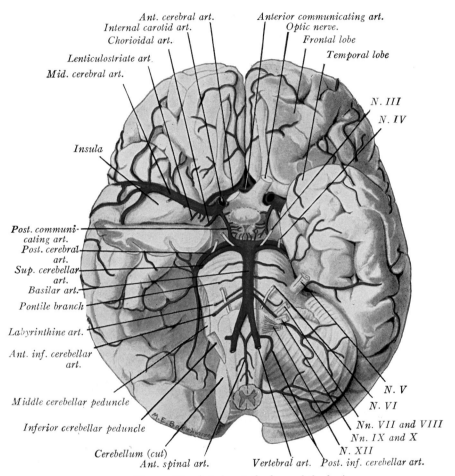

FIGURE 65.   Arteries at the base of the brain.

pons and parallel to the superior cerebellar arteries (Figs. 65, 68). Each posterior cerebral artery is continued back along the medial surface of the corresponding cerebral hemisphere beneath the splenium of the corpus callosum toward the occipital pole (Fig. 67). It supplies the medial surface of the occipital and the inferior surface of the temporal lobes of the cerebral hemisphere. The terminal branches wind around the borders of the hemisphere and can be seen on the

lateral surface. A comparison of Figs. 66 and 67 with Fig. 259 will show that
the posterior cerebral artery supplies practically all of the visual cortex.

The *internal carotid artery* passes through the carotid canal in the base of
the skull and enters the cranial cavity through the foramen lacerum. After a

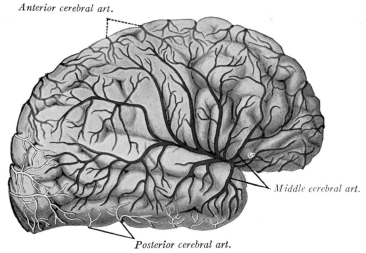

FIGURE 66.   Arteries on the lateral surface of the cerebral hemisphere

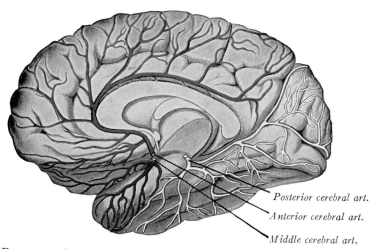

FIGURE 67.   Arteries on the medial surface of the cerebral hemisphere.

tortuous course along the lateral wall of the cavernous sinus, within which it
gives off an inferior hypophyseal artery to the posterior lobe of the hypophysis,
it reaches the brain near the medial side of the temporal lobe and divides close
to the anterior perforated substance into its two terminal branches, the *middle*
and *anterior cerebral arteries*. In addition to the terminal rami, other branches
arise from this part of the internal carotid artery. The *posterior communicating*

artery joins the internal carotid with the posterior cerebral artery. The *chorioidal artery* runs backward and laterally to the chorioid fissure through which it reaches the chorioid plexus of the lateral ventricle, with branches also to the cornu ammonis and globus pallidus. The superior hypophyseal artery leaves the carotid immediately after it passes through the dura over the cavernous sinus. This vessel supplies the stalk and anterior lobe of the hypophysis (McConnell, 1953).

The *middle cerebral artery* has been exposed on the left side of Fig. 65 by the removal of part of the temporal lobe. It runs lateralward between the temporal and frontal lobes in the stem of the lateral cerebral fissure which separates them. Near its origin it gives off several small *central* or *basal branches* which enter the brain through the anterior perforated substance and supply the corpus striatum and internal capsule. The majority of the branches from the middle cerebral artery ramify in the pia mater on the surface of the cerebral hemisphere and are known as *cortical branches*. These are distributed to the lateral part of the ventral surface of the frontal lobe, to the insula (Fig. 65), to the upper surface of the temporal lobe, and to the greater part of the convex dorsolateral surface of the hemisphere (Fig. 66). A comparison of Fig. 66 with Figs. 254, 259 and 258, 262 will show that the middle cerebral artery supplies the three cortical areas especially concerned with language, the auditory receptive center, and the greater portions of the motor projection center and the somesthetic area.

The *anterior cerebral artery*, the smaller of the two terminal branches of the internal carotid, runs forward and medially to the longitudinal fissure of the cerebrum (Fig. 65). Within this fissure it lies upon the medial surface of the cerebral hemisphere close to the genu and body of the corpus callosum. Its cortical branches supply the medial surface of the frontal and parietal lobes (Fig. 67). It is joined to its fellow of the opposite side by the short *anterior communicating artery* (Fig. 65), which may have a few branches that enter the hypothalamic region.

The *arterial circle of Willis* is a ring-shaped anastomosis formed at the base of the brain by the branches of the basilar and internal carotid arteries. The two anterior cerebral arteries are joined together by the anterior communicating artery. Each internal carotid anastomoses with the corresponding posterior cerebral by way of the posterior communicating. In this way there is formed an arterial ring into which there enters on each side the posterior cerebral, posterior communicating, internal carotid, anterior cerebral, and anterior communicating arteries. The circle surrounds the infundibulum and optic chiasma. This free anastomosis of the cerebral arteries provides for a collateral circulation in case one of the tributary vessels is occluded (Fig. 68).

The *cortical branches* of the cerebral arteries also anastomose, to a slight extent, upon the surface of the brain; but the anastomosis is not sufficient to provide adequate circulation in case a large branch is occluded. Neither do the *central* and *basal branches,* which are given off from the arteries forming the circle of Willis and which pierce the brain to ramify in its interior, anastomose sufficiently with each other or with the cortical branches. Although it is sometimes so stated they are not end arteries, but the occlusion of one of these small central branches always leads to the degeneration of the region supplied by it. The central branches arising from the middle cerebral artery supply the corpus striatum, internal capsule, and thalamus. A clot in or a hemorrhage from one of these small branches causes serious disability; and they have been called the "arteries of cerebral hemorrhage."

To speak of a single lenticulostriate artery is misleading. Several small vessels leaving the middle and anterior cerebral arteries and entering the anterior perforated substance may be termed striate arteries since they supply the striatum (Fig. 68). There is some variation in the source of these since all are derived from the middle cerebral in about a third of cases. The more medial ones (most often from the anterior cerebral artery) supply the head of the

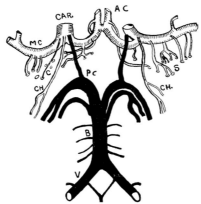

FIGURE 68.   The circle of Willis with the stumps of the carotid arteries turned forward to show branches beneath them. *Car,* carotid artery; *AC, MC, PC,* anterior, middle, and posterior cerebral arteries; *CH,* chorioid artery; *C,* "capsular" artery which runs to region of the genu of the internal capsule; *S,* striate arteries entering anterior perforate substance; *B,* basilar and *V,* vertebral artery.

caudate nucleus and part of the putamen, and the rest (from the middle cerebral) supply the remaining portion of caudate and putamen, with the exception of the recurved portion of the tail of the caudate which is supplied, along with adjacent structures, by the chorioidal artery. The medial segments of the globus pallidus and at times the lateral segment are supplied by the chorioidal artery, which also supplies the hippocampus and the ventral part of the posterior limb of the internal capsule. Small vessels from the internal carotid supply the genu of the internal capsule. The chorioidal artery has a longer free course in the subarachnoid space than other arteries of similar size and so is more subject to damage or thrombosis, which may explain the vulnerability of the medial portion of the globus pallidus and the cornu ammonis of the hippocampus.

Venous Drainage.   The blood from the brain drains through veins in the pia into venous sinuses, lined with endothelium, situated within the dura mater. Much of the blood from the interior of the brain drains through the *great internal cerebral vein* which joins the *inferior sagittal sinus* to form the *straight sinus* (Figs. 60, 69). The latter lies within the dura along the line of attachment of the falx cerebri to the tentorium cerebelli. Most of the veins on the lateral surface of the cerebral hemisphere drain upward into the *superior sagittal sinus* which is situated in the attached margin of the falx cerebri. The superior sagittal sinus commonly ends by turning slightly to the right and entering the right transverse sinus, but it occasionally joins the left transverse sinus or bifurcates and joins both transverse sinuses. Where it joins one of the transverse sinuses there is a dilatation called the *confluence of the sinuses*. The straight sinus forms a similar connection with the opposite transverse sinus and an anastomosing channel connects this junction with the confluence of sinuses across the internal occipital protuberance. The two *transverse sinuses* receive the blood from those previously mentioned and conduct it to the right and left internal jugular veins. In the first part of its course the transverse sinus runs lateralward in the attached margin of the tentorium. In the second part it curves ventrally

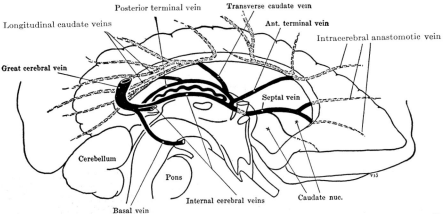

FIGURE 69. Diagram of the internal veins of the cerebrum. (From Mettler: Neuroanatomy, C. V. Mosby Co.)

as the sigmoid sinus and finally passes through the jugular foramen into the internal jugular vein. In this second part of its course it lies within the dura covering the mastoid portion of the temporal bone and leaves its impression on the bone in the form of the sigmoid groove. Because of this close proximity to the mastoid, middle ear infections sometimes spread to the transverse sinus.

The superficial middle cerebral vein drains downward into the *cavernous sinus*, a rather wide irregular space within the dura lateral to the sella turcica of the sphenoid bone (Fig. 194). The two cavernous sinuses are joined together by the anterior and posterior intercavernous sinuses (circular sinus). From the cavernous sinus the blood is drained downward through the *inferior petrosal sinus* into the internal jugular vein and backward through the *superior petrosal sinus* into the transverse sinus. *Emissary veins* place the venous sinuses in communication with extracranial veins. The most important of these communications are those formed by the ophthalmic veins with the nasal and other superficial veins of the face. Others are the mastoid, occipital, and parietal emissary veins. It is possible for superficial infections to travel along these channels and involve the intracranial sinuses.

Nervous tissue must be plentifully supplied with blood for proper functioning. To supply the brain with oxygen each minute a quantity of blood approximately equal to the weight of the brain is required. With the body at rest, the brain receives about one third of the blood leaving the left ventricle, though it represents only about two per cent of the body by weight. If the blood flow to the head is stopped instantaneously in man, unconsciousness occurs in six or seven seconds, and though irreversible changes occur in the brain after a few minutes without circulation, 100 seconds without blood supply has been followed by recovery of consciousness and no permanent damage (Rossen, Kabat,

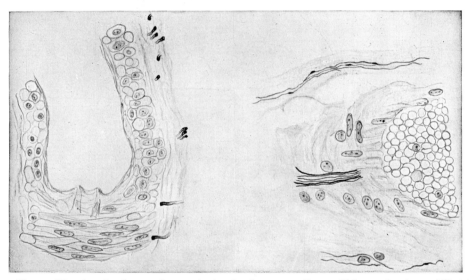

FIGURE 70. Arteries from a human brain showing nerve fibers which supply them. (Clark.) Nerve fibers as shown with a myelin sheath stain are on the vessel at the left, and with pyridine-silver at the right. Above and below the latter are nerve fibers of the adjacent brain substance. Between the vessel wall and the brain substance above is part of the perivascular space.

and Anderson, 1943). Lowering the temperature of the body allowed several periods of occlusion of the cerebral circulation for 12 to 15 minutes at a time in monkeys with recovery (McMurray et al., 1956). Young animals withstand cerebral anoxia better than adults (Grenell, 1953). Disturbances of circulation may be at the basis of many diseases of the nervous system the etiology of which is still obscure.

A cubic millimeter of human gray matter of the brain may contain over 1000 linear millimeters of capillaries. This is less than half the quantity of capillaries in striated and cardiac muscle, but three times that of the white matter.

Vessels of Spinal Cord.   The blood supply of the spinal cord, as described by Suh and Alexander (1939), is obtained from arteries entering the vertebral canal and passing to the cord by way of the nerve roots. They differ in size and are derived from intercostal and lumbar arteries.

In man the blood supply depends largely upon six to eight anterior radicular arteries and approximately the same number of posterior radicular arteries. The largest of these vessels is found in the lumbosacral region, the next in size in the cervical. In the thoracic region adequately sized vessels do not enter each segment and the supply of blood is reinforced from lumbar and cervical regions by the anastomosing channels. The anterior radicular arteries unite to form ventrally the anterior spinal artery, which at its upper end receives a supply from each vertebral artery and which varies in caliber as it meanders along the pia

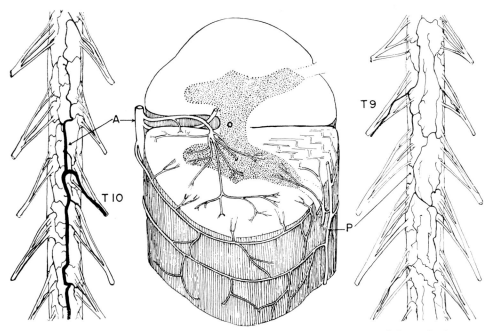

FIGURE 71. Arterial supply of the spinal cord. To the left of the central figure is shown an anterior (ventral) view of the low thoracic segments of the spinal cord, and to the right a posterior (dorsal) view, each with arteries injected. The contributing vessels passing to the *anterior spinal artery*—A and to the *posterior spinal artery*—P along the spinal nerve roots vary markedly in size. In the middle figure the separate branches of the anterior spinal artery passing through the anterior median fissure to the spinal gray matter are shown. (After Herren and Alexander, modified and redrawn.)

near the ventral median fissure; it is largest in the lumbosacral region, next in size in the cervical and smallest in the thoracic region. The posterior radicular arteries supply on each side a longitudinally running posterolateral vessel (posterior spinal artery), which connects with a branch of the posterior inferior cerebellar or occasionally the vertebral artery. From the anterior spinal artery, small branches enter the ventral median sulcus, passing into the cord at its deepest portion, with separate sulcal vessels passing to the right and left sides. These arteries supply neighboring structures, such as the anterior funiculus, the gray matter of the anterior horns, and the base of the posterior horn about the nucleus dorsalis; and they effectively reach much of the lateral funiculus, especially the area of the lateral corticospinal tract (Herren and Alexander, 1939). The posterolateral vessels and posterior radicular vessels supply branches to the posterior funiculus and posterior horn, which anastomose with the small branches from the anterior sulcal arteries. The pia mater between the posterior and anterior spinal vessels is supplied with vessels running around the circumference of the cord and from these, arterioles enter the periphery of the white matter.

The veins of the spinal cord generally resemble in pattern the arterial distribution, but, as is commonly true of veins, are more variable. The smaller venules appear to have single cusped valves at points of junction which can prevent backflow (Suh and Alexander, 1939).

It has been demonstrated experimentally that the more limited blood supply of the thoracic region of the spinal cord makes it subject to damage by vascular occlusion of the radicular arteries as with contrast media (Margolis, Tarazi and Grimson, 1956).

The blood vessels of the brain and spinal cord, as are those of the pia mater, are supplied with innervation (Clark, 1934), very much like blood vessels elsewhere (Fig. 70). By observation of pial vessels through a window set in the skull it has been shown that these vessels respond to stimulation of their nerve supply but their response is affected by the fact that they are in the closed, filled skull, and by other devices regulating the blood supply to the brain according to its needs (Wolff, 1938). It is interesting that the vessels cannot be seen pulsing when viewed through a glass window in the closed skull. The arteries of the pia and of the brain substance have plentiful muscle in their walls though the veins are without it. Capillaries, though abundant in the brain, are absent from the pia mater.

Cerebral Angiography.   With the development of methods of injecting radiopaque substances in the blood stream to visualize arteries and veins in their normal positions, cerebral angiography has revealed points about the blood vessels of the brain that were not clearly shown by dissections (Fig. 72). The fact that the skull is a closed compartment except for the relatively small foramina results in differences in position and prominence of certain vessels, and in their physiology. Blood passes more rapidly through the intracranial vessels than those in the face and neck. When x-ray pictures are taken in a series at intervals of one second following the injection of a solution of x-ray opaque substance in the common carotid artery, the branches of the internal carotid are revealed in the first picture, those of the external carotid a second later. If not more than 10 cc. of contrast medium is used, there follows after the visualization of the arteries a period in which no vessels are seen as the thorotrast is diffusely distributed in capillaries and the smaller arterioles and venules. About two seconds after injection the superficial intracranial veins show in the film, and after four seconds the deep veins and sinuses appear (Figs. 72, 73).

ARTERIAL SYSTEM.   In the first phase following injection of contrast medium, the internal carotid artery after its course in the cavernous sinus shows a curve forward and then backward, which caused Moniz to term this region the "carotid siphon." The siphon may be simple or may have a double curve or a transitional form, each condition occurring in about a third of the cases examined by Moniz (Lima, 1950).

From the carotid siphon three arteries arise, though seen without constancy in the films: the ophthalmic artery, which extends anteriorly toward the orbit: the chorioid artery, which extends posteriorly as almost a straight line; and the

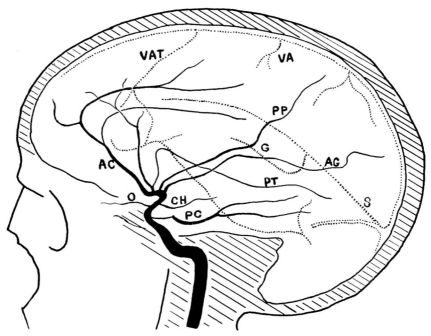

FIGURE 72. Composite diagram showing appearance of parts of some intracranial vessels displayed by intracarotid injection of an x-ray opaque medium. Arteries are shown in solid black, veins are dotted lines. The internal carotid is shown in its tortuous route through the cavernous sinus before branching. The posterior cerebral (*PC*) artery is seen connected with the carotid by the posterior communicating artery. Just above this are the anterior chorioid artery (*CH*) extending posteriorly and the ophthalmic (*O*) anteriorly. The next three vessels are branches of the middle cerebral artery which is foreshortened because its course is directed laterally: *PP*, posterior parietal; *AG*, artery of the angular gyrus; *PT*, posterior temporal. The anterior cerebral artery (*AC*) arches about the anterior end of the corpus callosum. The superior sagittal sinus is visible just beneath the cranial vault. The superior cerebral veins are sometimes called anastomotic (*VA*); one of these is associated with the name of Trolard (*VAT*). The straight sinus (*S*) shows its continuous line with the inferior sagittal sinus and the great cerebral vein (of Galen, *G*) entering it. Below the straight sinus is seen the transverse sinus.

posterior communicating, which connects with the posterior cerebral in such a way as to make an apparently continuous vessel. The posterior cerebral artery, though a branch of the basilar, arises ontogenetically with the internal carotid system, and receives its nerve supply via the internal carotid. It is not usually demonstrated with carotid injection. Injection of vessels in the posterior fossa shows the basilar artery to be vertical in position.

The terminal branches of the carotid siphon are the middle cerebral (Sylvian) and the anterior cerebral. Arising from the middle cerebral artery can be seen the posterior temporal, posterior parietal, and the artery to the angular gyrus extending along the lateral fissure (of Sylvius) as the source of supply to adjacent areas. In only about one fifth of the cases does the middle cerebral artery extend a long way without dividing. From its subdivisions ascending arteries supply the parietal and the frontal lobe, those in front of the motor area often resembling a branched candelabra; descending branches supply the temporal lobe.

The anterior cerebral artery passes toward the medial surface of the hemisphere, joining its fellow of the opposite side through the anterior communicat-

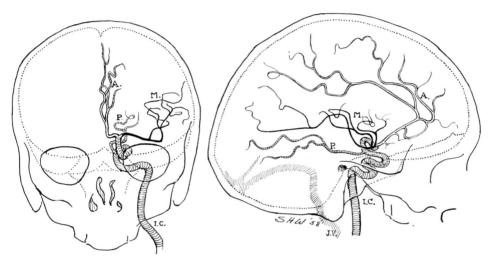

Figure 73. Anterior and lateral views of the head showing the main divisions of the internal carotid artery traced from x-ray plates of a patient following intra-arterial injection of a radio opaque suspension. *IC*, internal carotid artery (cross-banded); *A*, anterior cerebral artery (outlined); *P*, posterior cerebral artery (cross-banded); *M*, middle cerebral artery (solid black). In the lateral view posteriorly (shown in cross banding with no outline) are seen the transverse sinus and sigmoid sinus extending downward into the internal jugular vein, *JV*.

ing artery, and turns backward over the superior surface of the corpus callosum, where it usually divides into the callosomarginal and the pericallosal arteries. The latter marks the curve of the corpus callosum, gives off a sizable branch to the paracentral lobule, and extends to the splenium where it breaks up.

The anterior cerebral artery gives off central branches in the region of the anterior perforate space, which supply the anterior part of the caudate and lentiform nuclei and internal capsule, and, as it passes back over the corpus callosum, gives off collaterals to the medial aspect and superior margin of the hemispheres, thus supplying a significant part of the motor and sensory areas.

Venous System. In films showing the first phase of filling of superficial veins are seen several veins ascending to the superior sagittal sinus and others descending toward the lateral and cavernous sinuses. Two vessels are usually notable. The superior anastomotic vein (vein of Trolard) extends to the superior sagittal sinus anterior to or at the vertex; this vessel may or may not be in communication with a more posterior, horizontally placed vein which extends to the lateral sinus, and which is known as the vein of Labbé though this term is somewhat loosely used to indicate one or more veins in this region; it is typical in only about half the cases. A Rolandic vein in the region of the central sulcus is seen frequently but not always. Descending veins of the superficial group extend to the lateral, cavernous, and petrosal sinuses, and to the sinus confluens.

In the second phase of venous filling the dural sinuses are constantly seen, as well as the great vein of Galen with its tributaries. An interesting observation can be made that the inferior sagittal sinus and the straight sinus extend in a continuous smooth curve, the straight sinus lying nearly vertically (about 70 degrees) instead of bending like a sickle as usually depicted from dissections (Fig. 60). In certain pathologic conditions the normal pattern of the blood vessels is altered sufficiently to be displayed by angiography.

Baló (1950) has described a system of venous cavernous spaces within the dura surrounding the straight sinus, the confluence of sinuses, and the posterior part of the superior sagittal sinus which when engorged would appear to restrict the outflow of venous blood from the brain. Such a mechanism correlated with that of the carotid sinus and other controlling devices would aid in regulating the intracranial blood supply and pressure.

CHAPTER IV

Histogenesis of the Nervous System

The way in which the brain and spinal cord are constructed of neurons is made clearer by studying the development of these from the early neural tube stage. It should be kept in mind that the cells of the neural tube are laid down according to a definite hereditary pattern for each species, and it is to be expected that adequate quantities of mature nerve cells develop from the primitive ones to make the large masses of nervous tissue possessed by the adult. Furthermore the connections made by the growth of processes between distant collections of neurons are determined on a hereditary specific basis; but the active growth of these processes over any appreciable distance is subject to the hazards of the terrain. Growing like vines on a trellis, they exhibit stereotropism, following the fiber pattern or blood vessels in the region entered. Thus there is some variation in the connections of a pathway as between individuals, which may be reflected in functional differences.

Early Stages in the Differentiation of the Neural Tube.   The nervous system, including cerebrospinal and sympathetic nerves and their associated ganglia as well as the brain and spinal cord, is of ectodermal origin. At first the neural plate consists of a single layer of ectodermal cells (Fig. 74, *A*). These cells proliferate and at the time of closure of the neural tube several layers of nuclei can be seen, but each belongs to a cell reaching the inner and outer margins of the tube. In poorly fixed material the cell boundaries are indistinct. Terminal bars occur between the ends of the cells which line the cavity of the neural tube and the whole presents the appearance of a pseudostratified columnar epithelium (Fig. 74). Nuclei of cells undergoing mitosis migrate to a zone nearest the tubular lumen (Sauer, 1935). As proliferation continues the wall of the tube becomes thicker, the component cells begin to differentiate into both supporting cells and primitive nerve cells, and three zones may be distinguished: (1) An internal ependymal layer, which persists as the lining of the cavities of brain and spinal cord; (2) a middle *mantle layer* containing many cells which becomes the gray matter of the brain and cord; and (3) the outer *marginal layer,* which in the cord is the future white matter, but has not so conspicuous a role in the brain.

Golgi preparations of the developing neural tube reveal that some of the cells have long processes and extend between the inner and outer margins of the tubular wall (Fig. 75). These are *primitive spongioblasts* and those whose cell bodies remain in the ependymal layer develop into the ependymal cells which line the brain ventricles and the central canal of the spinal cord. Others, after losing their attachment to the internal margin and, later, in most instances also their attachment to the external margin, are transformed into neuroglia cells, the supporting elements of the nervous system. Even in the adult some ependymal cells in the region of the anterior median fissure of the spinal cord

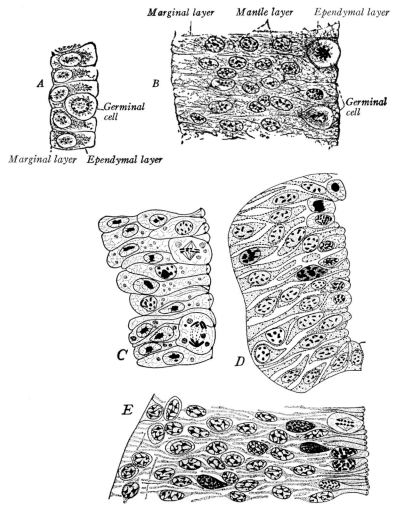

FIGURE 74. Early stages in the differentiation of the neural tube: *A,* From a rabbit embryo before closure of neural tube; *B,* from a 5 mm. pig embryo after closure of tube; (Hardesty, Prentiss-Arey.) *C,* neural plate of a chick embryo showing columnar shape of cells except when undergoing mitosis, and the terminal bars between adjacent cells; *D,* neural tube (one side) from a toadfish embryo showing independence of cells; *E,* alar plate of neural tube of a 10 mm. pig embryo showing columnar shape of cells, terminal bars, and mitoses near the lumen (*C, D,* and *E* from F. C. Sauer, 1935).

(Fig. 97) retain their superficial attachments, as do also the subpial neuroglia cells. Within the mantle layer, spongioblasts, neuroblasts, and indifferent cells fill the spaces between the primitive spongioblasts. Later the neuroblasts develop into neurons and the spongioblasts into neuroglia. The chart below shows the lineage of the cells derived from the medullary epithelium, including neurons, ependymal cells, and the different types of neuroglia (protoplasmic astrocytes, fibrillary astrocytes, and oligodendroglia). Mesodermal cells migrate into the

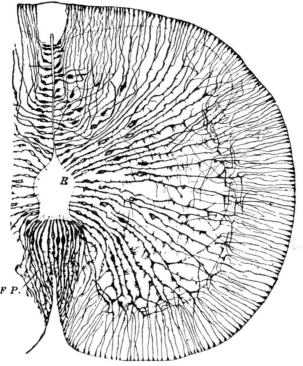

FIGURE 75. Neuroglia in the spinal cord of a ten weeks' human fetus: *E*, Central canal into which processes from ependymal cells project; *F.P.*, floor plate. (Cajal, Arey.)

central nervous system at about the time of birth and give rise to an additional element of the supporting tissue, microglia.

The Development of the Neuron. A neuron may be defined as a nerve cell with all its processes; each is derived from a single neuroblast. The young nerve cells, wherever they may be in the neural tube, in the neural crest, or ectodermal placodes, grow in characteristic manner which determines the histologic structure of nervous tissue. The processes sent out by the neuroblasts are of two types. The primary process, the future axon, grows away from the nerve cell. It is this sprout which forms the highly specialized axon (Fig. 76); the others developing later become dendrites, sometimes referred to as the protoplasmic extensions of the cell body.

The method of growth of the axon has been examined carefully by Cajal in fixed, stained preparations, by Harrison and his students in tissue cultures (Weiss, 1945), and by Speidel (1935) as the normal living nerve fiber in the tadpole's tail. All such observations serve to impress the principles of growth of young axons, which, incidentally, are the same as the principles of growth of axons regenerating after injury. Each newly growing nerve fiber bears upon its end an ameboid tip which projects small, searching pseudopodia into the interstices of the tissue through which the fiber is growing, and, while the general direction of growth is determined by other circumstances, the path of the individual fiber is influenced greatly by the terrain. As each ameboid tip moves along

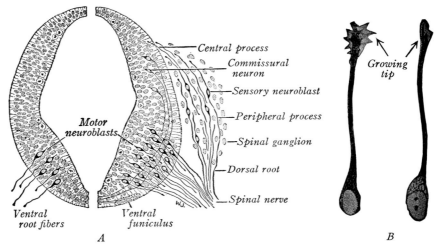

FIGURE 76.   Differentiation and growth of human neuroblasts. *A,* Drawings from transverse sections of the spinal cord of a 4 mm. embryo (on the left) and a 5 mm. embryo (on the right). (Arey.) *B,* Neuroblasts with enlarged growing tips. (Cajal, Arey.)

spinning its fiber behind it, it exhibits stereotropism, that is, the growing tip finds its way along by following previously laid down blood vessels, nerve fibers, or even connective tissue bundles. Once a few nerve fibers have traversed a region, many others may follow along these to form a nerve bundle. In the case of embryonic tissues where a certain orderliness prevails, the path of the nerve bundle will be reasonably straight, though obstacles such as blood vessels and supporting elements can cause temporary or permanent deviation. In the regrowth of a cut nerve through scar tissue the path may be quite devious.

The primary processes, or axons, of the neuroblasts of the neural tube (Fig. 76) grow into the marginal layer, within which they may turn and run up or down parallel to the long axis of the neural tube as association fibers; or they may run out of the neural tube in a ventrolateral direction as motor axons. In this way the motor fibers of the cerebrospinal nerves are laid down, each being the primary process which has grown out from a neuroblast in the basal plate of the neural tube.

CELL LINEAGE IN THE CENTRAL NERVOUS SYSTEM

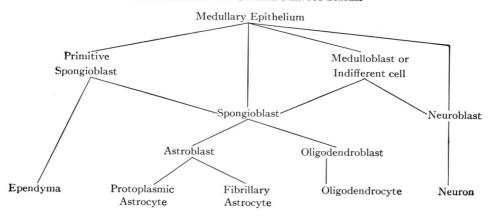

Development of Afferent Neurons. The sensory or afferent fibers of the spinal nerves take origin from neuroblasts which with few exceptions are from the beginning outside the neural tube. These neuroblasts are derived from the *neural crest,* a longitudinal ridge of ectodermal cells at the margin of the neural groove, where this becomes continuous with the superficial ectoderm. At first in contact with the dorsal surface of the neural tube, the neural crest soon separates from it and comes to form a band of cells lying in the angle between it and the superficial ectoderm (Fig. 12). Enlargements develop at intervals along this band due to the uneven proliferation of its cells and become the *sensory ganglia.* From neuroblasts located in these ganglia arise the sensory fibers of the cerebrospinal nerves.

Some exceptions to this general rule need to be mentioned. The fibers of the olfactory nerve arise from cells in the olfactory mucous membrane. The fibers of the mesencephalic root of the trigeminal nerve, which in all probability are sensory, arise from cells located within the mesencephalon. The optic nerve is also an exception, but this is morphologically a fiber tract of the brain and not a true nerve. An ingenious theory, advanced by Schulte and Tilney (1915), attempts to bring this mesencephalic root and the optic nerve into more obvious relation with the other sensory nerves. They assume that the part of the neural crest which lies rostral to the anlage of the semilunar ganglion fails to separate from the neural tube. From this part of the neural crest, retained within the brain, they would derive the mesencephalic nucleus of the trigeminal nerve and the optic vesicles.

On the other hand, there are observations which show that some of the cranial sensory ganglia are derived in part from other sources than the neural crest. Landacre (1910) observed that many of the sensory ganglion cells of the seventh, ninth, and tenth nerves are derived from thickened patches of the superficial ectoderm, known as placodes, with which the ganglia of these nerves come in contact at an early stage in their embryonic development. It has been demonstrated, at least in lower forms, that the visceral afferent neurons of the seventh, ninth, and tenth nerves are derived from cells of the epibranchial placodes, while the general somatic afferent fibers are derived from neural crest cells. However, such neural crest cells probably migrate from a more caudal source, the neural crest of the posterior medullary region entering into the formation of satellite cells, sheath cells and even cartilage (Yntema, 1944).

There is an interrelationship in their development and growth between the neurons and the peripheral field or structures with which they are connected. Removal of the field supplied in the young embryo results in diminution of the number and size of the nerve cells in centers and ganglia related to the fields.

Furthermore, the cytoplasmic differentiation within the nerve cells that would have supplied the lost structures is affected (Barron and Mottet, 1951).

The neuroblasts of the cerebrospinal ganglia become *bipolar* through the development of a primary process at either end (Fig. 77). Originally bipolar, a majority of these sensory neurons in the mammal become *unipolar* through the fusion of the two primary processes for some distance into a single main stem. Beyond the point of fusion this divides like a T into two primary branches, one of which is directed centrally, the other peripherally. The centrally directed branch grows into the neural tube as a sensory root fiber, the other grows

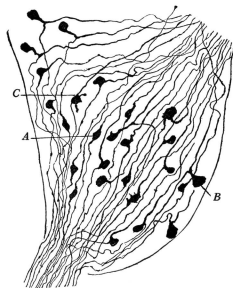

FIGURE 77. A section of a spinal ganglion from a 44 mm. fetus, showing stages in the transformation of bipolar neurons, *A*, into unipolar neurons, *B*, Golgi method. (Cajal.)

peripherally as an afferent fiber of a cerebrospinal nerve (Fig. 76, *A*). Some ectodermal cells, derived like the ganglion cells from the neural crest, form capsules surrounding these ganglion cells. It should be noted that the cells of the sensory ganglia of the acoustic nerve remain bipolar throughout life.

Nerve Fiber Sheaths. So far we have dealt only with the origin of the axis cylinders of the nerve fibers. But these soon become surrounded by protective *sheaths* which are also ectodermal in origin. In the path of the outgrowing axons there are seen numerous spindle-shaped ectodermal cells which have migrated from the neural tube and neural crest along the course of the ventral and dorsal roots. These cells form such a prominent feature in a developing nerve that it was once thought that the axons differentiate *in situ* from them. This theory, which gives to each axon a multicellular origin, has been known as the *cell chain hypothesis*. There are good reasons, however, for believing that each axon arises as an outgrowth from a single cell or neuroblast. This idea, which is in keeping with what is known of the structure and function of the neuron and which forms an integral part of the now generally accepted *neuron theory,* was first developed in the embryologic publications of His. Convincing experimental evidence has been furnished by Harrison (1906, 1935). Using amphibian larvae, this author showed that if the neural crest and tube are removed no peripheral nerves develop. He further showed that neuroblasts cultivated in lymph will give rise to long axons in the course of a few hours. The ectodermal cells, mentioned above, which are found along the course of the developing nerve, take an important part in the differentiation of the fibers. From them is derived the nucleated sheath or neurilemma of the peripheral nerve fiber. The myelin sheath, a lipoid covering often of some thickness, has been shown to develop around axis cylinders under the influence of the neurilemmal cells. Such interdependence between axis cylinder and neurilemma has been observed in living fibers by Speidel in the tadpole's tail, and in tissue cultures of spinal ganglia of chicks (Peterson and Murray, 1955).

Development of the Spinal Nerves. We have traced the development of the chief elements entering into the formation of the cerebrospinal nerves, and shall now see how these are combined in a typical spinal nerve. The spinal ganglion, derived from the neural crest, contains bipolar neuroblasts, which are transformed into unipolar neurons. The axons of such a nerve cell divides into a central branch, running through the dorsal root into the spinal cord, and a peripheral branch, running distally through the nerve to reach the skin or other sensitive portion of the body. Mingled with these afferent fibers in the spinal nerves are efferent axons which have grown out from neuroblasts in the basal plate of the spinal cord, through the ventral root, and are distributed by way of the spinal nerve to muscles.

The **sympathetic ganglia** consists of cells of ectodermal origin, derived like the cells of the neurilemma sheaths from the neural crest.

The exact origin of the cells which are found along the course of the developing nerves and give rise to the neurilemma sheaths, and of those which form the sympathetic ganglia, has been in dispute. It has been stated that some of both types migrate from the neural crests along the dorsal roots and that at a slightly later stage others come from the neural tube along the ventral roots. (Kuntz, 1934; Raybuck, 1956). According to Cowgill and Windle (1942) the cranial autonomic ganglia in the cat are derived from the neural crest cells associated with cranial nerves 5, 7, and 9 and receive no contribution from the neural tube.

Carefully controlled operative experiments in chick embryos show that the cells of the autonomic ganglia in all regions of the sympathetic trunk and the sacral parasympathetic ganglia are derived from the neural crest in the respective regions of the body and do not arise from the neural tube. Similarly, the intrinsic visceral ganglia of the thorax and abdomen are derived from neural crest near the origin of the vagus nerve. The experiments establishing these points and the literature can be traced through the papers of Yntema and Hammond (1945), 1954, 1955). Additional data in support of this interpretation are given by Nawar (1956).

Supporting cells other than those of mesodermal origin found in the ganglia of both autonomic and dorsal root ganglia are derived from the neural crest and possibly neural tube. They constitute sheath cells, capsular cells, and others resembling oligodendroglia (Brizzee, 1949).

The **spinal cord** of a 20 mm. human embryo presents well-defined ependymal, marginal, and mantle layers. Figure 78 should be compared with the appearance presented by a cross-section of the spinal cord in the adult (Fig.

126. The *mantle layer* with its many nuclei differentiates into the *gray matter* of the spinal cord, which contains the nerve cells and their dendritic processes. The *marginal layer* develops into the white substance as a result of the growth into it of the axons from neuroblasts located within the mantle layer. These form association fibers which ascend or descend through the marginal layer and serve to connect one level of the neural tube with another. It is not until these longitudinally coursing axons develop myelin sheaths that the *white substance* acquires its characteristis coloration.

The cavity of the neural tube is relatively large, and at the point marked "neural cavity" in Fig. 78 a groove is visible. This is the sulcus limitans. It

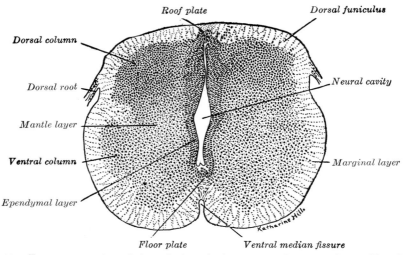

FIGURE 78. Transverse section of the spinal cord of a 20 mm. human embryo. (Prentiss-Arey.)

separates the dorsal or *alar plate* from the ventral or *basal plate*. The mantle layer of the alar plate develops into the *dorsal gray column* which, like the other parts developed from this plate, is afferent in function. The afferent fibers, growing into the spinal cord from the spinal ganglia, terminate in this dorsal column or ascend in the posterior part of the marginal zone to nuclei derived from the alar plate in the myelencephalon. Most of the association fibers which run in the marginal layer have grown out from neuroblasts located in the dorsal column. The mantle layer of the basal plate gives rise to the *ventral gray column*. From neuroblasts in this region grow out the motor fibers of the ventral roots and spinal nerves.

The spinal cord remains tubular in form, and the relationship of the parts developed from the alar and basal laminae can be distinguished in the completely developed cord. The position of the sulcus limitans can be traced as far forward as the diencephalon, and segregation of afferent neurons respectively dorsal and ventral to it is apparent in the brain stem. But with the development of the cranial nerves connected with the special senses and the motor side of the mechanisms for feeding, respiration, vocalization, and eye control, and with the acquisition of the large suprasegmental structures at the cranial end of the neural tube, the relative simplicity of the tubular pattern becomes obscured.

In the study of behavior, both prenatal and postnatal, many correlations with the appearance of neuronal structures and the histology of centers have been made. The elements of the various reflex arcs appear histologically at times in which the integrity of the reflex can be demonstrated physiologically. The complexity of both movement and central nervous system histology increases simultaneously. Windle, studying the cat, pointed out that at about four weeks of age the kitten's movements change from a slow clumsy waddling gait to the graceful, playful, rapid, agile manner characteristic of the species, and the complexity of the central nervous system neuropil likewise increases rapidly. His study of human prenatal behavior has been carefully reviewed by Hooker (1952) and compared with data from amphibia by Coghill and others, and birds and mammals by Windle and others. Hooker reviews the divergent points of view that have arisen concerning the pattern of appearance of mass movements and of individual reflexes. The researches of Coghill and others developed the concept that behavior starts as a total pattern out of which more or less specific reflexes appear. Windle (1940) has supported the concept that local reflexes appear individually as local responses in the fetus during development and later are brought together into more generalized movements.

This study extends naturally into that of postnatal behavior so completely observed in the human infant (Gesell and Amatruda, 1945) and to the differences in the behavior of various species described by such terms as instinctive, endogenous (Ewer, 1957) and conditioned (Pavlow, 1940).

CHAPTER V

Neurons and Neuroglia

In the study of the nervous system the purpose is to discover the underlying basis or mechanism by which the animal responds to stimuli. There are, of course, many directions from which this study could be approached. Although it is obvious that the function of the whole nervous system is more than the sum of the function of its parts, it is valuable to examine the shape and structure of the elements of which it is composed. From the earliest times the brain and spinal cord have been considered anatomically and the parts thereof named and described, but not until the development of the microscope and the technical methods of staining in the last century was sufficient analysis of the nervous system made to allow an interpretation of it on the basis of its ultimate units, which, it happens, are microscopic.

It was in 1838–39 that Schleiden and Schwann, making use of Brown's discovery of the nucleus (1831), developed the idea that all living substance was composed of separate small nucleated masses of protoplasm which they called cells; this was the term Hooke (1665) had applied to the empty box-like spaces he had seen with his simple microscope in thin slices of cork, and which had reminded him of the bare rooms of monasteries. Hooke was, of course, dealing with the cellulose walls of plant cells from which the protoplasm had disappeared, but the term cell has come to mean the original contents with its wonderful attributes of life.

As students of histology following Schleiden and Schwann went systematically through the body describing components of tissues, the nervous system resisted interpretation in terms of the cell theory because of the complex shape of its units. Ordinary staining procedures failed to disclose the processes of nerve cells although they did stain the cell body and nucleus. The way was prepared for the study of nervous tissue by the development of photography, for the process of precipitation of silver salts used by Daguerre (1839) was applied to the nervous system by Golgi (1880) and Cajal to reveal intricate details of nerve fibers and the shapes of neurons. As it became obvious that nerve cells were shaped quite differently from most other cells and included long extensions from the cell body the so-called *neuron doctrine* was formulated, and expressed by Waldeyer in 1891 as an application of the cell theory to nervous tissue.

98

Its chief tenets are as follows:

1. The neuron is the *genetic unit* of the nervous system—each neuron being derived from a single embryonic cell, the neuroblast.

2. The neuron is the *structural unit* of the nervous system, a nerve cell with all its processes. These cellular units remain anatomically separate, i. e., while they come into contact with each other at the synapses there is no continuity of their substance.

3. The neurons are the *functional units* of the nervous system and the conduction pathways are formed of chains of such units.

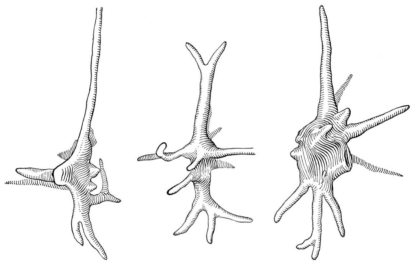

Figure 79. Drawings of reconstructions made by Weil of the bodies of three nerve cells from the ventral horn of gray matter of the spinal cord. Note that the craniocaudal diameter (vertical) is greater than the transverse. Only the stumps of the processes are shown. The cells from left to right were from cervical, thoracic, and lumbar segments respectively.

4. The neuron is also a *trophic unit*, as is seen (a) in the degeneration of a portion of an axon severed from its cell of origin, (b) in the phenomenon of chromatolysis or axon reaction, and (c) in the regeneration of the degenerated portion of the axon by an outgrowth from that part of the axon still in contact with its cell of origin.

5. Neurons are the only elements concerned in the conduction of nerve impulses. The nervous system is composed of untold numbers of such units linked together in conduction systems.

It has been pointed out that each neuron is the product of a single embryonic cell or neuroblast, and that, therefore, the nerve cell with all of its processes constitutes a genetic unit. In the present chapter, as the form and internal structure of the neurons and their relation to each other are examined it will be seen that they are also the structural and functional units of the nervous system.

Form. There is a wide variation in the shape of nerve cells but all present

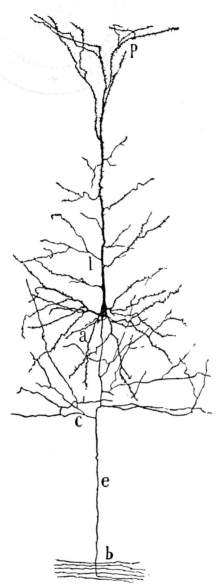

FIGURE 80. A pyramidal cell from the cerebral cortex of a mouse: *a*, Dendrites from the
base of the cell; *b*, white substance of the
hemisphere into which the axon, *e*, can be
traced; *c*, collateral from the first part of the
axon; *l*, apical dendrite; *p*, its terminal branches
near the surface of the cortex. Golgi method.
(Cajal.)

some features in common. About the
nucleus there is an accumulation of cytoplasm which together with the nucleus
forms what is often called the cell body,
or *perikaryon*. From the perikaryon,
cytoplasmic processes are given off.
These may be classified in two groups:
axons and dendrites.

From a histologic point of view
axons and dendrites differ. The dendrites
have much the same structure as the
perikaryon while the axons are more
specialized. From a functional point of
view it is often stated that axons conduct impulses away from the perikaryon
and dendrites toward it. Such a gen-
eralization creates a conflict with the
histologic distinction in some instances,
as for example, the neurons of the cerebrospinal ganglia. Furthermore, direct
stimulation of some dendrites, as the
apical ones of cortical pyramidal cells
(Bishop and Clare, 1953), results in conduction away from the cell body. The
histological distinction between axons
and dendrites is therefore the more
reliable.

Axons, of which each neuron has one
and very rarely more than one, are
usually longer than the dendrites and
some are very long, measuring as much
as 3 feet. Either naked or along with
their enclosing sheaths they are also
called nerve fibers and constitute the
bulk of the pathways of the central
nervous system as well as the various
nerves. Usually they show a conical
expansion at their point of attachment
to the cell body, the cone of origin or
axon hillock (Figs. 82, 86). One or more
side branches or *collaterals* may be given
off, usually at right angles to the fiber
(Fig. 80). Collaterals arise more commonly near than at great distances from
the cell body, while an axon terminates usually at considerable distance from
its cell of origin in a multitude of fine branches, called *teleodendria*. Such

collaterals extending from the axons of motor cells in the spinal cord (Fig. 84) apparently activate internuncial neurons of the adjacent gray matter, and these in turn act on other motor neurons, possibly to inhibit them or to bring them also into action, depending upon individual connections. Cells with long axons are classed in *Golgi's Type I*. Some cells have short axons that branch repeatedly and end in the neighborhood of the cell of origin and these belong to *Golgi's Type II* (Fig. 81). Axons are characterized by their

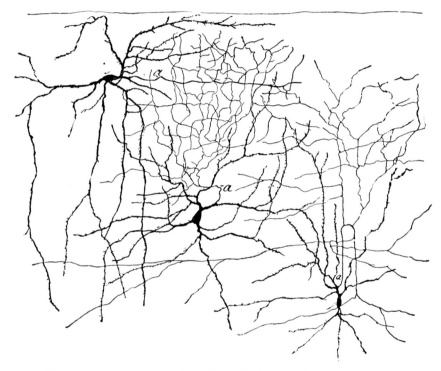

FIGURE 81.   Neurons with short axons (Type II of Golgi) from the cerebral cortex of a child: *a*, Axon Golgi method. (Cajal.)

uniform thickness, smooth contour, small diameter, relative freedom from side branches and usually also by their great length.

Several *dendrites* may and usually do arise from a single nerve cell. The origin is by a wide base, and near the cell dendrites may be much thicker than any axon, but they taper rapidly and form terminal arborizations at no great distance from their cell bodies. They are characterized by their repeated branching, short course, varying caliber, and irregular contour. They are often studded with short side branches which give them a spiny appearance. The feltwork formed by the interlacing arborizations of the dendrites of adjacent cells and the telodendria of axons from far and near form what is called the neuropil (Fig. 134).

The external form of the neuron depends on the shape of the perikaryon and on the number, shape, and ramification of the processes. Dependent upon the number of processes arising from the cell body, a neuron is termed unipolar, bipolar, or multipolar. The variety of forms is almost without limit, but a few typical examples will give an adequate picture of them.

The *pyramidal cells* of the cerebral cortex which are multipolar have the shape which the name implies (Fig. 80). One angle of the pyramid, that directed

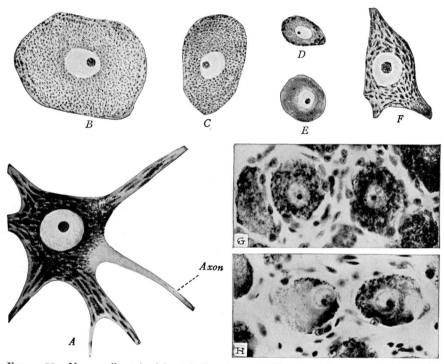

FIGURE 82.   Nerve cells stained by toluidine blue: *A*, Motor cell from anterior horn of spinal cord of a monkey (Schäfer); *B*, large sensory cell from spinal ganglion of a dog (Clark); *C*, sensory cell from the trigeminal mesencephalic nucleus of a dog (Clark); *D* and *E*, small sensory cells from spinal ganglion of a dog (Clark); *F*, motor cell from nucleus of trochlear nerve of a dog (Clark); *G*, photomicrograph of cells of spinal ganglion of a cat (Windle); *H*, photomicrograph of cells of cat's spinal ganglion, showing chromatolysis. (Windle.)

toward the surface of the cortex, is prolonged in the form of a long thick branching process, the apical dendrite. From the other angles and the sides of the perikaryon arise shorter branching dendrites, while from the base or from one of the basal dendrites arises a long slender axon which, after giving off collaterals, continues on its way to distant parts.

Another good example of multipolar cells (Fig. 79, 82, 84, 86) is furnished by the *primary motor neuron*. This is a large nerve cell with many rather long branching dendrites and an axon, which forms the axis cylinder of a motor nerve fiber and terminates by forming motor endings in a muscle. As illustrated in this figure, long axons tend to acquire myelin sheaths, and those which run in the cerebrospinal nerves are also covered by a nucleated membranous sheath—the neurilemma.

Examples of *unipolar* and *bipolar cells* are found in the cerebrospinal ganglia (Figs. 108, 188). These cells, which will be described in more detail in another chapter, are devoid of dendrites. The axon of such a unipolar cell divides dichotomously into a central and a peripheral branch, each possessing the characteristics of an axon.

It is not uncommon to regard the peripheral branch of a sensory neuron as a dendrite, because like the dendrites it conducts nerve impulses toward the cell body. But, since it possesses all the morphologic characteristics of an axon, and since any axon is able to conduct nerve impulses throughout its length in either direction, and since these peripheral branches of the sensory neurons actually convey impulses distally in the phenomenon of antidromic conduction, it seems best to consider both central and peripheral branches as divisions of a common axonic stem.

From what has been said it will be apparent that a neuron usually possesses several dendrites and a single axon, but some have only one process, which is then an axon. It may be added that some neurons have more than one axon.

Structure of Neurons.   Like other cells, a neuron consists of a nucleus surrounded by cytoplasm, and these possess the fundamental characteristics which belong to nuceus and cytoplasm everywhere, but each presents certain features more or less characteristic of the nerve cell. The *nucleus* is large and spheric, and, because it contains little chromatin, it stains lightly with the basic dyes (Fig. 82, *A*). It has a large spheric *nucleolus*, which contains ribose nucleic acid.

A nucleolar satellite of small size which contains desoxyribose nucleic acid is common in the nuclei of nerve cells, and it has been asserted that sex of the animal can be distinguished by it: the satellite in the female being conspicuous, and that in the male being small or absent. Although doubt has been expressed about this distinction, if proven it would be of great importance to the geneticist. This distinction is apparently not found in all orders of animals (Moore and Barr, 1953).

The *cytoplasm* is enclosed in a delicate cell membrane which may be nothing more than a surface film of protoplasm, but it has a fair degree of tensile strength and is functionally a very important part of the neuron. An examination of the cell body with appropriate staining methods shows that it possesses mitochondria, Golgi apparatus, occasionally pigment and other substances found in cells generally, but has in addition two structures which especially characterize the nerve cell, Nissl granules and neurofibrils.

Nissl Granules.   In properly prepared sections Nissl granules appear in the cytoplasm as fine basophilic granules which are usually grouped in dense clumps. Also known as tigroid masses, or chromatophilic substance, the Nissl bodies differ with the type of nerve cell studied (Fig. 82), and they tend to be larger in motor than in sensory neurons (Malone, 1913). While they are found in the larger dendrites, the axon and its cone origin are usually free from them. The material of which these granules is composed appears to be a product of the nucleus and is perhaps an iron-containing nucleoprotein. Where neurons are studied in stages of development, the Nissl substance is first seen to appear as fine particles lying close to the nuclear membrane, and it appears to increase as the nucleolus shows development (LaVelle, 1956). It has not been seen in the living cell where it is in a state of solution or uniform suspension and it is precipitated in the form of granules by the fixative used in preparing the tissue for microscopic study. Though it is highly probable that Nissl substance as it appears in fixed preparations represents a fixation artifact, similar cells always

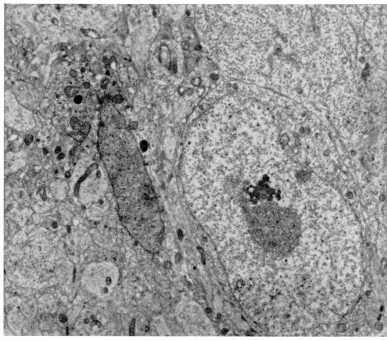

FIGURE 83. A small neuron from the medulla showing a large nucleus with a nucleolus. At the right of the nucleus is distinct neuronal cytoplasm with a definite membrane and granular complex of ergastoplasm. The clumping of the Nissl material is not seen so clearly in the thin sections of neurons in the medulla as it is in such cells as those of the posterior root ganglion. To the upper right of the neuron is cytoplasm of another neuron which is apparently in contact with the lower one. No nucleus is evident. To the left of the neuron is a microglial cell with a dense elongated nucleus. The complexity of the neuropil is evident elsewhere in the micrograph. (Luse.)

present similar Nissl pattern after fixation. It has been claimed that Nissl granules can be demonstrated in unstained, unfixed material by ultraviolet light, but it may be that the precipitation of such granules occurs at the moment of death. Ingvar (1923) was able to throw the Nissl substance to one side of the living cell by centrifuging while the neurofibrils remained nearer the center of the cell about the nucleus. Moulin (1923) simultaneously killed and stained nerve cells while watching them under the microscope, and observed first a diffuse staining succeeded by the appearance of clumps of basophilic staining material as the cell was fixed. Under electron microscopy Nissl substance is composed of thin laminae with granules about them resembling ergastoplasm (Fig. 83).

Morphologically, the pattern of distribution of Nissl substance varies in different nerve cells. Primary motor neurons are characterized by large flaky granules (Jacobsohn) arranged so that the long axis of the granules is parallel to the nearest margin of the cell. Malone pointed out that the somatic motor cells have larger granules than the visceral motor ones. On the other hand primary sensory neurons have quite a range of size in their Nissl granules. Those in the cerebro-spinal ganglia may be classified into four or five groups on the basis of the fineness and distribution of the Nissl substance, and while the most prominent cells in these ganglia are those large ones with fine evenly distributed Nissl granules there are at least a small number of others which have granules as large as some of the motor cells. It appears to be true then that a uniform stamp of Nissl granule arrangement is common to certain cells in the cerebrospinal ganglia. These cells may be of diverse functions but, perhaps, have a similar degree of specialization in their end organs. That is, neurons which receive impulses from the highly specialized tactile end organs have the same Nissl granule arrangement as those receiving impulses from proprioceptive end organs. And those in the 8th cranial nerve concerned with the reception of sound resemble those receiving impulses from the equilibratory apparatus of the internal ear (Clark, 1926).

One of the chief points of interest about Nissl substance is its capacity to re-act to injury of the neuron, for it is by this means that many paths and cell groups have been located in the nervous system. When the axon of a nerve cell is cut or injured, the cell body usually shows the phenomenon of **chromatolysis** during the week or two following the injury. The changes which occur include the gradual "dissolution" of the Nissl substance. At least, so it appears in stained sections, for the granules tend to disappear or recede to the periphery of the cell, leaving a diffusely stained or clear cytoplasm. The nucleus of the cell may be-come eccentric and show a cap of condensed chromophilic material. Mitochon-dria of the nerve cell showing chromatolysis increase in number, and may double in quantity by the tenth day after axon section (Hartman, 1948). The cell begins to show signs of repair after a week or two as the process of regene-ration of the cut axon goes on, unless the injury was too severe, in which case the neuron may undergo complete destruction.

While chromatolysis is a recognizable phenomenon when it occurs, it does not always follow injury to axons. The time of the peak reaction after injury varies somewhat with the distance of the injury from the cell, and with other conditions.

Better understanding of the Nissl substance in normal and damaged neu-rons has come through the work of Casperson and others who have used micro-chemical methods that involve identification of cell proteins by the selective absorption by specific proteins of definite spectral bands of ultraviolet light (microspectrophotometry). Such studies have revealed that the nerve cell in functioning normally continues to show protein synthesis like that of cells in rapid growth in developmental stages. It is stated that excessive neuronal activity, as in muscular work as related to motor nerve cells, or sensory stimu-lation, as in the effect of a prolonged sound on the neurons of the cochlear ganglion, resulted in diminution of the protein content of the cytoplasm to one-third its original quantity. Such work promises quantitative support of an idea long held that Nissl substance, which is rich in ribose nucleotides, is continually used up in normal function, and must be constantly replaced. There have been for years conflicting claims in the literature concerning the using up of Nissl substance in normal function. Quantitative studies will be necessary for proof, since there is normally as much variation in the Nissl pattern of similar cells in resting animals as that attributed to the effects of function (Liu, Bailey, and Windle, 1950).

Chromatolysis takes on a new interpretation as a result of microspectro-photometry. When the axon is severed normal action of the cell ceases, and the content of nucleotides and cytoplasmic proteins diminishes rapidly in the first two weeks. Then in the recovery stages as the cell activity returns there is

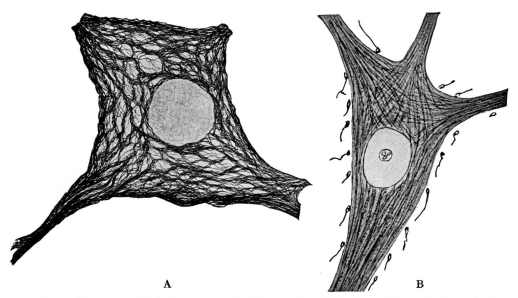

A   B

FIGURE 84. A, neurofibrils in a motor cell of the spinal cord (Maximow-Bloom). B, Neurofibrils in a nerve cell and synapses formed with it by looped endings of terminal branches of axons or boutons terminaux. (Cajal.)

noticeable increase in the substance of the nucleolus, the function of which is correlated with the synthesis of cytoplasmic protein. In the next stage of recovery large amounts of cytoplasmic nucleotides collect around the nuclear membrane, with a parallel increase in the cytoplasmic masses, and the nerve cell is gradually returned to its normal appearance.

It has been observed that a local constriction of nerve fibers which is maintained causes a kind of swelling of the axis cylinder proximal to the narrowing as if a flow of fluid were being dammed. Removal of the constriction is followed by movement distalward of the dammed up axoplasm at a slow rate. Such observations suggest that the perikaryon is the source of a supply of axoplasmic constituents which are used up in normal function and continuously supplied to the length of axon from the cell body (Weiss and Hiscoe, 1948).

NEUROFIBRILS. The neurofibrils are delicate threads which run through the cytoplasm in every direction and extend into the axon and dendrites (Fig. 84).

The appearance of the fibrillae differs according to the technique employed in preparing the tissue for microscopic examination. While in the preparations by Bethe's method the fibrils do not appear to branch or anastomose with each other, those seen in Cajal preparations divide, and by anastomosing form a true network. This network is present in the cell body; but, as the fibrils extend out into the processes, they become straight and run parallel to each other and to the long axes of the axons and dendrites in which they lie embedded in a viscous matrix. The neurofibrils can be traced to the terminations of the dendrites and axons. Their function is not known; but since they can be seen in living nerve fibres and nerve cells (de Rényi, 1929; Weiss and Wang, 1936), and in preparations made by the freezing-drying method (Hoerr, 1936), they cannot be regarded as artifacts produced by the reagents used in fixing the tissue.

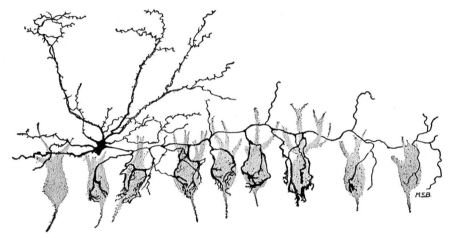

FIGURE 85. Basket cell from the cerebellar cortex of the white rat. The Purkinje cells are indicated in stipple. Branches of the axon of one basket cell form synapes with several Purkinje cells. Golgi method (Cajal).

Study of fixed axis cylinders with the electron microscope reveals nodose filaments of indefinite length and 75 to 200Å. in width which appear to be the basis of structure, but these are not identical with the much larger structures seen at ordinary magnification and termed neurofibrils (Schmitt, 1957).

OTHER CONTENTS OF NEURONS. *Pigment granules* are seen in the cytoplasm of some nerve cells and are of two kinds. Dark brown or almost black particles of melanin are found in the cells of certain regions (substantia nigra and locus caeruleus). Of a different nature are the yellow or orange colored granules which accumulate in nerve cells with advancing age. There is no reason to suppose that this pigment serves any useful purpose nor does it appear to interfere in any way with the normal function of the cell.

Small spheroids have been described in the nerve cells of the supraoptic and paraventricular nuclei, and even in Purkinje cells, which some have interpreted on morphologic grounds as evidence of a neurosecretion. Secretion products have been traced along the nerve fibers from the hypothalamus to the posterior lobe of the pituitary (Scharrer, 1944; Thomas, 1951; Smith, 1951; d'Angelo et al., 1956; Shanklin et al., 1957).

Other structures such as the internal reticular apparatus of Golgi and mitochondria are present in the cytoplasm.

Interrelation of Neurons. In the coelenterates, as we have learned, a single nerve cell may receive the stimulus and transmit it to the underlying muscle. But in vertebrates the transmission of a nerve impulse to an effector requires a

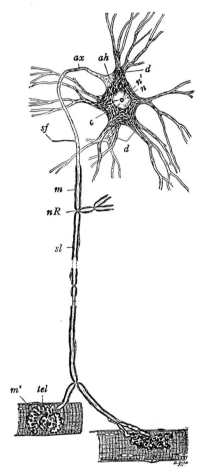

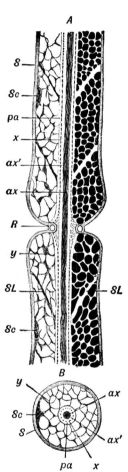

FIGURE 86. Primary motor neuron (diagrammatic): *ah*, Axon hillock; *ax*, axon; *c*, cytoplasm; *d*, dendrites; *m*, myelin sheath; *m'*, striated muscle; *n*, nucleus; *n'*, nucleolus; *nR*, node of Ranvier; *sf*, collateral; *sl*, neurilemma; *el*, motor end-plate. (Barker.)

FIGURE 87. Myelinated nerve fiber in *A*, longitudinal and *B*, transverse section (diagrammatic). On one side of the longitudinal section the myelin is black as after osmic acid fixation. Elsewhere the protoplasmic net, *y*, associated with the cytoplasm of the neurilemma cells, *Sc*, is shown as it appears after the myelin has been dissolved: *ax*, *ax'*, *x*, *pa*, somewhat shrunken axis cylinder; *SL*, Schmidt-Lantermann cleft; *S*, neurilemma sheath; *R*, node of Ranvier. (Nemiloff, Maximow-Bloom.)

chain of at least two neurons, the impulse passing from one neuron to the next along the chain. One of the most important problems in neurology, therefore, is this: How are the neurons related to each other so that the impulse may be propagated from one to the other? The place where two neurons come into such functional relation is known as a *synapse*. In a synapse the axon of one neuron terminates on the cell body or dendrites of another. It is not believed that functional connections are ever established between the dendrites of one neuron and the cell body or dendrites of another. The manner of termination of axons on cell bodies and dendrites of the cells varies in different localities (Figs. 84, 85).

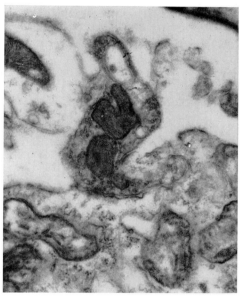

FIGURE 88. Synapse in medulla of rat. Within the synaptic ending there are numerous vesicular structures as well as mitochondria. In the cytoplasm of the neuron below on which the ending makes contact, there are both mitochondria and Nissl material. Note the distinct separation of the membrane of the synaptic ending and the plasma membrane of the neuron and also the increased density of the membrane at the point of contact. Electron micrograph. × 16,775. (Luse.)

There is the simple clasping of the nerve cell body by finger-like processes of the axon as in the trapezoid body, or the irregular expansions of collaterals meeting the cell body, as with the basket cells and their terminations on Purkinje cells of the cerebellum (Fig. 85). An incoming axon may break up in terminations which mingle with and end upon a tangled skein of dendrites from several cells as in autonomic ganglia (Fig. 118). Delicate branches of an axon may end on the surface of the cell body or dendrites of another neuron in the form of loops or *boutons terminaux* (Figs. 84, 88, 141). These terminal loops are the most common synaptic endings in the central nervous system. They vary in concentration and number in different parts of the brain (Smythies et al., 1957).

Although it has been maintained from time to time that there is protoplasmic continuity between neurons, there is no proof that the processes of one nerve cell are directly fused with those of others. On the contrary, *each neuron appears to be a distinct anatomic unit.* The most detailed study of Golgi and Cajal preparations, in which the finest ramifications of dendrites and axons are stained, has failed to demonstrate a structural continuity between neurons. In especially favorable material it has been shown that an axon and dendrite, entering into the formation of a synapse, are each surrounded by a distinct plasma membrane and that there is no direct protoplasmic continuity (Bodian, 1942). The electron microscope has disclosed finer details but the discontinuity is still evident (de Robertis and Bennett, 1955; Palay, 1956). There is close approximation of the limiting membranes of the presynaptic and postsynaptic neurons, the cleft between being in the neighborhood of 0.02 microns wide. The presynaptic expansion contains mitochondria and small vesicles which may be the source of neuro-

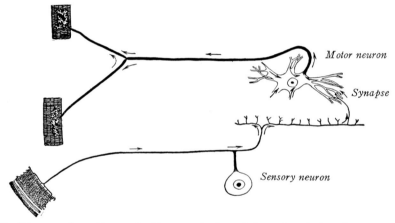

FIGURE 89.   Diagram of a reflex arc to illustrate the law of dynamic polarity. The arrows indicate the direction of conduction.

humoral substances. Studies of cholinesterase in the vertebrate brain point to a distribution specifically related to synapses (Shen et al., 1955). The conclusion that the relation between two neurons at a synapse is one of contact but not of continuity of substance, based primarily on histologic evidence, has been strongly reinforced by physiologic investigations (Eccles, 1957).

Nerve impulses are propagated across the synapse in one direction only, i.e., from the axon to the adjacent cell body or dendrite. As a corollary of this it is obvious that impulses must travel within the neuron from perikaryon out along the axon, as indicated by the arrow in Fig. 89. This is known as the *law of dynamic polarity.* The polarity, however, may not be dependent upon anything within the neuron itself, but upon something in the nature of the synaptic interval or the detailed arrangement of sensory and motor paths, which makes possible the propagation of an impulse in one direction only. There are many lines of evidence which show that when once activated a nerve fiber conducts equally well in either direction. When a motor fiber bifurcates, sending a branch to each of two separate muscles, stimulation of one branch will cause an impulse to ascend to the point of bifurcation, and then descend along the other branch to its motor ending (Fig. 89). This can often be demonstrated in regenerated nerves (Feiss, 1912), and is an example of antidromic conduction, i. e., conduction in the direction reverse to the usual one. It is also illustrated by dorsal root vasodilation and by the axon reflex (Bayliss, 1918).

Synaptic transmission, the propagation of a nerve impulse across a synapse, is not thoroughly understood. According to one view the incoming impulse causes an excitor substance, acetylcholine, to be liberated by the axonic terminals of the first neuron; and this substance excites the second neuron and initiates a nerve impulse in it. In contrast to this *chemical theory*, the *electrical theory* assumes that the second neuron of the synapse is excited by the action current potentials generated by the nerve impulse in the axonic terminals of the first neuron. In either case it is clear that the nerve impulse is not transmitted as such across the synaptic interval, but that it serves in some way to excite a new impulse in the second neuron (Gasser, 1939; Eccles, 1957).

There are those who support the idea that there is a neurochemical mechanism for transmission of nerve impulses at all synaptic junctions in both central and peripheral parts of the nervous system (Loewi, 1945). The evidence indicates that acetylcholine is released by the nerve endings which then acts on the next neuron in the chain but is promptly destroyed by cholinesterase. Such a mechanism has been demonstrated with reasonable certainty as occurring at the motor ending of skeletal muscle when it is excited by nerve impulses. And it seems fairly certain that the "Renshaw cells" in the medial portion of the ventral horn which receive collaterals from axons of the anterior horn cells are activated by the release of acetylcholine. This is implied since these same axons of anterior horn cells cause the release of acetylcholine at motor end plates on skeletal muscles. It has also been found that most postganglionic craniosacral autonomic nerves release acetylcholine at the junction with the effector muscle or gland, while most postganglionic thoracicolumbar autonomic fibers release epinephrine. (In a few instances the situation is reversed.) The terms "cholinergic" and "adrenergic" have been used to distinguish the fibers releasing acetylcholine and epinephrine respectively.

The use of microelectrodes has revealed potential changes in one neuron at a time (or its parts) produced by various methods of stimulation, and these have been studied with experimental alteration of the local environment.

From results of this and other types of experiment by many investigators, Eccles (1957) postulates that there are two types of neurons in the central nervous system, excitatory and inhibitory, and that each type releases a specific transmitter substance at its axonic terminals.

These in turn affect the ionic permeability of the appropriate subsynaptic membrane and there results the passage of specific sets of ions for each type of transmitter. (Permeability to all ions is supposed to occur with excitatory substance and only to small ions as chlorine and potassium, and *not* to sodium, with the inhibitory.) This process elicits the excitatory or inhibitory postsynaptic potential in the next neuron. Such an explanation demands, of course, proper specific arrangement of the intermediate neurons.

Within at least some neurons, differences occur in the type of response to stimuli applied to dendrites and cell body. For example, as described by Clare and Bishop (1955), when the dendrites of the pyramidal cells of the cerebral cortex are stimulated instead of the usual nerve impulse conducted toward the perikaryon, in all or none fashion, there is built up a relatively long lasting negative potential in the dendrite with a duration of 15 to 20 milliseconds, which can be added to or maintained by subsequent stimuli. During this period the cell body may be activated through other synaptic connections and fire an impulse along its axon, recover and continue to fire impulses repetitively, aided by the existing state of dendritic negativity. Such a principle, in which the parts of a neuron interact to maintain neural activity, adds to the generally accepted pattern of the interaction between neurons and has important implications on the function of the entire nervous system.

Nerve fibers are axons naked or ensheathed. The sheaths which may cover them are of two kinds: (1) a lipoid layer called the myelin sheath, which when present lies adjacent to the axis cylinder, and (2) a thin tubular covering with occasional nuclei. A nerve fiber may have neither, both, or either one of the sheaths upon it, so there are four possible types of nerve fibers according to the sheaths they possess. These may be presented readily by a diagram:

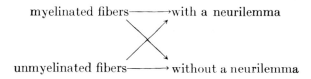

The neurilemma characteristically covers those nerve fibers found outside the central nervous system (except at some final terminations) and is lacking from those within it. Myelin is found on some fibers within and without the central nervous system but does not continue to the final terminations of the fibers. It is also found covering the bodies of the bipolar nerve cells upon the 8th cranial nerve (Fig. 91). The white glistening cerebrospinal nerves and the white matter of the brain and spinal cord owe their appearance to the presence of myelin.

The structure of a *myelinated peripheral nerve fiber* is shown in Figs. 86 and 87. The axon or *axis cylinder* is composed of delicate neurofibrils embedded in a semi-fluid neuroplasm. It is surrounded by a relatively thick *myelin sheath* and outside this a nucleated membranous *neurilemma sheath*. The myelin sheath consists of a fatty substance, myelin, supported by a reticulum. This net may perhaps be derived from the cytoplasm of the neurilemma cells or it may be a coagulation product developed during fixation. Thickened parts of the reticulum appear to correspond to the narrow clefts (Schmidt-Lantermann) that pass at irregular intervals obliquely through the myelin sheath. The highly refractive myelin gives to the myelinated fibers a whitish color. This sheath is interrupted at regular intervals by constrictions in the nerve fiber known as the nodes of Ranvier. Under electron microscopy the myelin sheath is seen as a series of parallel layers (Figs. 90, 91). At the constrictions is a dipping in of the neurilemma sheath toward the axon, which runs without interruption through the node. The part of a fiber between two nodes is an internodal segment, and each such segment possesses a nucleus which is surrounded by a small amount of cytoplasm and lies just beneath the neurilemma. In normal nerve fibers internodal segments are longer in larger than in smaller ones, although in newly regenerated fibers they are all about 300 micra in length regardless of caliber (Hiscoe, 1947). The neurilemma is a thin membranous outer covering for the fiber. Each segment of the neurilemma sheath, together with the cell which lies beneath, is the product of a single sheath cell of ectodermal origin.

The myelin is likewise considered to be at least in part the product of the activity of the sheath cell as it is deposited first in the neighborhood of the nucleus of this cell and then along the axon toward the next node of Ranvier. It has also been pointed out that the axis cylinder has part responsibility in the

FIGURE 90

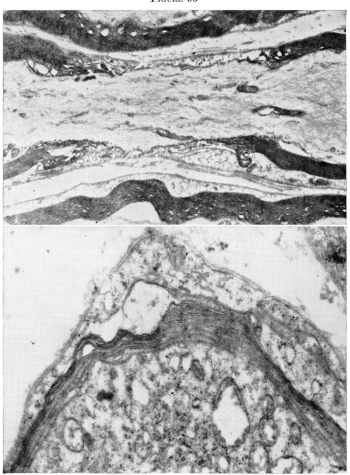

FIGURE 91

FIGURE 90. Peripheral node of Ranvier (from the trigeminal nerve) in which the neurofilaments are distinct in the axoplasm. The myelin lamellae are seen somewhat indistinctly at this magnification near their termination. The point of interest in this node is the covering of the axon by neurilemmal (Schwann cell) cytoplasm at the node and the continuation of the basement membrane of the cell. The endoneurium extends across the node external to the region in which the two neurilemmal cells meet. Electron micrograph × 6,000. (Luse.)

FIGURE 91. Portion of a neuron from the vestibular ganglion of the 8th nerve. The granular and membranous complex of the ergastoplasm are distinct. The mitochondria in this cell are somewhat swollen. The most distinctive feature of these cells is the myelin sheath which surrounds the ganglion cell body consisting here of about 12 lamellae. The outermost of these lamellae is continuous with the plasma membrane of a satellite cell, several satellite cells contributing to the sheath of the entire neuron. (Luse.)

deposition of myelin since, as Speidel has shown, sprouts of myelinated fibers develop myelin more commonly than sprouts of unmyelinated fibers, even though supplied with neurilemma by the descendants of the same sheath cells. That the neurilemma cells are not necessary for myelin production is shown by the presence of myelin about many of the nerve fibers of the central nervous system. The myelin sheath is known to impede diffusion of potassium from the nerve fibers, and perhaps has similar effect on other substances (van Harreveld, 1950).

The *myelinated fibers of the brain and spinal cord* differ from those of the peripheral nerves in the absence of neurilemma sheaths and sheath cells. Instead

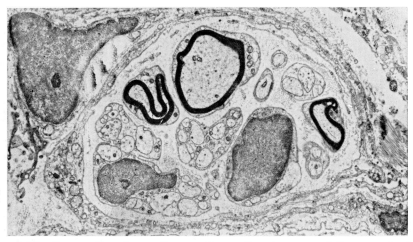

FIGURE 92.   Cross section of a small nerve. Surrounding the group of fibers are the flattened fibroblast-like cells of the epineurium. Three myelinated fibers are present and, although the neurilemmal nucleus is not present in the cross-section of any of these, the scant Schwann cytoplasm surrounding the fiber and its myelin sheath is distinct. Several groups of unmyelinated fibers in which no nucleus is evident are also seen. Nuclei of two neurilemmal cells are present. In the cytoplasm of the left one, numerous unmyelinated fibers are present, and in the right one there are three. Electron micrograph × 4,700. (Luse.)

there is an investment of neuroglia fibers and nuclei. It has been suggested that oligodendroglia cells may be concerned in the development of the myelin sheaths. The fibers of the brain and spinal cord have been shown to possess nodes of Ranvier, although this formerly was not thought to be true (Bodian, 1951; Pease, 1955).

Unmyelinated fibers are of two kinds, namely, naked axons and the fibers described by Remak that possess nuclei which may be regarded as belonging to a thin neurilemma. The latter are found in great numbers in the autonomic nervous system, and many of the fine afferent fibers of the cerebrospinal nerves also belong to this class (Ranson and Davenport, 1931). Naked axons are especially numerous in the gray matter and some paths of the brain and spinal cord, and every axon at its beginning from the nerve cell, as well as at its terminal arborization, is devoid of covering. Under electron microscopy it is seen that myelinated and unmyelinated axis cylinders have the same contents, and that more than one unmyelinated axon may be surrounded by a single neurilemmal sheath cell (Fig. 92).

By way of summary we may enumerate *four kinds of nerve fibers*: (1) myelinated fibers with a neurilemma, found in the peripheral nervous system, especially in the cerebrospinal nerves; (2) myelinated fibers without a neurilemma, found in the central nervous system; (3) unmyelinated fibers with a neurilemma (Remak's fibers), especially numerous in the autonomic system, and (4) naked axons, abundant in the brain and spinal cord.

Conduction of an impulse along a nerve fiber is accompanied by an alteration of the electrical potential of the tissues. By recording the potential with galvanometer or cathode ray oscillograph, the speed of conduction in nerve fibers can be determined. With such means it is possible to show that impulses pass

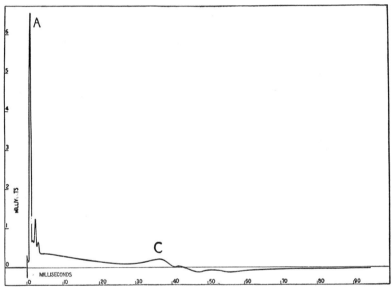

FIGURE 93. Form of action potential in the saphenous nerve of the cat, showing two spikes, *A* and *C*. (Gasser.)

over nerve fibers, at rates of from one to 100 meters per second. By measuring the speed of impulse transmission in selected bundles of nerve fibers it can also be shown that the larger fibers tend to transmit impulses at faster rates and smaller fibers at slower rates. By studying the fiber size and the speed of transmission in nerve bundles of known physiologic function, correlation of these items can be made.

An example of this type of analysis is shown in Fig. 93 which illustrates potentials recorded from the saphenous nerve of a cat following electrical stimulation. The nerve was stimulated at a point 5 cm. from the point where the potentials were picked up, and the stimulus was sufficiently strong to activate all the fibers in the nerve. The fastest fibers in this nerve, conducting at rates varying from 75 to 15 meters per second, had action potentials which were recorded as spike *A*, which includes a second smaller elevation. The third elevation, *C*, was produced by potentials from unmyelinated sensory and autonomic fibers having conduction velocities of 2 to 1 meters per second (Gasser, 1934, 1941). In motor nerves the large myelinated sensory and motor fibers with speeds up to 100 meters per second contribute to the *A* spike, which in the saphenous is formed by the sensory fibers to the skin. In records obtained from autonomic nerves an intermediate spike, *B,* appears, representing the action potentials of preganglionic visceral efferent fibers, with rates of conduction varying between 14 and 3 meters per second (Bishop and Heinbecker, 1930).

A relationship of acetylcholine metabolism and conduction in nerve fibers has been sought, but the content of acetylcholine in dorsal roots and postganglionic autonomic fibers as determined by extraction is said to be only about 1 per cent of the content of ventral roots. The surface of the axis cylinder, covered by a lipoid membrane, is apparently impervious to acetylcholine (Rothenberg, Sprinson and Nachmanson, 1948).

The Neuron as a Trophic Unit. All parts of a cell are interdependent, and a continuous interaction between the nucleus and cytoplasm is a necessary condition for life. Any part which is detached from the portion containing the nucleus will disintegrate. In this respect the nerve cell is no exception. When an axon is divided, that part which is separated from its cell of origin and therefore from its nucleus dies, while the part still connected with the cell usually survives. The degeneration of the distal fragment of the axon extends to its finest ramifications, but does not pass the synapse or involve the next neuron. In rare cases a slow atrophy of the secondary neurons may occur.

It must not be supposed, however, that after section of a nerve fiber the part of the neuron containing the nucleus remains intact, for as a result of the division of an axon important changes occur in the cell body. The Nissl substance undergoes solution and redistribution, the cell becomes swollen, and the nucleus perhaps more eccentric. This phenomenon is known as *chromatolysis,* or the axon reaction, and is illustrated in Fig. 82, *H.* If the changes have been very profound the entire neuron may completely disintegrate, but, as a rule, it is restored to normal again by reparative processes. The nucleus becomes more central, the Nissl bodies reform and usually become more abundant than before, while from the cut end of the axon new sprouts grow out to replace the part of the axon which has degenerated. From what has been said it will be apparent that the nucleus presides over the nutrition of the entire neuron, that the latter responds as a whole to an injury of even a distant part of its axon, that the immediate changes produced by such a lesion are limited to the neuron directly involved, and that nerve fibers are unable to maintain a separate existence or to regenerate when their continuity with the cell body has been lost. This is what is meant by the statement that the neuron is the trophic unit of the nervous system.

There is, however, an interrelationship between neurons that affects their integrity. If the afferent fibers synapsing with certain neurons are eliminated, a transneuronal atrophy occurs after several months. The phenomenon is apparently not universal, and partial deprivation of impulses to nerve cells may have no demonstrable effect, as, for example, in the case of those of the anterior horn of the cord following dorsal root section or cutting the tracts from higher levels of the brain (Cook, Walker, and Barr, 1951).

Degeneration and Regeneration of Nerve Fibers. When a peripheral nerve fiber is cut certain events follow in different parts of the neuron. The distal segment of a nerve fiber which has been removed from connection with its cell body undergoes degeneration which begins slowly, requiring days to be completed, and involves the separate parts of the nerve fiber differently. The axis cylinder gradually breaks up and the segments are digested and absorbed. If there is a myelin sheath it is gradually transformed into a chain of lipoid droplets, the larger of which may in the early stages contain degenerating fragments of the axis cylinder. These droplets of transformed myelin have a chemical composition which differs from the normal and which allows them to be stained specifically with the Marchi method. The neurilemmal sheath does not degenerate, but its constituent cells proliferate forming a band or tube with many nuclei evident. This neurilemmal tube may persist for months beyond the time of disappearance of the axis cylinder, the fragments of which disappear in a few days, or the degenerating myelin sheath, parts of which may (as droplets) persist for six months or more. The neurilemmal band awaits regenerating axons, but may diminish in diameter with time if not reached by regenerating axons. Regenerating nerve fibers of large size may be restricted in their growth in diameter if they enter smaller neurilemmal tubes (Hammond and Hinsey, 1945).

When a nerve fiber is cut the parts of the neuron centralward to the break (toward the cell body) show characteristic changes also. As previously stated the perikaryon is involved in chromatolysis. This change reaches its peak in 7 to 15 days and then the cell may recover, or if it is too badly damaged it may completely degenerate.

If the cell body completely degenerates, the nerve fiber between the cell body and the cut undergoes Wallerian degeneration just as the distal segment does. However, if the neuron survives only a small amount of destruction occurs at the distal end of the central stump of a cut nerve, the degeneration extending back along the nerve fiber to about the first node of Ranvier.

From each axis cylinder near the cut end a number of small sprouts grow out and make their way along, at first within the neurilemmal tube surrounding the fiber, (Fig. 94). Some of the sprouts may go centralward even as far as central nervous system or dorsal root ganglia (in case of sensory fibers), where they may form pericellular and periglomerular skeins about the ganglion cells.

Other sprouts grow distalward and eventually reach the cut end of the nerve. Here they leave their neurilemmal sheaths which have also been cut and grow into the scar tissue. The haphazard arrangement of connective tissue fibers has its influence on the ameboid growing tips of the nerve sprouts and they wander irregularly through the scar following bundles of connective tissue and tissue clefts and other nerve fibers. Some may even be turned back into the central stump. Eventually some of the sprouts find their way successfully across the scar tissue and enter the neurilemmal tubes persisting in the distal stump. Naturally there is confusion. Not all of the fibers get across the scar, and those that do are directed by chance into the available pathways. It is obvious that only a few would be likely to regain their original paths. Cajal was unable to demonstrate that a chemical attraction to growing fibers acted over any great distance.

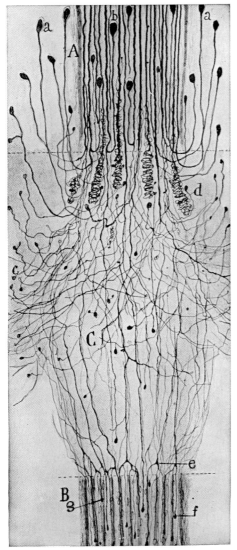

FIGURE 94. Diagrammatic drawing of a regenerating nerve: *A*, Central stump; *B*, distal stump; *C*, interval between stumps; *a*, *b*, bulbs on the ends of fibers growing centrally in and around the central stump; *f*, *g*, bulbs on the ends of fibers growing into the distal stump; *c*, bulb on the end of a fiber in the scar; *d*, coil formed by centrally growing fiber; *e*, expansion at point of bifurcation of a growing fiber sprouted from a cut axon. (Cajal.)

From a consideration of these principles of growth it is easy to see that the less the scar tissue between the cut ends of a severed nerve the more successful will be the restoration of fibers in the distal stump. Various artificial and natural channels have been placed between the cut ends of severed nerves with the idea of directing the growth of fibers to the distal stump.

The sprouts arising from the cut end of a nerve outnumber the fibers injured and it is possible, therefore, in particularly successful anastomosis or in the regrowth in the distal segment of a nerve crushed or injured but not separated from the central stump, to have finally a greater number of fibers distal to an injury than proximal.

When the sprouts of regenerating nerve fibers reach the distal segment and find their way into the neurilemmal tubes which act as conduits their rate of growth is considerably accelerated, some having been known to grow in this location several millimeters a day. When they have reached the site of the old endings there is another delay before the restoration of function while the endings become reorganized. Thus, while the neurilemma cells and the band fibers derived from them appear to be incapable of developing new nerve fibers by themselves in the peripheral stump, they play an important part in nerve regeneration in cooperation with the new axons from the central stump (Ranson, 1912; Cajal, 1928).

Speidel (1935) has shown that the fibers arising as sprouts from myelinated fibers have a greater tendency to become myelinated than those arising from unmyelinated ones, indicating a responsibility of the axis cylinder for the construction of the myelin sheath. New myelin has been seen to appear in regenerating mammalian nerves as early as 22 days after the original injury (Clark and Clark, 1947).

The amount and character of the function restored following regeneration of a cut nerve will depend upon the number of regrowing nerve fibers which reach the proper destination and perhaps upon those which reach the wrong destination. Sensory fibers will grow down the neurilemmal tubes of motor fibers but will not substitute functionally for the motor nerves (Weiss and Edds, 1945). There is evidence (but not conclusive) that preganglionic autonomic fibers may reinnervate skeletal muscle deprived of its nerve supply (Brown and Satinsky, 1951).

Somatic nerve fibers are apparently not limited to a length of growth since they will double in length if given the opportunity to regenerate through a sufficiently long distal nerve stump. Autonomic nerve fibers may not have this capacity for growth. Nerve fibers that do not reestablish connection with endings remain smaller than those which do.

It is important to note that the nerve fibers of the brain and spinal cord, which as has been stated before, are devoid of neurilemma sheaths, are incapable of regeneration sufficient to restore function. Abortive sprouts are put out from such central neurons which grow into the scar tissue at the site of injury. The amount of this scar tissue may be diminished under experimental conditions and the growth of axonal sprouts thus encouraged (Windle and Chambers, 1950).

Although further evidence is needed to establish the fact, there have been indications that partial restoration of function has occurred across the gap in the transected spinal cord, especially in young animals (Windle, 1955). It has also been shown that dorsal root fibers after entering the cord, when isolated by removal of neighboring dorsal roots, may sprout and spread terminals over a greater field of gray matter (Liu and Chambers, 1955). The severed spinal cords of lower forms such as fish and amphibia will regenerate and this gives hope to those who experiment with mammalian forms (Piatt, 1955).

Study of regeneration of nervous structures in lower forms has revealed many interesting points and, though only some of them apply to mammals, there are signifcant implications in others. For example, it has been reported that regeneration of the olfactory epithelium and nerves occurs in the frog after removal of the epithelium of the nasal cavity. This appears phenomenal when it is recalled that the primary olfactory neurons which give rise to the olfactory nerves are actually within the nasal epithelium (Smith, 1951).

Other equally surprising observations have been made by methods of tissue culture. Although it has been known for some time that mature nerve cells of dorsal root and autonomic ganglia will survive as transplants, it has been shown that mature human nerve cells from brain and autonomic ganglia can survive in tissue cultures for some time. The neurons cultured from fetal brains have survived when taken from refrigerated specimens even several days after therapeutic abortion (Hogue, 1947, 1953; Pomerat and Costero, 1956).

The fact that striated muscle which is not used undergoes atrophy is common knowledge; but it is surprising to find that some nerve cells may also change with disuse. The retinal ganglion cells of infant chimpanzees reared in darkness disappeared, though the bipolar cells of the retina persisted (Chow et al., 1957).

Neuron Chains. Though structurally its unit is the neuron, the functional activity of the nervous system is dependent upon the interconnection of various neurons and upon the ultimate connection of these with peripheral receptors and effectors. In fact, without intending any philosophical implications it can be stated that the entire activity of the nervous system is based on such connections. The simplest functional combination of neurons is seen in the *reflex arc*, and this again in its simplest form is illustrated in Fig. 95. Such an arc may consist of but two neurons, one of which is afferent and conducts toward the spinal cord;

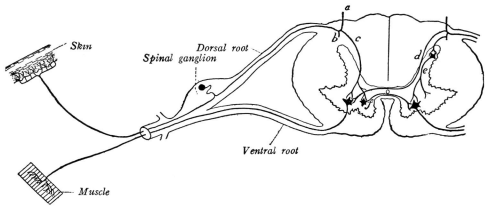

FIGURE 95. Diagrammatic section through the spinal cord and a spinal nerve to illustrate a simple reflex arc: *a, b, c,* and *d,* branches of sensory fibers of the dorsal roots; *e,* association neuron; *f,* commissural neuron.

the other is efferent and conducts the impulses to the organ of response. The arc consists of the following parts: (1) the receptor, the ramification of the sensory fiber in the skin or other sensory end organ; (2) the first conductor, which includes both branches of the axon of the spinal ganglion cell; (3) a center including the synapse; (4) the second conductor, which includes the entire motor neuron, with its cell body in the anterior gray column and its motor ending on the muscle, and (5) the effector or organ of response, which in this case is a muscle fiber. A wave of activation, known as the nerve impulse, is developed in the sensitive receptor and travels over the sensory fiber to the synapse where it activates the motor neuron. The resulting impulse travels along the motor fiber to the neuro-muscular ending and causes the muscle to contract. There is always a slight delay at the synapse, representing the time required for the new impulse to be generated. Although an impulse never crosses a synapse, it is convenient to follow the succession of impulses through a chain of neurons without mentioning the synaptic interruptions. A more common form of reflex arc involves a third, and purely central neuron, as illustrated on the right side of Fig. 95. Such central neurons may have short or long axons. In the latter case they may serve to connect distant parts of the central nervous system with each other. It is to the multiplication of these central neurons that we owe the complicated pathways within the mammalian brain and spinal cord.

Pathways through Higher Centers.   An idea of how the neurons of some of the centers in the brain are related to the primary motor and sensory spinal neurons is given by Fig. 96. It will be seen that many paths are open to an impulse entering the spinal cord by way of a dorsal root fiber. Ignoring the breaks

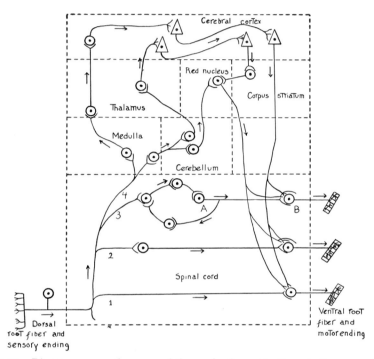

FIGURE 96.   Diagram representing some of the conduction paths through the mammalian central nervous system. An elaborate system of central or association neurons furnishes a number of alternative paths between the primary sensory and motor neurons. At the level of the spinal cord a closed neuron circuit is illustrated. (Redrawn and modified from Bayliss.)

at synapses we say that it can pass over one or all of the following paths: (1) by way of a collateral to a primary motor neuron in a two-neuron reflex arc. It may travel over an association neuron, belonging (2) to the same level of the spinal cord, or (3) to other levels, in reflex arcs of three or more neurons each; or (4) it may ascend to the brain along an ascending branch of a dorsal root fiber. Here it may travel over one or more of a number of paths, each consisting of several neurons, and be finally returned to the spinal cord and make its exit by way of a primary motor neuron. The figure illustrates but a few of the possible paths, many of which we shall have occasion to consider in the subsequent chapters.

The more elaborate the connections among the association neurons the greater the opportunity for variation in the response to a given stimulus. Thus it is apparent that the higher the development of the brain of a species of animal the less stereotyped its behavior may be. It might be added as a corollary that in a single species, man for example, any condition which limits the quantity of available internuncial neurons may result in more stereotypy in behavior. At the two extremes of life, infancy and old age, sterotyped behavior is common as a consequence of incompleteness of development of the nervous system at the one extreme and destruction of parts of it at the other, through aging or by disease.

Even when the most complicated paths through the brain are taken into consideration, the time required for an impulse to travel these paths from receptor to effector is very brief. But it is known that a stimulus to a sensory nerve may initiate a contraction that persists for a minute or more after the cessation of the stimulus. Throughout this period the motor neurons concerned are repeatedly discharging impulses along the motor fibers. Several theories have been offered to account for this prolonged activity. The most satisfactory explanation is offered by a conception of closed self-exciting neuron circuits. When once activated by an impulse reaching it along fiber 3 of Fig. 96, the closed circuit, which has been diagrammatically represented at the level of the spinal cord in that figure, would continue to be active, the impulse traveling around the circuit until interrupted by inhibition or fatigue. Each time neuron A was activated it would in turn activate the next neuron in the circuit and at the same time send an impulse to the primary motor neuron B, thus providing for continued activity in the muscle. The conception of closed circuits as an explanation for long continued activity in the central nervous system, though based on the work of Cajal and Forbes, was well supported by Ranson and Hinsey (1930). It is essentially similar to the circus movements described in heart muscle by Garrey. It has been put on a firm foundation by Lorente de Nó (1933) and has won wide recognition (Eccles, 1936; O'Leary, 1937).

There is reason to believe that activity can continue in the central nervous system in the absence of all afferent impulses. The goldfish brain, dissected free from the body, continues a rhythmical activity corresponding in tempo with the normal gill movements. This activity is probably located in the respiratory center. The waves of electrical potential, which travel over the cerebral cortex in man and animals, are independent of incoming sensory impulses. To explain such phenomena it has been assumed that neurons are endowed with the capacity for spontaneous rhythmical activity. Whatever one may think of this explanation, the existence of activity in the central nervous system which continues without reinforcement from incoming impulses cannot be doubted. It is quite possible that such a sustained rhythmic activity may be explained on the basis of conduction in closed self-exciting neuron chains (Eccles, 1936).

For an incoming impulse a variety of paths are open, one or more of which may be taken according to the momentary resistance of each. There is reason to believe that the resistance interposed by a synapse may vary from moment to moment, according to the physiologic state of the neurons involved. It is therefore not necessary that every impulse entering by a given fiber shall travel the same path within the central nervous system nor produce the same result. The pathways themselves are, however, more or less fixed, and depend upon the structural relations established by the neurons. Many of these synaptic connections are formed before birth, follow an hereditary pattern, and are approximately the same for each individual of the species. In the child these are illustrated by the nervous mechanisms involved in breathing and swallowing, which are perfect at birth. The newly hatched chick is able to run about and pick up food, acts which are dependent on nervous connections already established according to hereditary pattern. Though the original pattern of distribution of the cell bodies of embryonic neurons in separate individuals of a species is in general similar, these neurons must subsequently form the pathways of the nervous system by the growth of axons over long distances. Cajal suggested that the potentialities of the nervous systems of separate individuals differ because not all the nerve fibers as they grow stick to the predetermined paths. Also some may make aberrant connections or degenerate, or the ones remaining in the proper pathway may differ in quantity and connections. Even in identical twins this factor for variation is active, for though in twins the hereditary stamp of the nervous system must be more nearly the same than it is in any other two individuals, the axons of the neurons originally laid down must grow to make pathways. The variation here and there in the position and growth of blood vessels supplying the nervous tissue or the position of supporting structures must offer opportunities for diversification of connections because of the tendency of nerve fibers to grow like vines along a trellis, tending to follow the framework (stereotropism). The pattern of blood vessels and other structures, which can have an influence upon the pattern of growing fibers is not exactly the same in any two individuals. In man and to a less extent in other mammals the nervous system continues to develop long after birth. This postnatal development is influenced by the experience of the individual and is more or less individual in pattern.

The neurons which make up the nervous system of an adult man are therefore arranged in a system the larger outlines of which follow an hereditary pattern, but many of the details of which have been shaped by the experiences of the individual.

NEUROGLIA

Delicate strands of mesodermally derived connective tissue penetrate the central nervous system along the blood vessels but the chief supporting tissue of the brain and spinal cord is of an entirely different nature, a special tissue called *neuroglia*. Under this heading may be included: ependyma, neuroglia proper, including astrocytes and oligodendroglia, and microglia. Some authors also include under this heading the sheath and satellite cells of the peripheral nerves and ganglia.

The *ependyma* forms a single layer of columnar epithelial cells lining the ventricles of the brain and central canal of the spinal cord (Fig. 97). The cilia which project from the free surface in the embryo are almost entirely lost in the adult. From the base of the cell projects a long slender process which at one stage of embryonic development reached and was attached to the external limiting membrane. Some of these processes retain this attachment at the bottom of the anterior median fissure of the spinal cord in the adult. The cuticulae of the ependymal cells form the internal limiting membrane. In certain places such

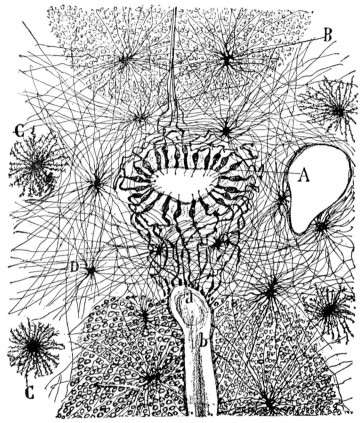

FIGURE 97. Ependyma and neuroglia in the region of the central canal of a child's spinal cord: *A*, Ependymal cells; *B* and *D*, fibrous astrocytes; *C*, protoplasmic astrocytes. Golgi method. (Cajal.)

as the roofs of the third and fourth ventricles the ventricular wall consists of a single layer of epithelium of ependymal origin.

Neuroglia in the restricted sense includes protoplasmic astrocytes, fibrous astrocytes, and oligodendroglia. *Protoplasmic astrocytes* are found in the gray matter of the brain and spinal cord. They are characterized by their numerous freely branching protoplasmic processes, which give them the characteristic appearance because of which they are often called mossy cells (Figs. 97, *C;* 98, *A*). *Fibrous astrocytes*, found chiefly in the white matter, differ from the preceding because of their long unbranched fibers. These run through the cytoplasm, project from the cell bodies in every direction and give them an appearance which has earned the name spider cells (Figs. 97, *D;* 98, *B*). Both types of astrocytes are attached to blood vessels by one or more processes that terminate in perivascular feet (Fig. 98, *B*). *Oligodendroglia* cells are smaller than the astrocytes. Their processes, which are few in number, are slender and relatively free from branches (Fig. 98, *D*). They are found in the white substance in rows between the nerve fibers, which are partly invested by their processes, and in the gray matter, closely applied as satellites to the nerve cells (Fig. 99). Others both in the gray and white matter lie with their cell bodies resting on small blood vessels. It is

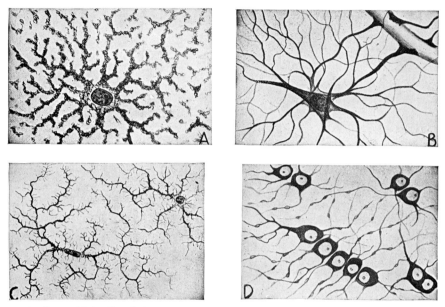

FIGURE 98.   Interstitial cells of the central nervous system: *A*, Protoplasmic neuroglia; *B*, fibrous neuroglia; *C*, microglia; *D*, oligodendroglia. (After Rio Hortega.)

not likely that oligodendrocytes offer much mechanical support for the nervous elements and it has been suggested that their function is chiefly a metabolic one, and that they act as intermediary agents in the exchange of metabolic products between ganglion cells and brain fluids. Study of the oligodendroglia in the rabbit spinal cord during myelin formation does not support the idea that they may assist in myelin formation (Dekaban, 1956). There has also been described an adendroglial cell, which has no processes and which is distributed like the oligodendroglia.

The *pia-glial membrane* which encloses the brain and spinal cord is composed of a condensation of neuroglia attached to the deep surface of the pia. Many astrocytes send processes considerable distances to terminate in expansions beneath the pia and there are numerous small astrocytes closely applied to its under surface. The pia-glial membrane accompanies the blood vessels into the brain and spinal cord forming tubular channels within which the vessels run (Fig. 62).

The space goes no further than arterioles, but the leptomeningeal sheath appears under electron microscopy as cytoplasm of cells in a thin layer partly surrounding the arteriole (Maynard, Schultz and Pease, 1957).

Along the route of blood vessels in the central nervous system, the ordinary connective tissue has within it the types of cells found in the same tissue else-

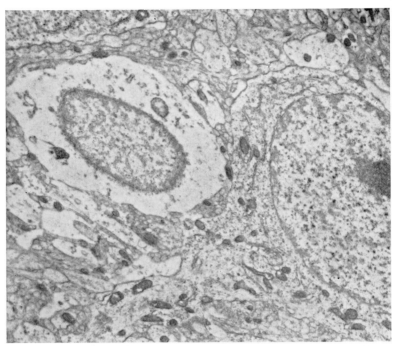

FIGURE 99. Oligodendroglial cell which is a satellite to a neuron. The oligodendroglial cell has clear cytoplasm which contains a scant amount of endoplasmic reticulum and a moderate number of mitochondria. It is adjacent to a neuron which has a much more dense cytoplasm containing a large amount of granular material associated with membranes. Within the large neuronal nucleus there is a distinct nucleolus and associated nucleolar chromatin. Surrounding the neuron and oligodendroglial cell are the intertwined cytoplasmic processes of other glial and neural elements, neuropil. × 7,400. (Luse.)

where. In addition to the connective tissue fibers and fibroblasts, there are a number of clasmatocytes and occasional mast cells. These are not to be confused with the true glial elements.

Microglial cells of mesodermal origin are found in both the gray and white matter. They are very small and, while the majority are multipolar, some are distinctly bipolar (Fig. 98, *C*). From the scanty cytoplasm surrounding the nucleus arise two, three or more spiny, frequently branching processes. A ground substance around and between the neurons of the central nervous system has been described (Hess, 1953).

There is evidence of difference in function of the various neuroglial cells. Whether or not microglial cells have any important function under normal conditions, when nervous tissue is damaged they assume the role of scavenger cells (compound granular corpuscles or gitter cells). When neurons disappear through slow processes, a collection of oligodendroglial cells may occupy the site. Larger areas of destruction are filled in by the proliferation of fibrous and protoplasmic astrocytes and even ordinary scar tissue.

The ependymal epithelial cells covering the chorioid plexuses constitute part of a semipermeable membrane through which much of the cerebrospinal fluid accumulates. Masses of neuroglial cells in the region of the area postrema have the peculiar quality of becoming vitally stained with trypan blue, a characteristic not common to normal neuroglia generally. It is possible this area and adjacent

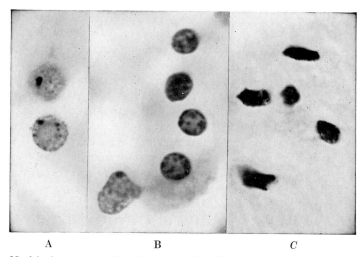

A   B   C

FIGURE 100.   Nuclei of astrocytes (A), oligodendroglia (B), and microglia (C). Stained with cresyl violet. Photographs by Weil.

similar structures may have a secretory function (Cammermeyer, 1949). The few nerve cells in the area postrema are pigmented in man, though not in lower animals.

In preparations stained with the basic dyes the nuclei of the different types of cells can be easily distinguished. The nerve cells have large, lightly staining vesicular nuclei with large round nucleoli (Fig. 82). The nuclei of astrocytes are about the size of those found in small nerve cells. They are irregularly oval, stain lightly, and contain granules of chromatin but no nucleolus (Fig. 100, A). Oligodendroglia nuclei are smaller than those of astrocytes and stain much darker (Fig. 100, B). The nuclei of microglia cells are the smallest and most darkly stained. They may be round, oblong, triangular, or curved like a "C" (Fig. 100, C).

CHAPTER VI

The Spinal Nerves

Since the nervous system is constructed of neurons related to each other as conductors of impulses, and since the action of the nervous system is dependent upon the course which impulses take that enter, and leave, and course about in the nervous system, it is important to analyze the pathways taken by such impulses. It is natural to begin by the study of the peripheral nerves by which impulses enter and leave the central nervous system, and follow this with the study of the internuncial paths and connections between the incoming or afferent neurons and the outgoing or motor ones. The central nervous system is made up of these internuncial neurons and it is through these neurons that connections are made between any source of afferent impulses and the appropriate effector mechanism. The functioning patterns of internuncial neurons therefore express the potential choice of responses to stimuli, and the more such patterns an animal type has developed the less stereotyped are its responses.

The incoming impulses may arise from external or internal environment and so may be conveyed in nerves from somatic or splanchnic areas, and the effects that follow any given stimulus may occur in voluntary muscle, involuntary muscle, or glands. There is thus complete interdependence between the cerebrospinal and autonomic (sympathetic) portions of the nervous system. These parts are named separately for convenience of description.

The sensory impulses conveyed to the central nervous system by spinal nerves are those familiar to everyday experience, and are interpreted as pain, temperature, touch, pressure, and proprioception. Proprioceptive impulses, or muscle sense, arises within the voluntary muscle and related structures. The other types of general sensibility come from both somatic and splanchnic areas. There are differences, however, in the sensitivity of parts. The skin of the fingers and palms is quite sensitive to touch, the tongue also. Other portions of the body covering are less sensitive to touch and this sensation is absent from the gastric mucosa and other visceral areas. Pain is felt from most normal skin on adequate stimulation by cutting, burning, stretching, and is apparently the chief sensation elicited from the cornea by contact. In the visceral area pain is not produced by cutting or burning or light pinching of normal mucosa, but does follow stimulation of a viscus which is inflamed or engorged.

Temperature sense in the skin allows discrimination of differences of a few degrees, but the visceral areas are relatively insensitive to heat or cold. In the stomach temperatures between 18° C. and 40° C. are not distinguished. Above 40° C. is interpreted as heat, and below 18° C. as cold. Pressure is appreciated in viscera and within the stomach may be roughly localized.

The spinal nerves are attached to the spinal cord by ventral and dorsal roots. On each dorsal root is a ganglion containing the cells of origin of the fibers of the dorsal root while the fibers forming the ventral root arise from cells in the ventral horn of gray matter of the spinal cord. The spinal nerve, made up of the fibers of the combined ventral and dorsal root, leaves the vertebral canal at the appropriate level by an intervertebral foramen and immediately branches into dorsal and ventral rami as the nerve begins its peripheral distribution. A short distance beyond its exit from the vertebral column the spinal nerve receives fibers

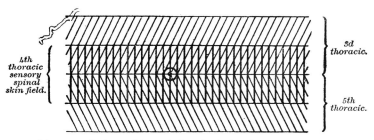

FIGURE 101. Diagram of the position of the nipple in the sensory skin fields of the fourth, third, and fifth thoracic spinal roots. The overlapping of the cutaneous areas is represented. (Sherrington.)

from the sympathetic trunk to be distributed, and some spinal nerves contribute fibers to the trunk, such fibers passing by way of the communicating rami.

Metamerism. That the spinal nerves are segmentally arranged, a pair for each metamere, is readily appreciated in the case of the typical body segments of the thoracic region. Here it is obvious that a nerve supplies the corresponding dermatome and myotome, or in the adult the skin and musculature of its own segment. While the *thoracic nerves* retain this primitive arrangement in the adult, the distribution of fibers from the other spinal nerves is complicated by the development of the limb buds and by the shifting of myotomes and dermatomes during the development of the embryo (Fig. 103).

Opposite the attachment of the limb buds the ventral rami of the corresponding nerves unite to form flattened plates, from which the *brachial* and *lumbosacral plexuses* are developed. Within these plexuses the fibers derived from a number of ventral rami are intermingled. Each nerve which extends from these plexuses into the limbs carries with it fibers from more than one spinal nerve. While it is not possible to follow by dissection the course of such fibers, the clinical neurologists through their study of paralyses and areas of anesthesia subsequent to lesions of one or more nerve roots within the vertebral canal have been able to demonstrate the areas of skin and groups of muscles supplied by specific spinal nerves.

Sherrington (1894) attacked the problem of the distribution of the sensory fibers by experimental methods on cats and monkeys; Head contributed much through the study of areas of skin involved in herpes zoster in which individual cerebrospinal ganglia were infected; and Foerster (1933) made use of his extensive neurosurgical practice to determine the distribution of sensory nerves in man. By injecting interspinous ligaments and separate muscles with strong salt solution

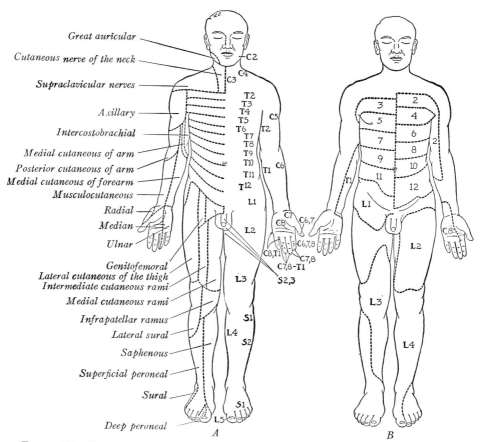

FIGURE 102. Dermatomes contrasted with the areas supplied by cutaneous nerves. A, Shows the distribution of cutaneous nerves on one side and on the other the general arrangement of the dermatomes. B, Shows the size, shape, and degree of overlapping of some of the dermatomes.

the segmental innervation of deeper structures has been demonstrated and patterns similar to dermatomal ones have been made (Lewis, 1942). Section of a single dorsal root does not cause complete anesthesia anywhere because of an overlapping of the areas of distribution of adjacent spinal nerves (Fig. 101), but either section of a nerve root or pressure upon it as by the herniation of the nucleus pulposus of an intervertebral disk produces sufficient alteration in the sensitivity of the primary area of skin supplied so that it can be mapped out (Keegan and Garrett, 1948). The zones so mapped are more delimited than those

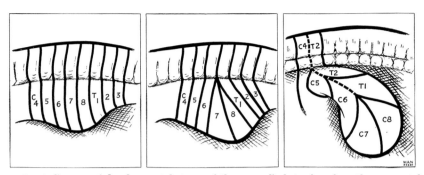

FIGURE 103. A diagram of developmental stages of the upper limb to show how the segmental inner-vation of the limb is derived. (Haymaker and Woodhall.)

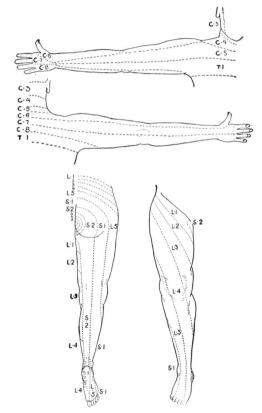

FIGURE 104. Diagram of skin areas of diminished sensitivity found by Keegan and Garrett in patients requiring operation for extruded intervertebral disks. The zones are labelled to show the segmental nerve supply.

obtained by other means, as the overlapping distribution of adjacent nerve roots is not shown (Fig. 104). The general arrangement of these sensory root fields in man is indicated on one side of Fig. 102, *A*. On the opposite side is indicated the distribution of the cutaneous nerves. The shape, size, and overlapping of some of the dermatomes is shown in Fig. 102, *B*. It will be seen that in the extremities

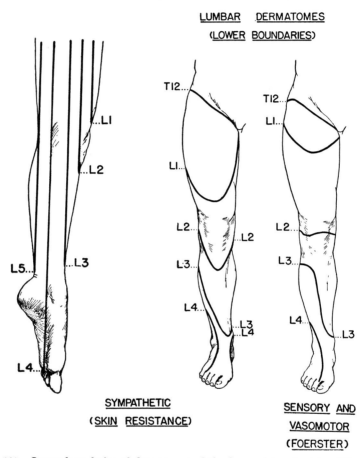

LUMBAR DERMATOMES
(LOWER BOUNDARIES)

SYMPATHETIC
(SKIN RESISTANCE)

SENSORY AND
VASOMOTOR
(FOERSTER)

FIGURE 105. Lower boundaries of dermatomes of the leg as determined by differences in skin resistance following lumbar sympathectomy are shown in the left and middle figures. In the figure on the right are dermatomes as described according to sensory and vasomotor patterns by Foerster. (Richter and Woodruff, 1945.)

there is no correspondence between the areas supplied by the peripheral nerves and those supplied by individual dorsal roots. It will also be evident that the fibers of a given dorsal root reach the corresponding sensory root field by way of more than one cutaneous nerve. Although in the plexuses associated with the innervation of the extremities each segmental nerve contributes sensory fibers to two or more peripheral nerves, the cutaneous distribution of the fibers from each root is not composed of disjointed patches, but forms a continuous field.

A knowledge of the cutaneous distribution of the various nerve roots is of great importance in enabling the clinician to determine the level of a lesion of the spinal cord or nerve roots within the vertebral canal. Dermatomes of the trunk show a regularity corresponding to successive spinal segments, but such a sequence is not so obvious in the cutaneous innervation of the limbs unless the embryologic history is considered (Fig. 103). With the gradual prolongation of the extremities the spinal nerves from segments supplying the middle portion of the limb bud are carried distally on the limbs, thus explaining the apparent apposition of remote segments, as C 5 and T 2 in the proximal part of the arm, for an example.

Evidence of the serial character of dermatomes in an extremity is shown by variations in skin resistance (Richter and Woodruff, 1945) of definite areas following removal of autonomic ganglia of the sympathetic trunk from which go postganglionic fibers to successive spinal nerves (Fig. 105).

During embryonic development the shifting of muscles has also been accompanied by corresponding changes in the spatial distribution of the *motor nerve fibers*. A familiar example is furnished by the diaphragm, the musculature of which is derived from cervical myotomes and which in its descent carries with it the phrenic nerve. This explains the origin of the phrenic from the third, fourth, and fifth cervical nerves.

If, as seems probable, the musculature of the extremities has not developed along metameric lines, there can be no true metamerism of the motor nerves to the limbs (Streeter, 1912). Yet the fibers from each ventral root are distributed in a very orderly manner. As is indicated in the diagram on page 28, almost every long muscle receives fibers from two or more ventral roots. It will be apparent that the muscles of the trunk are innervated from the roots belonging to the several metameres from the myotomes of which these muscles developed. The diagram shows in a general way the distribution of the fibers of the several ventral roots.

There are also *visceral afferent fibers* distributed to the thoracic and abdominal viscera by way of the white rami from the thoracic and upper lumbar nerves. These have their cells of origin in the spinal ganglia and are continued through the dorsal roots into the spinal cord (Fig. 109). Except for the distribution of their fibers to the visceral structures they innervate and from which they acquire the name visceral, they are like the somatic afferent neurons in location of cell bodies and other morphologic details. Many visceral afferent fibers run with some spinal nerves to reach glands and blood vessels in peripheral areas.

The Structure of the Spinal Nerves. A spinal nerve is composed of nerve fibers bound together by connective tissue, which may break it up into several fascicles (Fig. 106). Each fascicle, or the entire nerve if it is not fasciculated, is surrounded by a layer of dense connective tissue, the perineurium, from which fine strands of this tissue penetrate between the individual fibers, forming the endoneurium. Loose connective tissue, the epineurium, envelops the perineurium and, if several fascicles are present, binds these together. The cutaneous branches of the spinal nerves contain a high percentage of fine myelinated fibers and great numbers of unmyelinated fibers. In a preparation fixed with osmic acid the unmyelinated fibers remain unstained and in Fig. 106 the only evidence of their presence is the rather wide separation between the myelinated fibers. In cutaneous nerves the unmyelinated fibers, which are very numerous, are of two kinds: (1) sensory unmyelinated fibers with cells of origin in the spinal ganglia, and (2) post-ganglionic sympathetic fibers, which have entered the nerve by way of the gray ramus from the sympathetic ganglia. Nerves going to muscles are composed chiefly of large myelinated fibers, but also contain a few small myelinated and unmyelinated fibers.

The *ventral roots* of the spinal nerves contain somatic motor fibers most of which are large although a few are small (Fig. 107, *C*). In addition to the somatic

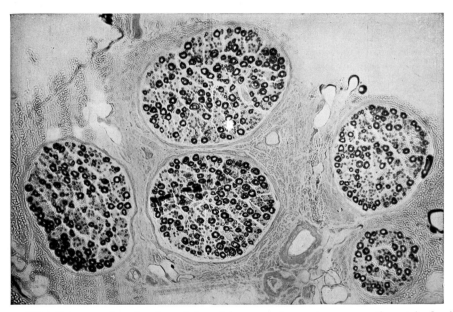

FIGURE 106. Cutaneous branch of an intercostal nerve of man in cross section stained with osmic acid.

components, the ventral roots of the thoracic and upper lumbar nerves, which are associated with white rami, and of the second, third, and fourth sacral nerves, which give off branches to the pelvic viscera, contain large numbers of fine myelinated preganglionic visceral efferent fibers. Relatively few myelinated fibers of medium size and few unmyelinated fibers are found in ventral roots as will be seen from a comparison of Fig. 107, *C*, in which the myelin sheaths are stained black with osmic acid, with Fig. 107, *D*, in which the axons are stained black with silver.

The *dorsal roots* contain myelinated fibers of all sizes and also great numbers of unmyelinated axons. In a cross section of such a root stained with silver (Fig. 107, *B*) one sees large and small darkly stained axons, corresponding to the myelinated fibers in the preparation of the same root stained with osmic acid (Fig. 107, *A*). The very numerous unmyelinated fibers are grouped in bundles which occupy the interstices among the myelinated fibers. In the photomicrograph of a cross section of the root stained with silver, the unmyelinated fibers appear as dots and the bundles as clusters of dots.

The Spinal Ganglia. The spinal ganglia are rather simple structures fundamentally. The ganglion is essentially a collection of nerve cells and fibers bound together by a covering of fibrous connective tissue and well supplied with blood vessels. It has long been known that the typical cells of the mammalian spinal ganglion are *unipolar*. The cell body is irregularly spheric. The axon, which is

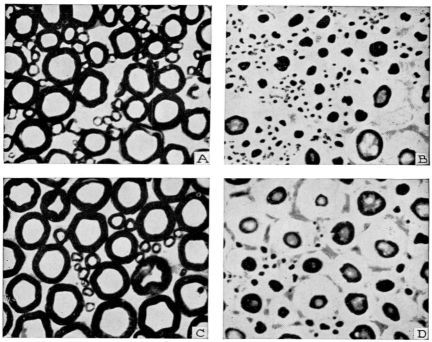

FIGURE 107. Sections of roots of the third sacral nerve of a dog: *A*, Dorsal root, osmic acid; *B*, same root, silver stain; *C*, ventral root, osmic acid; *D*, same root, silver stain. There are few if any preganglionic visceral efferent fibers in the ventral root of the third sacral nerve of the dog. (Davenport.)

attached to the perikaryon by an implantation cone, is coiled on itself in the neighborhood of the cell, forming what is known as a glomerulus (Fig. 108, *f*). Beyond the glomerulus the axon runs into one of the central fiber bundles of the ganglion and divides in the form of a **T** or **Y** into two branches, one of which is directed toward the spinal cord in the dorsal root. The other and somewhat larger branch is directed distally in the spinal nerve. The cells vary greatly in size and the diameter of the axon varies with that of the cell from which it springs. An axon arising from a *large cell* usually forms a very pronounced glomerulus and soon becomes ensheathed with myelin, and this myelin sheath is continued along both branches into which it divides. The branching occurs at a node of Ranvier.

As was originally pointed out by Cajal (1907) and Dogiel (1908) and strongly emphasized by Ranson (1912), the *small cells* of these ganglia give rise to fine unmyelinated fibers. These coil but little near the cell, or the glomerulus may be entirely lacking (Fig. 108, *a*). They divide dichotomously, just as do the myelinated fibers, into finer central and coarser peripheral branches. At the point of bifurcation there is a triangular expansion in place of the constriction so characteristic of a dividing myelinated fiber. It has been shown that the small cells are considerably more numerous than the large cells, though because of their small size they constitute a less conspicuous element.

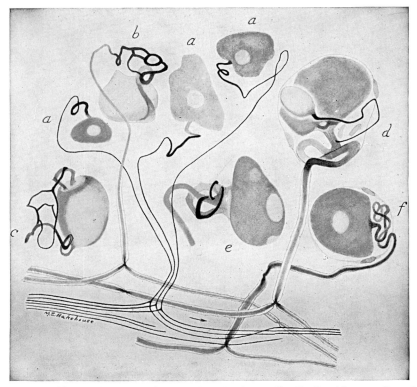

FIGURE 108.   Neurons from the spinal ganglion of a dog: *a*, Small cells with unmyelinated axons; *b*, *c*, *d*, *e*, and *f*, large cells with myelinated axons; *f*, typical large spinal ganglion cell showing glomerulus and capsule. The arrow points toward the spinal cord. Pyridine-silver method.

A few cells retain the *bipolar* form characteristic of all the spinal ganglion cells at an early stage of development (Fig. 77).

The spinal ganglion cells are each surrounded by a *capsule* or membranous sheath with nuclei on its inner surface (Fig. 108, *d*, *f*) which is continuous with the neurilemma sheath of the associated nerve fiber. The cells forming the capsule are of ectodermal origin, being derived like the spinal ganglion cells themselves from the neural crest.

Beneath the capsule are small *satellite* cells which appear to be embedded in the sides of the ganglion cells. The function of these is obscure. Their relation to the ganglion cells is similar to that of certain oligodendroglial cells about neurons of the central nervous system.

In good methylene blue preparations and in sections stained by the newer silver methods it is possible to make out many additional details of structure. The axon may split into many branches, which subdivide and anastomose, forming a true network in the neighborhood of the cell (Fig. 108, b). From this network the axon is again assembled and passes on to a typical bifurcation. Or the axon may be assembled out of a similar plexus which, however, is connected with the cell by several roots (Fig. 108, c). Some of the fibers give off collaterals terminating in spheric or pear-shaped end bulbs. Such an end bulb may rest upon the surface of its own perikaryon (Fig. 108, d) or elsewhere in the ganglion. From the body of some cells short, club-shaped dendrites arise, which, however, terminate beneath the capsules which surround the cells.

Under pathologic conditions the number of unusual cell types is greatly increased. This can best be seen in tabetic ganglia and after the transplantation of the spinal ganglion in animals. Under such conditions pericellular plexuses are formed around many of the cells as a result of the growth in circles around the cells of new-formed fibers, which have sprouted from the cell body or the adjacent portion of the axon or from an adjacent cell. It now seems probable that the atypical cells seen in normal ganglia represent proliferative activity on the part of a few isolated neurons in response to some disturbing influence. Pericellular plexuses are rare in strictly normal ganglia and it is doubtful if any of them represent the termination of fibers entering the ganglion from the sympathetic system (Cajal, 1928; de Castro, 1932; Barris, 1934). In fact pericellular plexuses were found to be more elaborate and more numerous than normal in animals from which the sympathetic chains had been previously removed (Clark, 1933).

The *fiber bundles of the ganglia* are composed of both myelinated and unmyelinated fibers representing the branches of the axons of the spinal ganglion cells. Both types of fibers can be followed through the dorsal roots into the spinal cord, as well as distally into the nerves. In the latter they mingle with the large myelinated fibers coming from the ventral roots. When traced distally in the peripheral nerve the unmyelinated fibers are found to go in large part to the skin, though a few run in the muscular branches (Ranson and Davenport, 1931; Duncan, 1938). Their ultimate termination is in the various sensory endings of the skin and deeper structures. By knowing the function of a particular nerve its histologic picture in terms of fiber types may be predicted and conversely some knowledge of the function of a particular nerve may be obtained by examining its fiber content.

Functional Classification of Nerve Fibers. Many years ago Sir Charles Bell (1811, 1844) showed that the dorsal roots are sensory in function and the ventral roots motor; this has been known since then as Bell's law. He recognized that sensory and motor fibers are distributed to the viscera as well as to the rest of the body. But Gaskell (1886) was the first to make a detailed study of the nerve fibers supplying the visceral and vascular systems. We now recognize in the spinal nerves elements belonging to four functionally distinct varieties, namely, *visceral afferent, visceral efferent, somatic afferent,* and *somatic efferent* fibers (Fig. 109), all of which are classed as *general* in contrast to certain special ones in cranial nerves.

The terms visceral and somatic refer to different areas of the body which are not sharply defined. It is customary to refer to areas about the endodermally derived alimentary tract and respiratory system as visceral as well as other obviously visceral structures derived from mesoderm, as the parts of the urogenital system. Custom also has included in the term all the vascular system with its involuntary muscle, and most if not all glandular structures. Somatic refers primarily to the ectodermally derived covering of the body and the voluntary muscle derived from myotomes. Naturally those areas overlap and a few conflicts arise. For example, the sweat glands are derived from ectoderm but are "visceral" in nerve supply. The terms are useful for description in spite of such conflicts.

Visceral Components.   Visceral efferent fibers are those innervating involuntary muscle and glands. Between the central nervous system and the visceral effector there extends a two-neuron chain, the limbs of which are named in relation to the peripheral ganglion, and according to the direction taken by the nerve impulses, as *pre-* and *postganglionic* neurons. The cell body of the preganglionic neuron lies within the central nervous system. Its axon is small and

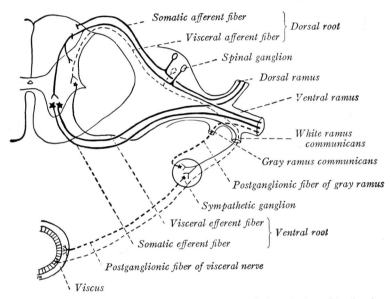

FIGURE 109.   Diagrammatic section through a spinal nerve and the spinal cord in the thoracic region to illustrate the chief functional types of peripheral nerve fibers.

myelinated and extends out through one of the spinal nerves to an autonomic ganglion to synapse there with one or more *postganglionic* neurons, the axons of which extend to the particular structures innervated. Visceral efferent fibers leave the spinal cord by all of the thoracic and the upper four lumbar nerves (i. e., those spinal nerves possessing white rami communicantes) and by way of the second, third, and fourth sacral nerves. Those from thoracic and lumbar nerves enter the sympathetic trunk, and those from the sacral nerves are carried by visceral branches to the pelvic plexuses.

The neurons of the sympathetic ganglia with which the preganglionic visceral efferent fibers synapse give rise to unmyelinated postganglionic visceral efferent fibers some of which run in visceral nerves to the smooth muscle and glandular tissue of viscera and some of which enter each spinal nerve via the gray rami communicantes. These fibers are distributed through the peripheral branches of the spinal nerves to smooth muscle and glandular tissue, especially to the sweat glands and to the smooth muscle in blood vessels and about hair follicles. The visceral components of the spinal nerves will be considered further in the chapter on the Autonomic Nervous System.

Somatic Efferent Components. The skeletal muscles are innervated by myelinated fibers, which are, for the most part, of large caliber. The axis cylinders of these fibers are the axons of cells located in the ventral part of the gray matter of the spinal cord, and they end on the muscle fibers in special *motor end plates.* Such a primary motor neuron is illustrated in Fig. 86. A motor fiber undergoes repeated division as it approaches its termination, and each anterior horn cell may innervate therefore as many as 100 to 200 individual muscle fibers

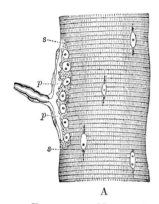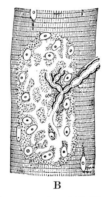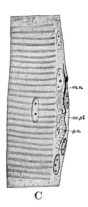

FIGURE 110. Nerve endings in striated muscle. *A* and *B,* Motor end plates in muscle fibers from a lizard in profile and surface views: *s,* sarcolemma; *p,* branch of axon. Beneath this is a layer of granular sarcoplasm containing a number of nuclei. In *B* the ramifications of the unstained axon are seen spreading from the termination of the medullated fiber (Kühne in Quain's Anatomy). *C,* Motor end plate on a muscle fiber of a mole: *m.n.* Ramification of axon; *so.pl.,* specialized sarcoplasm containing nuclei and the periterminal net, *p.n.* (Boeke in Penfield's Cytology and Cellular Pathology of the Nervous System, Paul B. Hoeber, Inc.)

which can be considered as physiologic motor units. The muscle fibers constituting one of these units are intermingled with fibers of adjacent units (Feindel, 1954). Incidentally each voluntary muscle fiber is supplied with one and except in rare instances only one motor nerve ending.

In the nerves to skeletal muscles that possess muscle spindles there are also some myelinated fibers smaller in caliber than the usual large ones to the motor end plates of the main mass of muscle fibers. These smaller fibers innervate the small intrafusal muscle fibers of the spindle which through their varying tensions aid in giving proprioceptive information to the central nervous system (Kuffler, Hunt, and Quilliam, 1951).

The idea that skeletal muscle fibers are innervated by nerve fibers from sympathetic ganglia, which had supporters for a time, has been successfully disproved (Hinsey, 1927). Each branch of a motor nerve fiber retains its myelin sheath until it reaches the muscle fiber to be innervated. At this point this sheath terminates abruptly, and the neurilemma becomes continuous with the sarcolemma (Fig. 110). The terminal branches of the axon are short, thick, and irregular. They lie immediately under the sarcolemma in a bed of specialized sarcoplasm containing a number of large clear nuclei. The wave of activation, which travels down an axon as a nerve impulse, is transmitted through these motor nerve endings to the muscle and initiates a contraction.

Since the branching axon of the anterior horn cell is the only source of stimuli to skeletal muscle fibers, destruction of an anterior horn cell or disruption of its axon results in paralysis of the muscle fibers supplied by it. In poliomyelitis the anterior horn cells are attacked. If an anterior horn cell is destroyed its axon dies and no regeneration of this neuron occurs. Disruption of motor fibers in peripheral nerves, however, may be followed by regeneration from the point of section distalward and restoration of nerve supply to the affected muscles. If muscle fibers are permanently deprived of their nerve supply they undergo atrophy. But a denervated muscle may have its function restored any time before complete atrophy by the ingrowth of motor nerve fibers arising from the original or some other motor nerve cells.

Classification of the Somatic Afferent Fibers According to Function. Sherrington (1906) in an instructive book on "The Integrative Action of the Nervous System" has furnished us with a useful classification of the elements belonging to the afferent side of the nervous system. He designates those carrying impulses from the viscera as *interoceptive,* and subdivides the somatic afferent elements into exteroceptive and proprioceptive groups. The *exteroceptive fibers* carry impulses from the surface of the body and from such sense organs, as the eye and ear, that are designed to receive stimuli from without. These fibers, therefore, are activated almost exclusively by external stimuli. The *proprioceptive fibers,* on the other hand, respond to stimuli arising within the body itself and convey impulses from the muscles, joints, tendons, and the semicircular canals of the ear. Each group has receptors or sensory endings designed to respond to its appropriate set of stimuli, and for each there are special connections within the brain and spinal cord.

All are of value to the individual in keeping the body oriented in its environment. The proprioceptive or kinesthetic system of receptors is oriented to tensions on muscles, tendons and related structures within the body. The vestibular system is oriented to changes in the gravitational field while the visual and auditory systems are oriented to stimuli arising more or less at a distance from the body.

Exteroceptive fibers and **sensory endings** are activated by changes in the environment, that is to say, they are stimulated by objects outside the body. The impulses, produced in this way and carried by these fibers to the spinal cord, call forth for the most part reactions of the body to its environment; and, when relayed to the cerebral cortex, they may be accompanied by sensations of touch, heat, cold, or pain. The receptors are, for the most part, located in the skin; yet it is convenient to include in the exteroceptive group the pressure receptors which are closely allied to those for touch, but which lie below the surface of the body. At this point it should be noted that sensibility to those forms of contact which include some slight pressure, such as the placing of a finger on the skin, is not abolished by the section of all of the cutaneous nerves going to the area in question, since the deeper nerves carry fibers capable of responding to such contacts (Head, 1905). This deep contact sensibility, which for lack of a better name we may call "pressure-touch," must not be overlooked in the analysis of cutaneous sensations.

The balance of evidence is in favor of the assumption that each of the varieties of cutaneous sensation is mediated by a separate set of nerve fibers. We know that both myelinated and unmyelinated fibers of dorsal root origin are present in the cutaneous nerves (Ranson and Davenport, 1931). It is well established that the larger myelinated fibers mediate touch and that even when

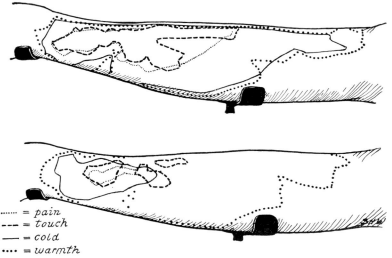

```
...... = pain
--- = touch
—— = cold
•••• = warmth
```

FIGURE 111. Two diagrams of the same forearm showing areas of anesthesia following alcohol block of peripheral nerves and subsequent partial return of innervation. The dissociation of specific sensitivities is indicated by the outlined areas. The upper figure represents the state a few weeks after the nerve injection and the lower figure the same arm seven weeks later. (After Lanier, Carney and Wilson.)

these fibers are made to function at their maximum capacity the impulses which they carry do not give rise to pain. Information concerning the fibers mediating temperature sensation is less definite, but they are probably of the small myelinated variety. Temperature changes have been shown to excite nerve fibers, cooling causing excitation of the large ones, and warming activating the non-medullated and the d-afferent fibers. According to the best available evidence, pain is conveyed by the fine myelinated and unmyelinated fibers.

Observations on the restoration of function by the regeneration of injured peripheral nerves support the belief that specific nerve fibers and endings are responsible for reception of impulses of specific sensations. For example in the carefully controlled experiments upon nerves in their own arms, Lanier, Carney, and Wilson (1935) demonstrated the selective return of specific sensations of touch, pain, and temperature independently of each other (Fig. 111).

All sensory nerve endings in the skin subserve exteroceptive functions. On structural grounds they may be divided into three principal groups: (1) endings in hair follicles, (2) encapsulated nerve endings, and (3) free terminations in the epidermis.

Free Nerve Endings. Some of the myelinated fibers as they approach their terminations divide repeatedly. At first the branches retain their sheaths, but after many divisions the myelin sheaths and finally the neurilemma are lost and only the naked axis cylinders remain. These enter the epidermis, where, after further divisions, they end among the epithelial cells (Fig. 112). This type of nerve ending is found in the skin, mucous membranes, and cornea. Similar endings are also found in the serous membranes and intermuscular connective tissue.

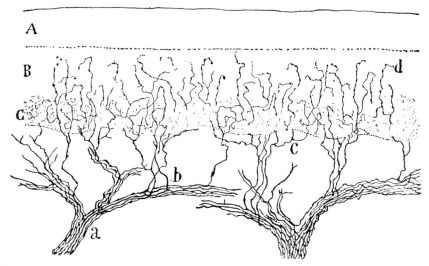

FIGURE 112. Free nerve endings in the epidermis of a cat's paw. *A*, Stratum corneum; *B*, stratum germinativum Malpighii, and *C*, its deepest portion; *a*, large nerve trunk; *b*, collateral fibers; *c*, terminal branches; *d*, terminations among the epithelial cells. Golgi method. (Cajal.)

We do not know what form the endings of the afferent unmyelinated fibers may take, but it is not unlikely that they also ramify in the epidermis like the terminal branches of the myelinated fibers just described. It seems certain that at least a part of the free nerve endings in the epidermis are pain receptors. In the central part of the cornea, the tympanic membrane, and the dentine and pulp of the teeth, such free nerve endings alone are present, and pain is the only sensation that can be appreciated. It seems probable that pain is mediated also by unmyelinated fibers that give accessory innervation to encapsulated endings which are supplied primarily with myelinated fibers for reception of sensation other than pain.

It appears that pain fibers in the skin can be stimulated by being stretched. A cut which breaks the integrity of the epidermis allows distortion of the relations more readily; movement of the edges of even a slight cut gives rise to pain, and though cutting through a viscus is painless, stretching its tissues may give rise to severe pain.

Pain perception in the skin usually results from the stimulation of more than one nerve ending since there is an overlapping mosaic of nerve terminals. In regions partially denervated, as in scars or where the nerve fibers have partially regrown after injury, the sensation of pain in response to needle-prick may have an unnatural unpleasant quality. This is said to be due to the stimulation of pain endings that were isolated from neighboring ones (Weddell, Sinclair and Feindel, 1948; Bishop, 1949). For additional discussion of the characteristics of pain see pp. 425–430.

Some of the nerve fibers which enter the epidermis end in disk-like expansions in contact with specialized epithelial cells. The expansions have been known as Merkel's tactile disks, and there is evidence that these also are touch receptors.

Encapsulated Nerve Endings.   Among the encapsulated nerve endings are the *corpuscles of Meissner* (Fig. 113, *A*). These have quite generally been regarded as tactile end organs and are located in the corium or subepidermal connective tissue of the hands and feet, forearms, lips, and certain other regions. They are of large size, oval, and possess a thin connective tissue capsule. Each receives one or more large myelinated fibers (two to nine according to Cauna, 1956), which lose their myelin sheaths as they enter the capsule. They make a variable number of spiral turns and break up into varicose branches which form a complex network. The spiral turns give the corpuscle a striated appearance under low magnification. There is also an accessory innervation of the corpuscle by one or more unmyelinated branches of thin myelinated fibers. To another type of encapsulated end organ belong those known as the *end bulbs of Krause*. One of these is illustrated in Fig. 113, *B*. They are found in the conjunctiva, edge of the cornea, lips and some other localities.

Histologic observation does not allow the determination of function of a nerve ending but may give evidence of it when used with other data. Study of specific points of sensitivity on the human skin and subsequent histologic search for nerve endings of various types in the same piece of skin has resulted in associating end organs like those of Ruffini with heat perception, and those of Krause with cold perception. By careful recording of the time of conduction of thermal changes through tissue and the appearance of impulses in the nerve fibers activated by cooling and rewarming, it was shown that the endings responsive to cooling lie 0.18 mm. below the surface (in the cat's tongue), which is in accord with histologic studies (Hensel et al., 1951).

The *Pacinian corpuscles,* two of which are illustrated in Fig. 113, have a very wide distribution in the deeper parts of the dermis of the hands and feet, and in association with tendons, intermuscular septa, periosteum, peritoneum, pleura, and pericardium. They are also numerous in the neighborhood of the joints. Because of their deep location and frequent association with the joints and tendons they probably serve for the perception of movement (proprioceptive function) and of pressure as distinct from light touch (exteroceptive function). They are large oval corpuscles, made up in great part of concentric lamellae of connective tissue. The axis of the corpuscle is occupied by a core containing the termination of a nerve fiber. Each corpuscle receives in addition to one or more unmyelinated fibers a single thick fiber that loses its myelin sheath as it enters the core, through which it passes from end to end, and terminates in a slight expansion. Side branches are also given off within the core.

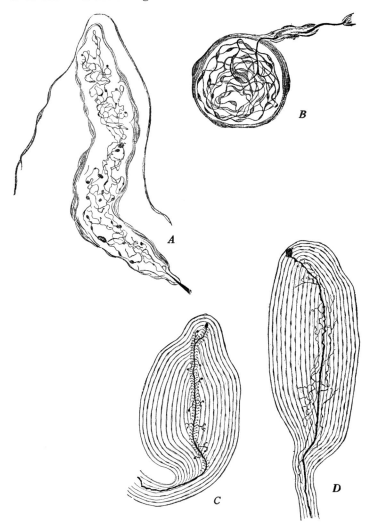

FIGURE 113.   Encapsulated sensory endings, A, Meissner's tactile corpuscle; B, end bulb of Krause from conjunctiva of man; C and D, Pacinian corpuscles. Methylene blue stain. (Dogiel, Sala, Böhm-Davidoff, Huber.)

Tissues vary somewhat in the nerve endings supplying them both as to location and types of endings. Details of the arrangement and distribution of neurotendinous endings, Pacinian corpuscles and bare endings in the neighborhood of tendons and muscles have been worked out by Stillwell (1957) and in the retroperitoneal tissues by Takashi et al. (1955).

Nerve Endings in the Hair Follicles.   It has long been known that the *hairs* are delicate *tactile organs*. The hair-clad parts lose much of their responsiveness to touch when the hair is removed. As would be expected on these grounds, the hair follicles are richly supplied with nerve endings. Just below the opening of the sebaceous gland into the follicle myelinated nerve fibers enter it, losing their myelin sheaths as they enter. They give off horizontal branches, which encircle

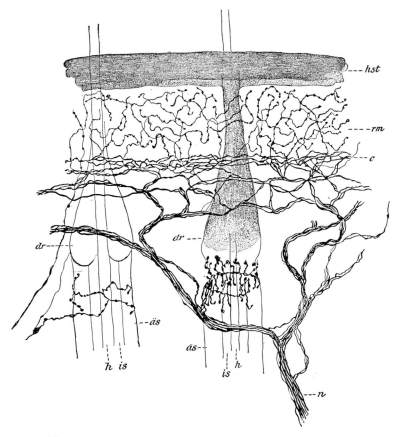

FIGURE 114.   Nerves and nerve endings in the skin and hair follicles: *hst*, Stratum corneum; *rm*, stratum germinativum Malpighii; *c*, most superficial nerve fiber plexus in the cutis; *n*, cutaneous nerve; *is*, inner root sheath of hair; *äs*, outer root sheath; *h*, the hair itself; *dr*, glandulae sebaceae. (Retzius, Barker.)

the root of the hair, and from these arise ascending branches (Fig. 114). Some of these are connected with leaf-like expansions, associated with cells resembling Merkel's touch cells.

Proprioceptive Fibers and Sensory Nerve Endings.   To this group belong the afferent elements which receive and convey the impulses arising in the muscles, joints, and tendons. Changes in tension of muscles and tendons and movements of the joints are adequate stimuli for the receptors of this class and excite nerve impulses which, on reaching the central nervous system, give information concerning tension of the muscles and the relative position of the various parts of the body. For the most part, however, these impulses do not rise into consciousness, but serve for the subconscious control of muscular activity. The unsteady gait of a tabetic patient illustrates the lack of muscular control that results when these impulses are prevented from reaching the central nervous system.

The proprioceptive fibers are myelinated and are associated with motor fibers in the nerves to the muscles. Some follow along the muscles to reach the tendons. Three types of end organs belong to this group, Pacinian corpuscles, muscle spindles, and neurotendinous end organs. Many *Pacinian corpuscles* are found in the neighborhood of the joints. They have been described in a preceding paragraph.

NEUROMUSCULAR END ORGANS. The afferent fibers to the muscles end on small spindle-shaped bundles of specialized muscle fibers (Fig. 115). These *muscle spindles* are invested by connective tissue capsules, and within each of them one or more large myelinated nerve fibers terminate. Within the spindle the myelin sheath is lost and the branches of the axis cylinders wind spirally about the specialized muscle fibers, or they may end in irregular disks. These muscle fibers receive also a somatic motor innervation (Hinsey, 1927). The motor nerve fibers innervating the intrafusal muscle fibers are of the smaller myelinated variety and are quite numerous, constituting as much as one-fourth of the outflow in the lumbosacral ventral roots (Kuffler, Hunt, and Quilliam, 1951). Where muscle spindles are few in number or entirely absent, as for example in the ocular muscles, the sensory fibers terminate in non-encapsulated endings upon the surface of ordinary muscle fibers. Structures somewhat analogous to the muscle spindles are the *neurotendinous end organs* or tendon spindles where myelinated nerve fibers end in relation to specialized tendon fasciculi.

Analysis of afferent impulses passing by way of muscular nerves to the dorsal root ganglia reveals two types. Afferent impulses from the muscle spindles are set up on contraction of the muscle but diminish in number as the muscle contraction is maintained, while impulses from stretch receptors in tendons increase during contraction of the muscle.

Sensation. Some generalizations may now be made concerning the functions of the different types of sensory nerve endings found in or immediately beneath the skin. Pain is almost certainly mediated by free nerve endings in the epithelium. The most important tactile receptors are the hair follicles and Meissner's corpuscles. For most of the skin covering the body and extremities the hair-follicles are said to be the only end organs serving this purpose, and each spot sensitive to touch is situated at the base of a hair. The hairless skin of the palmar surface of the hand and fingers is supplied with specialized tactile end organs in the form of Meissner's corpuscles. In other places, such as the skin of the pig's snout and the human prepuce, unencapsulated plates and disks in contact with epithelial cells serve the same purpose. Firm contacts producing some deformation of the skin may stimulate Pacinian corpuscles giving rise to sensations of pressure. In certain regions at least, cold seems to be mediated by Krause's end bulbs

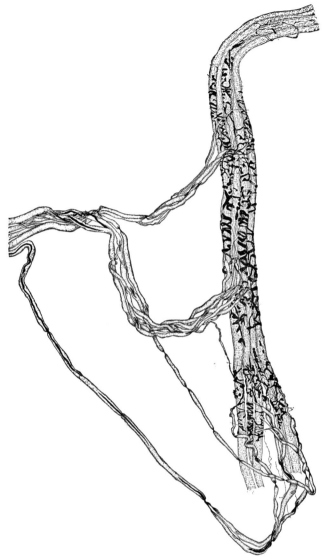

Figure 115. Neuromuscular nerve end organ from a dog. The figure shows the intrafusal muscle fibers, the nerve fibers and their terminations, but not the capsule nor the sheath of Henle. Methylene blue stain. (Huber and De Witt.)

and there is some evidence that the corpuscles of Ruffini may be sensitive to warmth. In the skin by punctate stimulation (and penetration) with a sharp needle different points may be found which when stimulated yield sensations of touch, pressure, cold, warmth, and pain like those elicited by contact with ordinary objects. Temperatures within 5° C. of the skin's temperature are not recognized as different.

While a carefully controlled stimulus to a pain spot on the skin of the arm and hand seems to elicit a single sensation, painful puncture of the skin is characterized by two sensations. The first is abrupt, brief, and only slightly painful and is elicited when the skin is penetrated only a quarter of a millimeter; the second is a delayed pain of increasing intensity, giving the sensation of stinging, occurring after penetration of about 1 mm. and reaching its maximum a second or two after the stimulus. In different areas these two portions of the painful stimulus may be blended or recognized separately (Weddell, Guttmann, and Guttmann, 1941). In tabetics there may be quite a long delay in the perception of a painful sensation on peripheral stimulus, Gowers having observed a delay as long as seven seconds. Two types of pain have also been described for deep fascia, tendons and periosteum (Weddell and Harpman, 1940).

As Gasser (1937) has pointed out, because of the different rates of conduction in large and small fibers the times of arrival at the spinal cord of various sensory impressions of a painful injury to the foot are very different. The first impulse in terms of contact, travelling over the rapidly conducting large fibers connected with tactile endings, would arrive at the spinal cord in a little over one hundredth of a second; the impulses over the fastest pain fibers would reach the cord in about four hundredths of a second; and over the slowest conducting fibers in about one and a half seconds. The first feeling of pain as judged by the time of arrival of the impulse in conscious regions would not occur until half a second after the stimulus. Incidentally, by this time reflex responses of skeletal muscle in the limb could have occurred.

The interpretation of particular sensations is a central, probably cortical, phenomenon. The paths in the cord and brain stem, though mingling their fibers in instances, convey the impulses received from the specific peripheral endings and nerves. Section of separate pathways in cord and brain stem can abolish specific sensations over restricted areas, leaving other types of sensation intact.

Specific sensations are conveyed from the periphery by separate nerve fibers and indeed can be elicited by stimulation of a sensory nerve trunk (with greater intensity in one regenerating after peripheral section), but the sensation is referred to the area of distribution of the nerve. A single sensory nerve fiber derived from a cell of a cerebrospinal ganglion divides at its peripheral end and supplies several endings spread over a macroscopic area on the surface and occupying appreciable depth of tissue.

The arrangement of such a sensory unit and its relation to adjacent similar units concerned with other sensory modalities is important in the interpretation of ordinary sensations. Tactile localization and discrimination, for example, for which there are no specific end organs, may depend upon the geometric pattern of tactile and other endings stimulated.

It may well be that the endings and nerve fibers are not so specific as have been considered. For example, it is possible that there are no specific types of endings for cold perception as compared with warmth. Touch also is used loosely to mean evidence of contact or pressure, or disturbance of a hair. For interpretation, more exact clinical observations are needed (Sinclair, 1955).

Visceral afferent fibers are found in the ninth and tenth cranial nerves and in many of the spinal nerves, especially in those associated with the white rami

the work of King (1939) would imply it was generously supplied with nerve fibers ending in knobs and loops. Special portions of it at least show numerous endings, which may be sensory. It is stated by Stotler and McMahon (1947) that only the conducting bundles of Purkinje fibers are innervated with motor fibers.

Gland cells in many places show knobbed endings upon them but these have not been universally demonstrated. Stormont (1926) has distinguished between endings arising from the cranial division of the autonomic and others from the thoracicolumbar division in the salivary glands of rabbits, but these are on separate groups of cells, an arrangement comparable to the innervation of the intrinsic muscles of the iris.

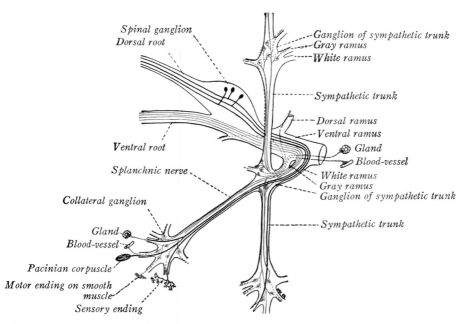

FIGURE 122.   Diagram showing the composition of visceral nerves. Black lines, visceral afferent fibers; unbroken red lines, preganglionic visceral efferent fibers; dotted red lines, postganglionic visceral efferent fibers.

Blood vessels receive numerous autonomic fibers and yet the terminations seem to be confined to those regions of vessels possessing muscle.

The action of visceral effectors in most instances is that of large groups of cells, and, in the absence of direct innervation to each unit cell in gland and muscle, there is implied a method of spread of influence to the units not in contact with nerve endings. This need is supplied in some instances by the release of humoral substances in the tissue juice and other body fluids which activates or prolongs the action of visceral effectors. Epinephrine produced by the cells of the medulla of the adrenal gland is the best known example of such a substance.

In the literature there is considerable discussion of a "sympathetic end formation" or "ground-plexus" which includes "periterminal net," which is regarded by its exponents as the ultimate connection between the nervous system and various tissues (Boeke, 1949; Kuntz and Napolitano, 1956; Honjin, 1956). The identification of these structures with nervous tissue has never been generally accepted.

The two **sympathetic trunks,** extending from the level of the second cervical vertebra to the coccyx (Figs. 117, 123), are symmetrically placed along the anterolateral aspects of the bodies of the vertebrae. There are 21 or 22 ganglia in each chain; and of these, 3 or 4 are associated with the cervical spinal nerves,

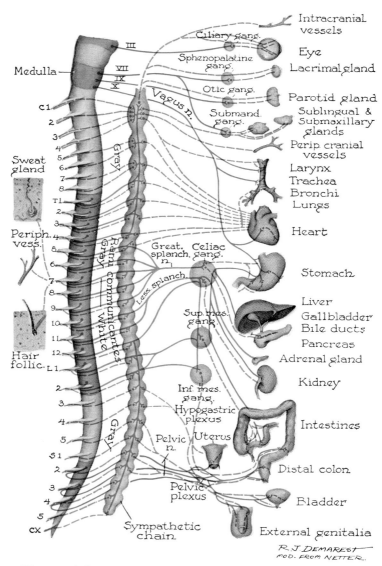

FIGURE 123. Diagram of the autonomic nervous system. Red lines indicate thoracicolumbar, blue lines craniosacral outflow; solid lines preganglionic, broken lines postganglionic fibers.

10 or 11 with the thoracic, 4 with the lumbar, and 4 with the sacral spinal nerves. Every spinal nerve is connected with the sympathetic trunk of its own side by one or more delicate nerve strands, called rami communicantes (Figs. 117, 123).

To each spinal nerve there runs a *gray ramus* from the sympathetic trunk. The *white rami,* on the other hand, are more limited in distribution and unite the thoracic and upper four lumbar nerves with the corresponding portion of the sympathetic trunk. Each sympathetic trunk gives off branches to blood vessels and viscera. These branches enter into the formation of plexuses, most of which bear the names of the arteries they accompany. Those illustrated in Fig. 117 are the pulmonary, esophageal, cardiac, coronary, aortic, celiac, gastric, superior and inferior mesenteric, hypogastric, pelvic, and vesical plexuses. These all receive directly or indirectly fiber bundles from the sympathetic trunk.

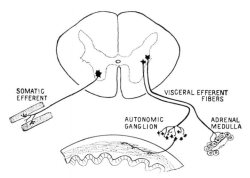

FIGURE 124.   Diagram to show the pattern of innervation of visceral structures in comparison with somatic muscle. One somatic motor fiber supplies directly 100 to 200 muscle fibers; one preganglionic visceral efferent fiber supplies 10 to 20 or more cells in an autonomic ganglion, each of which supplies several smooth muscle cells, from which the impulse for contraction spreads to other muscle cells. The adrenal medulla receives fibers directly from the spinal gray matter, and by its secretion into the blood stream produces widespread sympathicomimetic action.

The **white rami** consist of visceral afferent and preganglionic visceral efferent fibers directed from the central into the sympathetic nervous system. They contribute the great majority of the ascending and descending fibers of the sympathetic trunk (Fig. 122). While some of the fibers may terminate in the ganglion with which the white ramus is associated, and others run directly through the trunk into the splanchnic nerves, the majority of the fibers turn either upward or downward in the trunk and run for considerable distances within it (Fig. 123). The fibers from the upper white rami run upward, those from the lower white rami downward, while those from the intermediate rami may run either upward or downward. The cervical portion of the sympathetic trunk consists almost exclusively of ascending fibers, the lumbar and sacral portions of the trunk largely of descending fibers from the white rami. The *afferent fibers* of the white rami merely pass through the trunk and its branches to the viscera. The *preganglionic fibers,* with the exception of those which run out through the splanchnic nerves, end in ganglia of the trunk. Here they enter into synaptic relations with the postganglionic neurons. The majority of the postganglionic neurons, located in the ganglia of the sympathetic trunk, send their axons into the *gray rami* (Figs. 122).

The **gray rami** are composed of postganglionic fibers directed from the sympathetic trunk into the spinal nerves. These unmyelinated fibers, after joining the spinal nerves, are distributed with them as vasomotor, secretory, and pilomotor fibers to the blood vessels, the sweat glands, and the smooth muscle of the hair follicles. None go to skeletal muscle (Hinsey, 1927; Wilkinson, 1929).

The **cervical portion of the sympathetic trunk** consists of three ganglia bound together by ascending preganglionic fibers from the white rami. The *superior cervical ganglion* is the largest of the three ganglia and from it there are given off numerous gray nerve strands. These are all composed of postganglionic fibers which arise in this ganglion. They run to the neighboring cranial and spinal nerves, to which they carry vasomotor, pilomotor, and secretory fibers, and to the heart, pharynx, and the internal and external carotid arteries (Figs. 117, 123, 124). The most important of these branches of the superior cervical ganglion are the three following: (1) The superior cervical cardiac nerve, which runs from the superior cervical ganglion to the cardiac plexus, carries fibers to the heart. (2) The internal carotid nerve runs vertically from the ganglion to the internal carotid artery, about which its fibers form a plexus, known as the internal carotid plexus (Fig. 123). It is by the way of this nerve and plexus that the pupillary dilator fibers reach the eye (Fig. 280). (3) The branch of the superior cervical ganglion to the external carotid artery breaks up in a plexus on that artery. Continuations of this plexus extend along the branches of that artery to the parotid, sublingual, and submaxillary salivary glands (Fig. 285).

The middle and inferior cervical sympathetic ganglia are smaller. Among the branches from these ganglia we may mention the gray rami to the adjacent spinal nerves and the middle and inferior cardiac nerves to the cardiac plexus (Figs. 117, 123).

The **thoracic portion of the sympathetic trunk** is connected with the thoracic nerves by the gray and white rami. In addition to the rami communicantes and some small branches to the aortic and pulmonary plexuses, there are three important branches of the thoracic portion of the sympathetic trunk known as the splanchnic nerves. These run through the diaphragm for the innervation of abdominal viscera (Figs. 117, 123). The *greater splanchnic nerve* is usually formed by branches from the fifth to the ninth thoracic sympathetic ganglia and after piercing the diaphragm joins the celiac ganglion. The *smaller splanchnic nerve* is usually formed by branches from the ninth and tenth thoracic sympathetic ganglia and terminates in the celiac plexus. The *lowermost splanchnic nerve* arises from the last thoracic sympathetic ganglion and terminates in the renal plexus. These splanchnic nerves, although they appear to be branches of the thoracic sympathetic trunk, are at least in major part composed of fibers from the white rami, which merely pass through the trunk on their way to the ganglia of the celiac plexus (Fig. 122).

The Autonomic Plexuses of the Thorax. In close association with the vagus nerve in the thorax are three important visceral plexuses. The *cardiac plexus* lies in close relation to the arch of the aorta, and from it subordinate plexuses are continued along the coronary arteries. It receives the three cardiac sympathetic nerves from the cervical portion of each sympathetic trunk, as well as branches from both vagus nerves (Figs. 117, 123). The preganglionic fibers of the vagus terminate in synaptic relation with the cells of the cardiac ganglia. They convey inhibitory impulses which are relayed through these ganglia to the cardiac musculature (Fig. 124). The cardiac sympathetic nerves contain postganglionic fibers which take origin in the cervical sympathetic ganglia; and they relay accelerator impulses, coming from the spinal cord by way of the upper white rami and sympathetic trunk, to the heart (Fig. 123). The *pulmonary* and *esophageal plexuses* of the vagus are also to be regarded as parts of the autonomic system (Fig. 123).

The **celiac plexus** (solar plexus) is located in the abdomen in close relation to the celiac artery (Figs. 117, 123). It is continuous with the plexus which surrounds the aorta. Subordinate portions of the celiac plexus accompany the branches of the celiac artery and the branches from the upper part of the abdominal aorta. These are designated as the phrenic, suprarenal, renal, spermatic or ovarian, abdominal aortic, superior gastric, inferior gastric, hepatic, splenic, superior mesenteric, and inferior mesenteric plexuses. The celiac plexus contains a number of ganglia which in man are grouped into two large flat masses, placed one on either side of the celiac artery and known as the celiac ganglia. These ganglia are bound together by strands which cross the median plane above and below this artery. Somewhat detached portions of the celiac ganglion, which lie near the origin of the renal and superior mesenteric arteries, are known respectively as the *aorticorenal* and *superior mesenteric ganglia*. In addition, there is a small mass of nerve cells in the inferior mesenteric plexus close to the beginning of the inferior mesenteric artery. This is known as the *inferior mesenteric ganglion*. The larger collateral ganglia do not contain all the postganglionic neurons since scattered ganglion cells occur in the periarterial plexuses accompanying branches of celiac and mesenteric arteries (Kuntz and Jacobs, 1955).

Preganglionic fibers reach the celiac plexus from two sources: namely, from the *white rami* by way of the sympathetic trunk and *splanchnic nerves* and from the *vagus nerve* (Fig. 123). Most if not all of the preganglionic fibers contained in the splanchnic nerves terminate in the ganglia of the celiac plexus. At the lower end of the esophageal plexus the fibers from the right vagus nerve become assembled into a trunk which passes to the posterior surface of the stomach and the celiac plexus. The fibers of the left vagus pass to the anterior surface of the stomach and to the hepatic plexus (Fig. 123). It is probable that the preganglionic fibers of the vagus do not terminate in the ganglia of the celiac plexus, but merely pass through that plexus to end in the terminal ganglia, such as the small groups of nerve cells in the myenteric and submucous plexuses of the intestine (Fig. 123).

The *myenteric plexus* (of Auerbach) and the *submucous plexus* (of Meissner), located within the walls of the stomach and intestines, receive filaments from the gastric and mesenteric divisions of the celiac plexus. They also receive fibers from the vagus either directly, as in the case of the stomach, or indirectly through the celiac plexus (Fig. 123). Unfortunately, very little is known concerning the synaptic relations established in the ganglia of these plexuses. According to Langley, the postganglionic fibers from the celiac ganglia run through these plexuses without interruption and end in the muscular coats and glands of the gastrointestinal tract. The preganglionic fibers from the vagus probably end in synaptic relation to cells in these small ganglia; and the axons of these cells serve as postganglionic fibers, relaying the impulses from the vagus to the glands and muscular tissue. As was indicated in a preceding paragraph, the enteric plexuses must also contain a mechanism for purely local reactions, since peristalsis can be set up by distention in an excised portion of the gut. But as yet we are entirely ignorant as to what that mechanism may be.

The **hypogastric plexus** is formed by strands which run into the pelvis from the lower end of the aortic plexus and are joined by the visceral branches of the second, third, and fourth sacral nerves and by branches from the sympathetic trunk (Figs. 117, 123). As the hypogastric plexus enters the pelvis it splits into two parts, which lie on either side of the rectum and are sometimes called the pelvic plexuses. From these plexuses branches are supplied to the pelvic viscera and the external genitalia. Though called plexuses there are scattered ganglia throughout the bundles of nerve fibers, evidently like the collateral ganglia about the aortic branches.

The Cephalic Ganglionated Plexus. In close topographic relation to the branches of the fifth cranial nerve are four autonomic ganglia, known as the ciliary, sphenopalatine, otic, and submaxillary ganglia. Each of these is connected with the superior cervical sympathetic ganglion by filaments derived from the plexuses on the internal and external carotid arteries and their branches (Fig. 123). These filaments are designated in descriptive anatomy as the sympathetic roots of the ganglia. Each ganglion receives preganglionic fibers from one of the cranial nerves by way of what is usually designated as its motor root (Fig. 123). Thus the ciliary ganglion receives fibers from the oculomotor nerve; the sphenopalatine ganglion receives fibers from the facial nerve by way of the great superficial petrosal nerve and the nerve of the pterygoid canal; the otic ganglion receives fibers from the glossopharyngeal nerve, and the submaxillary ganglion receives fibers from the facial nerve by way of the nervus intermedius and the lingual nerve. Postganglionic fibers arising in these ganglia are distributed to the structures of the head. From the ciliary ganglion, fibers go to the intrinsic musculature of the eye. Some of the fibers arising in the sphenopalatine ganglion go to the blood vessels in the mucous membrane of the nose. Fibers from the otic ganglion reach the parotid gland. Those arising in the submaxillary ganglion end in the submaxillary and sublingual salivary glands.

Visceral Reflexes. The purely local reactions, which occur in the gut wall after section of all of the nerves leading to the gastrointestinal tract, are known as *myenteric reflexes* and depend upon a mechanism entirely contained within the enteric wall. With this exception the evidence strongly indicates that all visceral reflex arcs pass through the cerebrospinal axis. It seems certain that no reflexes occur in the ganglia of the sympathetic chain (Bolton, Williams, and Carmichael, 1937; Hare, 1941); but the possibility cannot be excluded that the collateral ganglia may serve as reflex centers, controlling to some extent the viscera which they supply (Kuntz, 1940). The visceral reflex arc represented in Fig. 116 is an over-simplification, since in most cases the impulses travel up the cord to higher centers and back again.

Postganglionic thoracicolumbar autonomic (sympathetic) fibers are widely distributed through the body. Under this heading are included vasoconstrictor fibers to the blood vessels, secretory fibers to the sweat glands, pilomotor fibers to the hair follicles, dilator fibers to the iris, dilator fibers to the bronchioles, accelerator fibers to the heart, inhibitory fibers to the gastrointestinal musculature, constrictor fibers to the spleen, and inhibitory fibers to the bladder.

Vasodilator fibers are said to run in the dorsal roots, but the neurons producing vasodilator impulses generally have not been identified. It has been suggested that adequate vasodilation occurs as a result of blocking or inhibition of vasoconstrictor impulses (Warren, Walter, Romano and Stead, 1942). However, Lindgren et al. (1956) described a central vasodilator path which was demonstrated by electrical stimulation. The path extends from the hypothalamus to the spinal cord where it lies in the lateral funiculus near the corticospinal tract. Stimulation of the path activates cholinergic fibers which cause vasodilation in skeletal muscles, accompanied by vasoconstriction in the skin. It is apparently represented in the cerebral cortex in the posterior part of the motor area (Eliasson et al., 1952).

Specific structures receive innervation from specific segmental levels of the outflow of thoracicolumbar autonomic fibers. For example, the pupils dilate in man when preganglionic fibers leaving the cord between the 8th cervical and the 4th thoracic segment are stimulated. The vessels and sweat glands in the hand of man may receive fibers from thoracic levels one to ten (Ray, Hinsey, Geohegan, 1943). By measuring skin resistance after lumbar and sacral sympathectomies Richter and Woodruff (1945) were able to map out areas of skin containing sweat glands supplied from different levels of postganglionic outflow. The skin areas or dermatomes mapped on this basis agreed closely with dermatomes mapped by Foerster on the basis of sensory representation (Fig. 105).

The medullary cells of the adrenal gland are derived embryologically from neural crest cells, just as are the cells of autonomic ganglia, and stand similarly in relation to the central nervous system. That is, axons of nerve cells in the intermediolateral cell column of the spinal cord terminate about the chromaffin cells of the adrenal medulla and there is no postganglionic neuron involved, this being the one known exception to the principle that a two-neuron chain exists between central nervous system and visceral effector (Fig. 124).

When the fibers in the splanchnic nerve to the adrenal medullary cells are stimulated, the gland secretes epinephrine, which is carried by the blood stream to all parts of the body and produces an effect like that resulting from generalized stimulation of the thoracic autonomic system. The epinephrine therefore prolongs the effect of "sympathetic" stimulation producing a sympathicomimetic action. This diffuse action is not uncommon as it is characteristic of the thoracicolumbar autonomic system itself that it tends to function as a unit. A familiar example is the widespread activity manifested during emotional excitement—

dilation of the pupils, erection of hair, rapid beating of the heart, etc. These visceral effects which accompany emotional excitement are eliminated by removal of the thoracicolumbar outflow as Cannon showed in his sympathectomized animals. A cat without its sympathetic chain will growl and defend itself from attack by a dog but its hair does not stand on end, its heart does not speed up, its pupils do not dilate, and its blood sugar does not rise.

It is of interest that these observations enabled Cannon to make critical commentary upon the James-Lange theory of emotions which stated that the emotion followed the visceral activity. Without the visceral effects, however, the animals appear to express fear and anger in appropriate circumstances.

Simultaneous activation of widely separated parts of the thoracicolumbar system is brought about by discharges of impulses from special centers in the medulla oblongata and the hypothalamus. Stimulation of the dorsolateral part of the reticular formation in the upper part of the medulla oblongata causes a generalized activation of "sympathetic" effectors (Chen, Lim, Wang, and Yi, 1936; Wang and Ranson, 1939). Most reflex responses are mediated through this medullary center. There is a descending path in the ventral part of the lateral funiculus of the cord from these centers to the intermediolateral cell column (Wang and Ranson, 1939).

There is no similar unified control of the *craniosacral autonomic* (parasympathetic) system and the several parts of this system function independently. The "parasympathetic" system includes fibers from widely separated sources. The oculomotor nerve supplies motor fibers for the ciliary muscle and the sphincter of the iris. The facial and glossopharyngeal nerves supply secretory and vasodilator fibers for the salivary glands and the mucous membrane of the mouth and pharynx. The vagi contain inhibitory fibers for the heart, constrictor fibers for the bronchioles, and motor and secretory fibers for the stomach and intestines. The visceral branches of the sacral nerves supply motor fibers to the colon, rectum, and bladder.

Surgery of the autonomic system has shown increasing value and promise. Treatment of hypertension by removal of the thoracicolumbar outflow which supplies the vasoconstrictor fibers to the blood vessels of the splanchnic area and kidneys as well as the innervation of the adrenal medulla has been successful in certain cases. Section of the vagus nerves supplying the areas of stomach and duodenum subject to ulcers has at times afforded relief. Injections designed to block the thoracicolumbar ganglia supplying an area in which thrombophlebitis exists have often shown immediate as well as continued improvement. For details of these and other procedures in common practice the literature should be consulted.

To leave the autonomic system with a discussion of its peripheral structure and the location of its preganglionic neurons is not to complete its study. Beyond these basic peripheral connections centers related to autonomic function are found at all levels of the nervous system, especially in the medulla, mesencephalon, and hypothalamus; furthermore a significant representation occurs in the cerebral cortex, especially in the precentral and the orbital region of the frontal lobe, the temporal pole, insula, and some of the olfactory regions. Autonomic representation in the cerebellum also occurs.

The autonomic outflow is under control of suprasegmental central mechanisms to such an extent that lesions of the spinal cord may interfere seriously with the regulation of basic autonomic reflexes. For example, when the urinary bladder is distended in the patient with cervical cord damage, responses of visceral character occur, as sweating, flushing, pilomotor responses, and marked rise of blood pressure; and the changes are much greater than would occur in a normal individual, who retains the connections with higher levels necessary for inhibitory and excitatory control of visceral neurons at spinal level (Pollock et al., 1951). While descending visceral paths are not well known it appears likely that one such pathway concerned with sweating descends in the cord just ventral to the lateral corticospinal tract.

CHAPTER VIII

The Spinal Cord

Thus far the story of the nervous system has been taken up with its phylogenetic history, its development in man, its gross anatomy, and some necessary details of the histologic elements in its parts. The next task involves locating groups and clusters of nerve cells within the nervous system and tracing bundles of nerve fibers to and from these cellular aggregations, keeping in mind the function of the impulses that pass over them. Almost as a by-product of this process certain conclusions can be drawn concerning the function of larger portions of the nervous system. This part of the account begins with the spinal cord because of its basic connections and segmental simplicity.

The Spinal Cord in Section. A cut through brain or spinal cord shows two conspicuous zones which are called gray and white matter, although neither term is an exact description of the color shown in either the fixed or the unfixed conditions. The white matter, which forms the outer portion of the spinal cord and the inner portion of the cerebral hemisphere, is white because of the predominance of myelinated fibers in it. The gray matter is darker in shade and has fewer myelinated fibers, but more nerve cells, unmyelinated nerve fibers, and blood vessels.

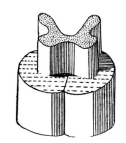

FIGURE 125. Diagram of gray columns of spinal cord.

The **gray section** (substantia grisea) of the spinal cord is centrally placed and forms a continuous fluted column, which is everywhere enclosed by the white matter (Fig. 125). In cross-section it has the form of a letter H (Fig. 126). There is a comma-shaped gray field in each lateral half of the cord, and these are united across the middle line by a transverse gray bar. The enlarged anterior end of the comma has been known as the ventral horn, the tapering posterior end as the dorsal horn, and the transverse bar as the *gray commissure*. But, when it is remembered that the gray substance forms a continuous mass throughout the length of the spinal cord, it will be seen that the term "column" is more appropriate than "horn." The long gray mass in either lateral half of the cord is convex medially and concave laterally.

166

As seen in a cross-section of the cervical cord, the *posterior column* is relatively long and narrow and nearly reaches the dorsolateral sulcus (Fig. 126). It is derived from the alar lamina and its cells receive afferent fibers of the dorsal roots. The posterior column presents a constricted portion known as the

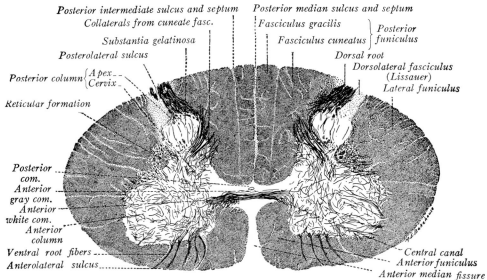

FIGURE 126. Section through seventh cervical segment of the spinal cord of a child. Pal-Weigert method.

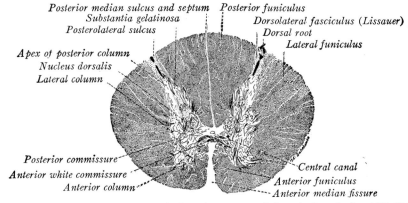

FIGURE 127. Section through the seventh thoracic segment of the spinal cord of a child. Pal-Weigert method.

cervix, a pointed dorsal extremity or *apex,* and between the two an expanded part sometimes called the *caput.* The apex consists largely of a special variety of gray substance, gelatinous in appearance in the fresh condition and very difficult to stain by neurologic methods, which in sections has the shape of an inverted V. It is known as the *substantia gelatinosa.* In the thoracic portion the posterior column, which is here very slender, does not come so close to the surface, and in the lumbosacral segments it is much thicker (Figs. 127, 128).

The *anterior column* is relatively short and thick and projects toward the anterolateral sulcus. It contains the cells of origin of the fibers of the ventral roots. From its lateral aspect nearly opposite the gray commissure there projects a triangular mass, known as the *lateral column* (columna lateralis). This is prominent in the thoracic and upper cervical segments, but it blends with the expanded anterior column in the cervical and lumbar enlargements.

The *reticular formation* (formatio reticularis), situated just lateral to the cervix of the posterior column in the cervical region, is a mixture of gray and white matter (Fig. 126). Here a network of gray matter extends into the white

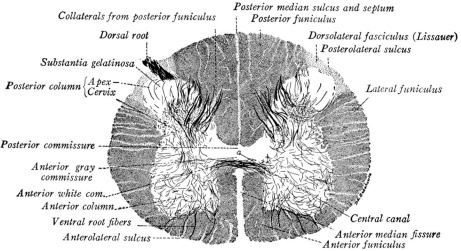

FIGURE 128. Section through the fifth lumbar segment of the spinal cord of a child. Pal-Weigert method.

substance, breaking it up into fine bundles of longitudinal fibers. The reticular formation is most evident in the cervical region, but traces of it appear at other levels.

The gray commissure contains the central canal, and by it is divided into the *posterior commissure* (commissura posterior) and the *anterior gray commissure* (commissura anterior grisea). Ventral to the latter, many medullated fibers cross the midline, constituting the *anterior white commissure*.

The cavity of the neural tube persists as the *central canal,* which lies in the gray commissure throughout the entire length of the cord. The canal is so small as to be barely visible to the naked eye. It is lined with ependymal epithelium and the lumen is often blocked with epithelial débris. The canal, which is narrowest in the thoracic region, expands within the lower part of the conus medullaris to form a fusiform dilatation, the *ventriculus terminalis.*

The White Substance. The long myelinated fibers of the cord, arranged in parallel longitudinal bundles, constitute the white substance which forms a thick mantle surrounding the gray columns. In each lateral half of the cord it is divided into the three great strands or funiculi, which have been described on the surface of the cord. The *anterior funiculus* (funiculus anterior) is bounded by the anterior median fissure, the anterior column, and the emergent fibers of the ventral roots. The *lateral funiculus* (funiculus lateralis) lies lateral to the gray substance between the anterolateral and posterolateral sulci, i. e., between the lines of exit of the ventral and dorsal roots. The *posterior funiculus* (funiculus posterior) is bounded by the posterolateral sulcus and posterior column on the one side, and the posterior median septum on the other. The septum, just mentioned, completely separates the two posterior funiculi from

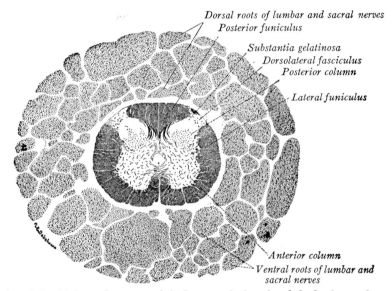

FIGURE 129. Section of the third sacral segment of the human spinal cord and the lumbosacral nerve roots of the cauda equina. Pal-Weigert method.

each other. Incomplete septa project into the white substance from the enveloping pia mater. One of these, more regular than the others, enters along the line of the posterior intermediate sulcus. It is restricted to the cervical and upper thoracic segments, is known as the *posterior intermediate septum,* and divides the posterior funiculus into two bundles, the more medial of which is known as the *fasciculus gracilis,* while the other is called the *fasciculus cuneatus.*

Characteristics of the Several Regions of the Spinal Cord. It will be apparent from Figs. 126–129 that the size and shape of the spinal cord, as seen in transverse section, varies greatly at the different levels and that the relative proportion of gray and white matter is equally variable. Two factors are primarily responsible for these differences. One of these is the variation in the size of the nerve roots at the different levels, for where great numbers of nerve fibers enter, they cause an increase in the size of the cord and particularly in the volume of the gray matter. It has already been pointed out that the cervical and lumbar enlargements are directly related to the large nerves supplying the extremities. The second factor is this: Since all levels of the cord are associated with the brain by bundles of long fibers, it is obvious that such long fibers must increase in number and the white matter increase in volume as we follow the cord from its caudal end toward the brain. All this is well illustrated in a diagram reproduced in Fig. 130.

Characteristic Features of Transverse Sections at Various Levels of the Spinal Cord

LEVEL	CERVICAL	THORACIC	LUMBAR	SACRAL
Outline	Oval, greatest diameter transverse	Oval to circular	Nearly circular	Circular to quadrilateral
Volume of gray matter	Large	Small	Large	Relatively large
Anterior gray column	Massive	Slender	Massive	Massive
Posterior gray column	Relatively slender, but extends far posteriorly	Slender	Massive	Massive
Lateral gray column	Absorbed in the anterior except in the upper three cervical segments	Well marked	Absorbed in the anterior column	Present
Processus reticularis	Well developed	Poorly developed	Absent	Absent
White matter	In large amount	Less than in the cervical region but relatively a large amount in comparison to the gray matter	Slightly less than in the thoracic region; very little in comparison to the large volume of the gray	Very little
Sulcus intermedius posterior	Present throughout	Present in upper seven thoracic segments	Absent	Absent

The outline of a section of the spinal cord at the *fourth sacral segment* is somewhat quadrilateral. The total area is small and the greater part is occupied by the thick gray columns (Fig. 131). The size of the cord is much greater at the level of the *first sacral* and *fifth lumbar segments,* as might be expected from the large size of the associated nerves (Figs. 128, 131). There is both an absolute and a relative increase in the white substance, which here contains the long paths connecting the sacral portions of the spinal cord with the brain. Both the anterior and posterior columns are massive, and the anterior presents a prominent lateral angle. The large nerve cells in the lateral part of the anterior column give rise to the fibers which run to the muscles of the leg. At the level of the *seventh thoracic segment* (Figs. 127–131) the cross-sectional area is less than in the lumbar enlargement. Corresponding to the small size of the thoracic nerves the gray matter in this region is much reduced, both anterior and posterior columns being very slender. The apex of the latter is some distance

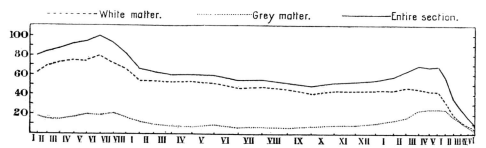

FIGURE 130. Curves showing the variations in sectional area of the gray matter, the white matter, and the entire cord in the various segments of the human spinal cord. (Donaldson and Davis.)

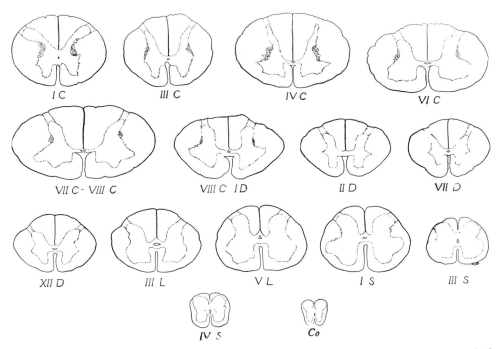

FIGURE 131. Outline drawings of sections through representative segments of the human spinal cord: *C*, cervical; *D*, dorsal or thoracic; *L*, lumbar; *S*, sacral; *Co*, coccygeal.

from the surface and its cervix is thickened by a column of cells known as the nucleus dorsalis. The columna lateralis is prominent. The white matter is some-what more abundant than in the lumbar region, and increases slightly in amount as we follow the cord rostrally through the thoracic region (Fig. 130).

    A transverse section at the level of the *seventh cervical segment* is elliptic in outline and has an area greater than that of any other level of the cord (Figs. 126, 131). The white matter is voluminous and contains the long fiber tracts connecting the brain with the more caudal portions of the cord. The gray matter is also abundant, as we might expect from the large size of the seventh cervical nerve. The ventral column is especially thick and presents a prominent lateral angle. The large laterally placed nerve cells of the anterior column are associated with the innervation of the musculature of the arm. The posterior column is relatively slender, but reaches nearly to the dorsolateral sulcus. The spinal cord at the largest point in the cervical enlargement measures approximately 13 $\times$ 7 mm., at the smallest point in the thoracic portion 8 $\times$ 6.5 mm., and at the largest point in the sacral region 9.6 $\times$ 8 mm.; but the variation is large (Elliott, 1945).

MICROSCOPIC ANATOMY

Neuroglia.   Occupying the interstices among the true nervous elements of the spinal cord is a peculiar supporting tissue, neuroglia, the structure of which has been described in a preceding chapter. *Ependymal cells* line the central canal. Some of them send processes to terminate beneath the pia in the anterior median fissure and others send similar processes dorsally along the midline in the posterior median septum (Fig. 97). A special condensation of neuroglia surrounds the central canal and is known as the *substantia gelatinosa centralis.* Unlike the rest of the gray matter it contains many fibrous astrocytes, which elsewhere are found chiefly in the white matter while the protoplasmic astrocytes are confined to the gray substance. Beneath the pia mater and closely investing the spinal cord externally is a thin stratum of neuroglia, the *glial sheath,* which is adherent to the under surface of the pia and with it forms the pia-glial membrane. The blood vessels, which penetrate the spinal cord, are surrounded by tubular prolongations of this membrane with the pial layer separated from the vessels only by perivascular spaces which communicate with the subarachnoid space (Fig. 62). The *posterior median septum* is composed of neuroglia and greatly elongated ependymal elements and is in no part formed by the pia mater.

White Substance.   The white matter of the spinal cord consists of longitudinally coursing bundles of nerve fibers, bound together by a feltwork of neuroglia fibers, a majority of which run in a direction transverse to the long axis of the nerve fibers. The neuroglia fibers are associated with the fibrous astrocytes which are scattered through the white columns. Oligodendrocytes are found in rows between the longitudinally coursing nerve fibers. The longer expansions of these oligodendroglia cells run parallel to the myelinated nerve fibers and with their side branches form closely woven tubular nets around them. Blood vessels enter the cord from the pia mater and are accompanied by connective tissue from the pia and by the subpial neuroglia. It has been generally supposed that the white fascicles of the cord were composed almost exclusively of myelinated fibers; and it is true that these, partly because of their size, are the most conspicuous elements. In cross-sections stained by the Weigert method the myelin sheaths alone are stained; and since the fibers are cut at right angles to their long axes, they appear as rings. Cajal (1909) has shown that there are also great numbers of unmyelinated fibers in the longitudinal fascicles of the cord (Fig. 132). The different fascicles differ not only in the size of their myelinated fibers but also in the proportion of unmyelinated fibers which they contain. The fasciculus dorsolateralis or tract of Lissauer (Fig. 133) contains fine myelinated fibers and great numbers of unmyelinated axons. Close to it

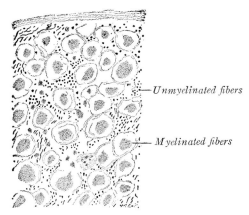

Unmyelinated fibers

Myelinated fibers

FIGURE 132. From a cross-section through the spinal cord of a rabbit showing the structure of the white matter as revealed by the Cajal method. (Cajal.)

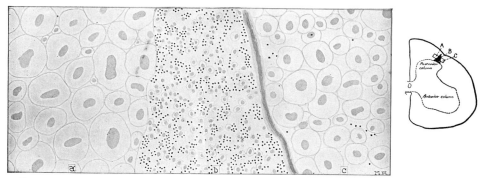

FIGURE 133. From a cross-section of the spinal cord of the cat; a narrow strip extending across the dorsolateral fasciculus in the position indicated by the sketch on the right: *a*, Fasciculus cuneatus; *b*, fasciculus dorsolateralis (Lissauer); *c*, dorsal spinocerebellar tract. The unmyelinated fibers appear as black dots. Pyridine-silver method.

lies the dorsal spinocerebellar tract which is composed almost exclusively of large myelinated fibers. Only in special regions, however, can separate fascicles such as these be observed. The various tracts are not sharply separated from each other in the cord, but where they lie adjacent the fibers intermingle at the edges as a rule, and in some instances overlap greatly.

Gray Substance. The gray matter is composed of nerve cells, including their dendrites, and of unmyelinated axons and smaller numbers of myelinated fibers—all supported by a neuroglia framework and richly supplied with capillary blood vessels. The axons of some cells (Golgi's Type I) are very long and run out into the white substance or into the ventral roots, while those of others (Type II) are short and end within the gray matter. In addition, great numbers of collaterals from the dorsal root fibers and from the longitudinal fibers of the cord, as well as terminal branches of these fibers, enter the gray substance and ramify extensively within it, entering into synaptic relations with the neurons which it contains. The branches of the myelinated fibers soon lose their sheaths, and it is this relative scarcity of myelin which gives to this substance its gray appearance. The ramification of dendrites and unmyelinated fibers forms a very intricate feltwork throughout the gray substance (Fig. 134), which in fetal life

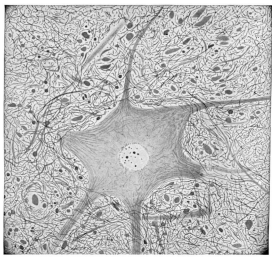

FIGURE 134. From a section through the spinal cord of a monkey, showing part of the anterior gray column including a multipolar nerve cell and the surrounding neuropil. Pyridine-silver method.

can be seen to increase in density as development proceeds. In early life, as the behavior pattern increases in complexity, the nerve fibers in this neuropil continue to become more numerous, as pointed out previously.

Nerve Cells. The nerve cells of the spinal cord vary in form, size, and connections. They are multipolar and each possesses a single axon. For convenience the cells may be described in four groups which differ in the location of the cell body and the course of their axons: (1) There are small cells of Golgi's Type II with short axons branching about in the gray substance not far from the cell body. These are not numerous in the spinal cord and are found mostly in the posterior horn, and especially in the substantia gelatinosa Rolandi. (2) Cells of a second group, which incidentally are the most conspicuous cells in the cord, are the large motor cells in the anterior horn of gray matter the axons of which pass out of the cord as ventral root fibers to reach skeletal muscle, where each supplies motor end plates to a number of muscle fibers. (3) Cells of a third group somewhat smaller in size than the anterior horn cells lie in the intermediolateral cell column and send their axons out of the cord via the ventral roots to reach the autonomic ganglia as preganglionic fibers (Fig. 109). (4) Cells of the fourth group are generally of small or medium size, although some are large, and are quite numerous, especially in the posterior horn where they are related synaptically to fibers that enter the cord from the dorsal roots. They are of great significance since they constitute the means of connection

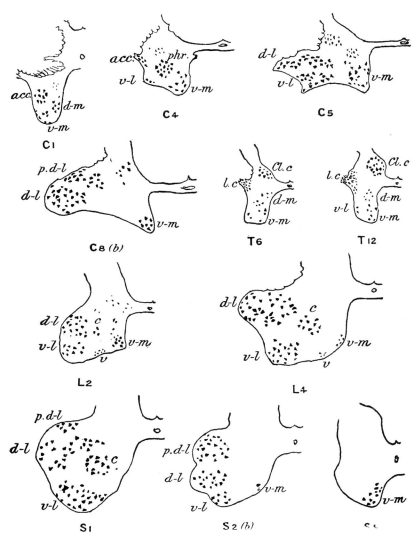

FIGURE 135. Outline sketches of ventral horn and ventral part of the dorsal horn of left side of cord at different levels, showing the relative number and position of the chief cell-groups: C_1, C_4, T_6, etc., indicate the segments—e.g., first cervical, fourth cervical, sixth thoracic; C_8 (b), lower part of eighth cervical. The following letters designate the cell-groups: v-m, Anteromedian; d-m, posteromedian; v-l, anterolateral; d-l, posterolateral; p.d-l, retroposterolateral; v in L_2, L_4, ventral; c in L_2, L_4, S_1, central; l. c. in T_6, T_{12}, intermediolateral; acc. in C_1, C_4, accessorius; phr. in C_4, phrenic; Cl.c. in T_6, T_{12}, nucleus dorsalis. (Bruce, Quain's Anatomy.)

between different regions of the nervous system (Fig. 139). The axons of some of these cells as they enter the white matter turn cranialward and form long ascending pathways which reach the brain at different levels. The axons of other cells divide into ascending and descending branches which extend different distances, sending collaterals and terminal branches into the gray matter of the cord to make connection between its various segments. These fibers constitute the *fasciculi proprii* which border the gray matter in each funiculus of the cord. The nerve fibers which connect different levels of the cord are called *association* fibers, while those which cross the midline are known as *commissural* ones. The ventral white commissure is made of such fibers.

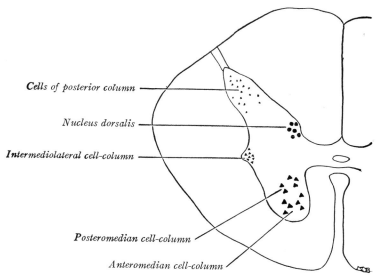

Cells of posterior column

Nucleus dorsalis

Intermediolateral cell-column

Posteromedian cell-column

Anteromedian cell-column

FIGURE 136. Diagrammatic drawing showing the arrangement of nerve cells in the thoracic spinal cord.

The nerve cells of the gray matter of the cord are not uniformly distributed, and so more or less specific groups are visible in each section (Figs. 135, 136). It has been customary in the past to refer to these groups seen in cross-section as "columns," with the implication that they extend through many segments of the cord. It is true that there is continuity in some groups. For example, the *substantia gelatinosa* and its contained cells form a long column at the tip of the posterior horn; the *nucleus dorsalis* at the medial part of the base of the posterior horn extends through the thoracic region and a little beyond, as does also the intermediolateral column of cells which are preganglionic visceral efferent neurons for the thoracicolumbar division of the autonomic system.

The *nucleus dorsalis,* or column of Clarke, is a group of large cells in the medial part of the base of the posterior column (Fig. 136). It extends from the last cervical or first thoracic to the first or second lumbar segments. It is a prominent feature in cross-sections of the thoracic cord, appearing as a well defined oval area richly supplied with collaterals from the dorsal roots. The cells have an oval or pyriform shape; each has several dendritic processes and an axon which enters the lateral funiculus, within which it runs toward the cerebellum in the dorsal spinocerebellar tract. While this column of cells extends only through the thoracic and upper lumbar segments, the dorsal root fibers entering it come from forelimb, trunk, and hindlimb. There is considerable spread of the collaterals of the primary afferent neurons upward and downward from the point of entrance. The tenth thoracic dorsal root, for example, supplies fibers to nearly the entire column of cells (Liu, 1956).

In the ventral or anterior horn of gray matter groups of nerve cells can be seen but the attempt to subdivide these into numerous columns appears not to

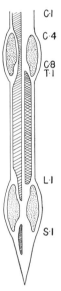

FIGURE 137. Diagram of groups of motor cells of the spinal cord of the monkey. The stippled groups of cells supply the lumbosacral and brachial plexuses; the area of diagonal lines represents cells entering the dorsal primary rami; cross-hatched area contained cells passing into intercostal and abdominal nerves (after Sprague, 1948).

be justified. Sprague's (1951) analysis of these in the monkey has shown that there are two types of cells in the anterior horn: large multipolar cells (greater than 25 μ diameter) and smaller cells. The larger ones give rise to the motor fibers of skeletal muscle, the smaller ones appear to innervate the small intrafusal muscle fibers of the muscle spindles.

The larger cells form three nuclear groups in the gray matter, especially in the cervical and lumbar enlargements, a lateral, a medial, and a ventral group. In the thoracic region, the medial and lateral groups send fibers through both dorsal and ventral primary rami of the spinal nerves; the ventral group supplies fibers only to the dorsal rami. The lateral groups, which chiefly are responsible for the wideness of the ventral horns in the lumbar and cervical enlargements, here supply the ventral rami only, while both medial and ventral groups supply dorsal rami. In the thoracic region there is no segregation; the cells supplying fibers to the dorsal and the ventral rami of the thoracic nerves are intermingled. Sprague also observed that the motor cells sending out fibers through the dorsal ramus of a single thoracic nerve are located not only in the corresponding segment but in the one above and below as well. The cells sending fibers through the ventral ramus tend to be confined to the same segment. While it is customary to separate gray and white matter in the cord rather arbitrarily, many nerve cells occur scattered in the white matter, especially near the intermediolateral column and the reticular formation; and they are more numerous in the region of the cervical and lumbar enlargements (Duncan, 1953).

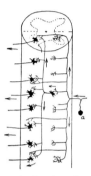

FIGURE 138. Diagram of the spinal cord, showing the elements concerned in a diffuse unilateral reflex: *a*, Spinal ganglion cell giving origin to a dorsal root fiber, one branch of which enters the cord and divides into an ascending and a descending branch; *b*, motor cell in anterior column; *c*, association neuron with axon in the lateral fasciculus proprius (Cajal).

The Spinal Reflex Mechanism.   In the next chapter is considered at length the long ascending and descending paths in the white substance of the cord by which afferent impulses from the spinal nerves reach the brain, and those through which the motor centers of the brain exert in return a controlling influence over the spinal motor apparatus. But these would be without function except for the purely intraspinal connections—the spinal reflex mechanism. The dorsal root fibers subserving tactile, thermal, painful and proprioceptive sensations enter into synaptic relations within the gray matter of the spinal cord, not only with secondary sensory neurons that relay the impulses onward toward the cerebral cortex but also with association and commissural neurons, which are connected with motor neurons and are concerned with spinal reflexes (Fig. 139).

A **reflex arc** in its simplest form may be made up of only two neurons, the primary sensory and motor neurons, with a synapse in the gray matter of the anterior column (Fig. 95). It consists of the following parts: (1) a receptor, the peripheral sensory ending; (2) a conductor, the afferent nerve fiber; (3) a center, including the synapse in the anterior column; (4) a second conductor, the efferent nerve fiber; and (5) an effector, the muscle fiber. Usually, however, there are interposed between the primary sensory and motor elements one or more intermediate neurons, the axons of which may extend only a short way or for long distances in the central nervous system in one of the named pathways. These, when restricted to one side of the cord, are known as *association* *neurons;* when their axons cross the median plane, as many of them do through the anterior white commissure, they are called *commissural neurons.* When the circuit is complete within a single neural segment it may be said to be intrasegmental (Fig. 96); if it extends through two or more such segments it is an intersegmental reflex arc.

Intersegmental Reflex Arcs. Impulses enter the spinal cord through dorsal root fibers from which they may pass to motor neurons of the same or opposite side at the same or some other level. The *fibers of the dorsal root* divide, soon

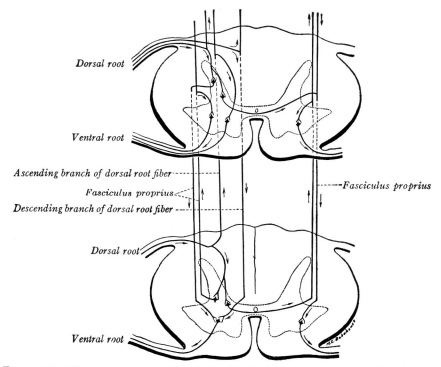

FIGURE 139.   Diagram of the spinal cord, showing fibers of the fasciculi proprii and other elements concerned in intersegmental reflexes.

after their entrance into the cord, into long ascending and shorter descending branches, which together form the greater part of the posterior funiculus and give off many collaterals to the gray matter of the successive levels of the cord (Fig. 138). Many of the ascending branches reach the brain; but the others terminate, as do the descending branches and all the collaterals, in the gray matter of the cord about cells, among which are some whose axons form the secondary pathways known as fasciculi proprii. The *fasciculi proprii* immediately surround the gray columns and consist of ascending and descending fibers of various lengths, which arise and terminate within the gray substance of the cord (Fig. 139). Most of these fibers remain on the same side as *association fibers* concerned in unilateral reflexes. Others cross in the anterior white commissure and are *commissural fibers* concerned in crossed reflexes. Afferent impulses may be transmitted along the cord in either direction by the branches of the dorsal root fibers; or by a means of synapses in the gray matter they may be transferred to the long association and commissural fibers just described and conveyed to the primary motor neurons of the same or opposite side in more or less distant segments. The course of a nerve impulse in a unilateral intersegmental reflex is indicated on the left side of Fig. 139, while on the right side of the same figure are shown the elements concerned in crossed reflexes.

The observations of Coghill (1913 and 1914) and of Herrick and Coghill (1915) tend to show that the simple form of reflex arc illustrated in Fig. 95 is not the primitive type. In larval Amblystoma the first arcs to become functionally mature are composed of chains of many neurons, so arranged that every effective cutaneous stimulus elicits the same complex response of the entire somatic musculature, i. e., the swimming movement. It is of particular interest to note that in this primitive reflex mechanism the sensory root fibers arise from giant cells located within the spinal cord and that the motor root fibers are collaterals from a central motor tract. In adult Amblystoma these sensory and motor elements are replaced by the usual type of primary sensory and motor neurons. The primitive reflex system characteristic of larval Amblystoma is not found in mammals. In the cat embryo it has been shown that individual reflexes can be elicited before mass responses, and the time of first appearance of these reflexes coincides with that of the completion of the reflex arcs through the development of collaterals from the dorsal root fibers. (Windle, O'Donnell, and Glasshagel, 1933; Windle, 1934, 1940.)

We may mention as an example of a reflex arc involving many segments of the cord the "scratch-reflex" of the dog, which has been very carefully investi-

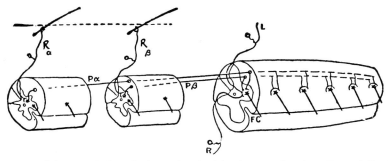

FIGURE 140. Diagram of the spinal arcs involved in the scratch reflex: $R\alpha$ and $R\beta$, Receptive paths from hairs in the dorsal skin of left side; $P\alpha$ and $P\beta$, association neurons; FC, motor fibers of ventral root. (Sherrington.)

gated by Sherrington (1906). If, some time after transection of the spinal cord in the low cervical region, the skin covering the dorsal aspect of the thorax is stimulated by pulling lightly on a hair, the hind limb of the corresponding side begins a series of rhythmic scratching movements. By degeneration experiments it was shown that this reflex arc probably includes the following elements: (1) a primary sensory neuron from the skin to the spinal gray matter of the corresponding neural segment; (2) a long descending association neuron from the shoulder to the leg segments, and (3) a primary motor neuron to a flexor muscle of the leg (Fig. 140).

A **primary motor neuron** seldom, if ever, belongs exclusively to one arc, but serves as the final channel to which many streams converge. Its perikaryon gives off widespread dendritic processes, through which it comes into relation with the ramifications of axons from many different sources. In this way impulses reach it from the dorsal roots, and from the fasciculi proprii of the spinal cord, as well as from a number of tracts which descend into the spinal cord from centers in the brain (the corticospinal, rubrospinal, tectospinal, and vestibulospinal tracts). The primary motor neuron is, as Sherrington has said, "*the final common path.*" Actual connections to the anterior horn cells from the long pathways may be by internuncial neurons. In turn, some of the internuncial cells may be fired by recurrent collaterals of axons of anterior horn cells involved in a kind of "feed-back" principle.

Functional Considerations. It is customary to speak of the reflex arcs in the spinal cord as if they were isolated phenomena of importance only in the laboratory or during a physical examination. The extent to which reflexes form the basis of much of ordinary action is often difficult to demonstrate in the normal situation, but in the presence of lesions which interrupt pathways of voluntary action part of the reflex background is more readily brought out.

Reflex mechanisms exist which depend on pathways through the spinal cord but have centers between the afferent and efferent side at higher levels, even in the cerebral cortex itself. The fanning reaction of toes to stroking the sole (Babinski response) is produced on interruption of the corticospinal tract at any point in its course, and so even in the cortex where many of its cells of origin are found.

The immediate response to spinal transection is "shock," more marked in the portion of the cord caudal to the point of transection. This may last from a few minutes in lower forms to a day or two in the higher ones including man, and is characterized by lack of responsiveness to stimulus, that is, a high threshold across the synapses in the isolated region of the cord. This state of spinal shock is not identical with traumatic shock from fluid loss; in fact the blood pressure may remain normal throughout the period of shock.

As recovery occurs, the reflexes in the isolated portion of cord reappear and are exaggerated in their response, presumably from release from the inhibiting controls of higher levels. A spinal cat placed on its feet will stand temporarily if supported laterally, and extra stimuli such as pinching its tail, though not felt consciously, prolong the standing response. A stimulus to a sensory nerve on one side results in withdrawal, that is flexion, of the homolateral limb and extension of the contralateral one. Simultaneous stimuli of the nerves of two sides result in rhythmic flexion alternating with extension. Thus it can be seen that the basic mechanisms for standing and for rhythmic stepping are in the spinal cord. Cells lying in the medial part of the ventral horn of gray matter, termed "Renshaw cells," are supplied by collaterals of the motor cells supplying skeletal muscle. When excited (by the release of acetylcholine from the motor neuron collaterals) they inhibit all types of motor neurons at that segmental level. Such a mechanism must be part of the quick control of rhythmic movement (Eccles, 1957).

Visceral mechanisms allow the development of automatic bladder and rectal emptying, which is of significance to the human cases of spinal transection.

In cases of cervical spinal transection or severe damage, the ascending and descending pathways concerned with visceral control are interrupted, and the effects show evidence of lack of both excitatory and inhibitory control from suprasegmental centers comparable to the effects on voluntary muscle. In that part of the body below the spinal cord damage, defects occur in regulation of sweating and vasomotor control. Patients with such defects will have abnormal changes in temperature when the surrounding medium becomes hot or cold. When such a patient is changed from a horizontal to a vertical position the blood pressure may fall as much as 80 or more mm. of mercury and precipitate unconsciousness from cerebral anemia. Patients with spinal injuries not so severe as complete transection may show marked retention of functions and improvement in motor ability with the passage of time. In lower animals the recovery is greater than that observed in man (Pollock et al., 1951).

CHAPTER IX

Fiber Tracts of the Spinal Cord

The fibers composing the white substance of the spinal cord are not scattered and intermingled at random, but, on the contrary, those of a given function are grouped together in more or less definite bundles. A bundle of fibers all of which have the same origin, termination, and function is known as a *fiber tract*. The *funiculi* of the spinal cord are composed of many such tracts of longitudinal fibers, which, while occupying fairly definite areas, blend more or less with each other, in the sense that there is considerable intermingling of the fibers of adjacent tracts. The topography of these at different levels of the spinal cord is slightly variable also (Smith, 1957). It is convenient to have a name for certain obvious subdivisions of the funiculi which contain fibers belonging to more than one tract. Such a mixed bundle is properly called a *fasciculus*. Many tracts have names which indicate their origin, destination, and the direction in which impulses pass. For example, the spinocerebellar tract carries impulses which ascend from the tract's origin, the spinal gray matter, to its destination, the cerebellar cortex. It would be helpful if all tracts were named in this manner, but others have names descriptive of their location, as fasciculus dorsolateralis; or shape, fasciculus gracilis; and a number under the old terminology were designated by the names of investigators who first described them, as tract of Lissauer, now known as the fasciculus dorsolateralis.

Functionally, the conspicuous tracts in the cord are distinguished as *motor* or *sensory*, but there are a number of paths which interconnect different portions of the central nervous system whose functions are not exactly described in these terms. Some of these are referred to as *association* bundles. For convenience of interpretation of injury to the spinal cord, a knowledge of the course and distribution of the main motor and sensory paths is valuable.

In order to trace the tracts of interest in the spinal cord it is convenient to follow them in the direction the impulses travel, so the course of the fibers of the dorsal roots that enter the cord will be considered and with them the paths of the various types of sensory impulses conveyed from peripheral end organs.

THE INTRAMEDULLARY COURSE OF THE DORSAL ROOT FIBERS

The central end of a dorsal root breaks up into many rootlets or filaments (fila radicularia), which enter the spinal cord in linear order along the line of the posterior lateral sulcus. As it enters the cord each filament can be seen to separate into a larger medial and a much smaller lateral division. The fibers of the *medial division* are of relatively large caliber and run over the tip of

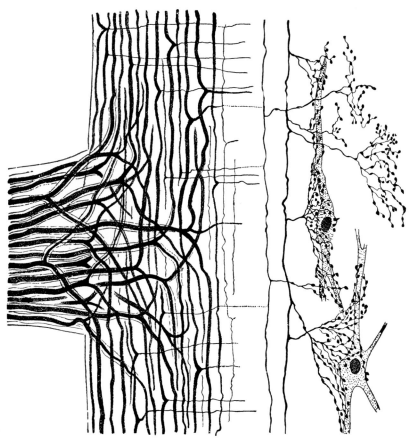

FIGURE 141. Bifurcation of the dorsal root fibers within the spinal cord into ascending and descending branches, which in turn give off collaterals; the termination of some of these collaterals in synaptic relation to cells of the posterior gray column. (Cajal, Edinger.)

the posterior column into the posterior funiculus (Fig. 143). Those of the *lateral division* are fine and enter a small fascicle which lies along the apex of the posterior column, the fasciculus dorsolateralis or tract of Lissauer. Very soon after its entrance into the cord each dorsal root fiber divides in the manner of a Y into a longer ascending and a shorter descending branch (Fig. 141). The large fibers in the medial division are those associated in the periphery with large encapsulated or elaborate forms of ending, as the tactile corpuscles of Meissner, Pacinian corpuscles, muscle and tendon spindles, and so forth. They are therefore concerned with touch, pressure, and proprioception. The smaller fibers of the lateral division terminate peripherally in endings concerned with pain and temperature sense.

The **ascending branches of the fibers of the medial division** of the dorsal root run for considerable but varying distances in the posterior funiculus; some from each root reach the medulla oblongata (according to Glees and Soler, 1951, only about 25 per cent reach the medulla in the cat), others terminate at different levels in the gray matter of the spinal cord. At the level of their entry into the cord these fibers occupy the lateral portion of the *posterior*

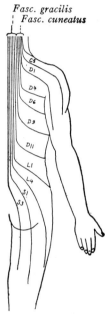

Fasc. gracilis
Fasc. cuneatus

FIGURE 142. Diagram to illustrate the arrangement of the ascending branches of the dorsal root fibers within the posterior funiculus of the spinal cord.

funiculus; but in their course cephalad, as each successive root adds its quota, those from the more caudal roots are displaced medianward. In this way the longer fibers come to occupy the medial portion of the posterior funiculus (Fig. 142). In the cervical and upper thoracic regions the long ascending fibers from the sacral, lumbar, and lower thoracic roots constitute a well defined medially placed bundle, the *fasciculus gracilis,* separated from the rest of the posterior funiculus, called the *fasciculus cuneatus,* by the posterior intermediate septum. Those of the long ascending fibers, which finally reach the brain, terminate in gray masses in the posterior funiculi of the medulla oblongata (nucleus of the funiculus gracilis and nucleus of the funiculus cuneatus). Since the number of these long ascending branches must increase from below upward, it is easy to understand the progressive increase in size of the posterior funiculus from

the sacral to the cervical region (Fig. 131). The fasciculus cuneatus and fasciculus gracilis are not recognizable as separate parts of the posterior funiculus
below the level of the sixth thoracic segment.

The **descending branches of the fibers of the medial division** of the dorsal
root are all relatively short. The shortest terminate at once in the gray matter
of the posterior column. Others descend in the *fasciculus interfascicularis,* or
comma tract of Schultz, which is situated between the fasciculus gracilis and
the fasciculus cuneatus; and still others run near the posterior median septum
in the *septomarginal fasciculus* (Figs. 147, 149). In both of these fascicles they
are intermingled with descending fibers, arising from cells within the gray
matter of the spinal cord.

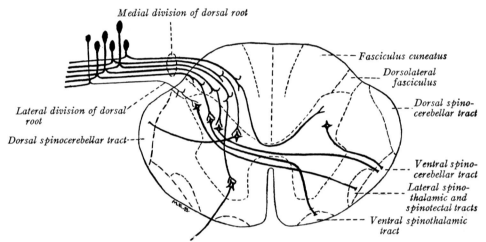

FIGURE 143.   Diagram of the spinal cord and dorsal root, showing the divisions of the dorsal root,
the collaterals of the dorsal root fibers, and some of the connections which are established by
them.

Collaterals.   At intervals along both ascending and descending branches
collaterals are given off which run ventrally to end in the gray matter (Fig.
141). They are much finer than the fibers from which they arise, and the total
number arising from a given fiber is rather large. As has been mentioned
earlier, fibers from one dorsal root may extend to many adjacent segments
of the cord. Some of them end in the ventral gray column; others, in the
posterior gray column, including the substantia gelatinosa and the nucleus
dorsalis; still others run through the dorsal commissure to the opposite side of
the cord, where they appear to end in the posterior columns (Fig. 143). In
Fig. 141 there are illustrated the arborizations formed by some of these collaterals about cells of the posterior column.

The *terminals* of the descending branches and of those ascending branches,
which do not reach the brain, end as do the collaterals within the gray matter
of the spinal cord.

The **fibers of the lateral division** of the dorsal root are all very fine. The

majority are unmyelinated and can be recognized only in preparations in which
the axons are stained. In Weigert preparations one must look carefully to find
the fine myelinated fibers contained in this division. But in pyridine-silver
preparations great numbers of delicate axons can be seen to turn lateralward
as the root filament enters the cord. These constitute the lateral division of
the root and enter the *dorsolateral fasciculus* or tract of Lissauer (Fig. 143). The
medial division, on the other hand, consists exclusively or almost exclusively
of myelinated fibers and all of the large fibers from the root enter it. The
fibers of the lateral division of the root divide into ascending and descending
branches, both of which, however, are very short. The ascending branch, which
is the longer of the two, does not extend more than the length of one or two
segments in the long axis of the cord (Ranson, 1913, 1914).

The **dorsolateral fasciculus,** or tract of Lissauer, lies between the apex of
the posterior column and the periphery of the cord, and varies greatly in shape
and size at the different levels (Figs. 126–129). It is composed of unmyelinated
and fine myelinated fibers, which are derived in part from the lateral division
of the dorsal root and in part arise from cells in the neighboring gray matter
(Fig. 133). Though called a tract most of its fibers end within a segment or two
of the point of entrance into the cord.

AFFERENT PATHS IN THE SPINAL CORD

All afferent impulses which reach the cord are carried by the dorsal root
fibers, and so their course and distribution are of great significance. Interoceptive fibers from the viscera, proprioceptive fibers from the muscles, tendons,
and joints, as well as exteroceptive fibers from the skin are included in these
roots; among the latter group are several subvarieties, mediating the afferent
impulses out of which the sensations of touch, heat, cold, and pain are
elaborated. While the fibers carrying these various impulses were intermingled
in the nerves, they showed in the medial and lateral divisions of the dorsal roots
a beginning of segregation. In the paths of the cord there is further segregation
of functional groups of fibers.

The **proprioceptive fibers,** which terminate at the periphery in neuromuscular and neurotendinous spindles and in Pacinian corpuscles, are known
to be myelinated. They must, therefore, pass through the well myelinated
medial division of the dorsal root into the posterior funiculus. As shown by
Brown-Séquard in 1847 by a study of patients with unilateral lesions of the
spinal cord, sensations from the muscles, joints, and tendons reach the brain
without undergoing a crossing in the spinal cord. This and other evidence
points unmistakably to the long ascending branches of the dorsal root fibers,
which are continued uncrossed in the posterior funiculus to the medulla
oblongata, as the conductors of this type of sensation. When these fibers are
destroyed by a tumor or other lesion confined to the posterior funiculus,
muscular sensibility and the recognition of posture are abolished, while crude
touch, pain, and temperature sensations remain intact.

No better exposition of the *proprioceptive functions* could be furnished
than by describing the sensory deficiencies found in cases of tabes dorsalis or

locomotor ataxia, a disease in which there is degeneration of the posterior funiculi. Lying in bed, with eyes closed, a tabetic may not be able to say in what position his foot has been placed by an attendant because afferent impulses from the muscles, joints, and tendons fail to reach the cerebral cortex to arouse sensations of posture. Not only are the sensations of this variety lacking, but the unconscious reflex motor adjustments initiated by proprioceptive afferent impulses are also impaired. Standing with feet together and eyes closed, the patient loses his balance and sways from side to side. In walking his gait is uncertain and the movements of his limbs poorly coordinated. All of this motor incoordinaton is explained by a loss of the controlling afferent impulses from the muscles, joints, and tendons.

Some of the fibers which ascend in the posterior funiculus to reach the nucleus gracilis and cuneatus convey a peculiar form of sensation, a sense of vibration such as is produced by the handle of a tuning fork resting upon subcutaneous bone, and in addition the fibers conveying impulses of tactile localization and discrimination have a similar course. Sensitiveness to vibration is lost along with muscle sense in degeneration of the posterior funiculus.

The long ascending fibers of the posterior funiculus, which reach the brain and end in the nucleus gracilis and cuneatus, are for the most part proprioceptive in function (Fig. 269). The connections which they make there can best be considered in another chapter. Collaterals and many terminal branches end in the gray matter of the cord, entering into *synaptic relations with the neurons of the spinocerebellar paths* and with neurons belonging to spinal reflex arcs.

Proprioceptive Paths to the Cerebellum. The spinocerebellar tracts are concerned with the transmission to the cerebellum of afferent impulses from the muscles, joints, tendons, and skin, which remain, however, at a subconscious level. The primary afferent neurons conveying these impulses are the same whether the impulses go eventually to the cerebrum or cerebellum.

The **dorsal spinocerebellar tract** (fasciculus spinocerebellaris dorsalis, direct cerebellar tract of Flechsig, fasciculus cerebellospinalis) is a well defined bundle at the surface of the lateral funiculus just ventral to the posterior lateral sulcus (Figs. 143, 149). In cross-section it has the form of a flattened band, situated between the periphery of the cord and the lateral corticospinal tract. It begins in the upper lumbar segments, is prominent in the thoracic and cervical portions of the cord, and transmits impulses to the cerebellum from the muscles of the trunk and legs. It consists of uniformly large fibers, which take origin from the cells of the nucleus dorsalis of the same side and perhaps to a slight extent from those of the opposite side (Strong, 1936). This nucleus forms a prominent feature of the sections through the thoracic portion of the cord, but is not found above the eighth cervical nor below the second lumbar segments. A conspicuous bundle of myelinated collaterals from fibers of the fasciculus cuneatus run to this nucleus where their arborizations form baskets about the individual cells of the nucleus. *The fibers arising from the cells of the nucleus dorsalis run to the periphery of the lateral funiculus, where they turn* *rostrally and form the dorsal spinocerebellar tract*, which reaches the cerebellum by way of the inferior cerebellar peduncle (Fig. 269).

The **ventral spinocerebellar tract** constitutes the more superficial portion of a large ascending bundle of fibers, known as the fasciculus anterolateralis superficialis or Gowers' tract, which also includes the spinotectal and lateral spinothalamic tracts (Fig. 143). It is situated at the periphery of the lateral funiculus ventral to the tract we have just considered. It is said to consist of *fibers which arise from the cells of the posterior gray column and intermediate gray matter of the same and the opposite side*. These fibers reach the cerebellum by way of the medulla, pons, and anterior medullary velum (Fig. 269).

From what has been presented above, it will be apparent that collaterals and terminal branches of proprioceptive dorsal root fibers enter into synaptic relations with certain intraspinal neurons, the axons of which run to the cerebellum by way of the ventral and dorsal spinocerebellar tracts. The entire path from periphery to cerebellum, therefore, consists of two neurons with a synaptic interruption in the gray matter.

Exteroceptive Sensations. There is good reason for believing that there are separate fibers for each of the four modalities of cutaneous sensation: touch, warmth, cold, and pain. In the spinal nerves these fibers are intermingled so that an injury to such a nerve usually affects all four modalities simultaneously, but in the spinal cord there is a segregation of the sensory pathways. Separate points on the skin can be located which respond to stimulation with these separate sensations, specific nerve endings have been identified in the body coverings for each of them, and the types of nerve fibers supplying these can be distinguished. The nerve fibers supplying large encapsulated endings sensitive to touch and pressure are large and myelinated. Those supplying the endings believed to be responsible for pain and temperature sense are small myelinated or unmyelinated. When these fibers enter the cord they become segregated as described above. The large myelinated ones conveying touch and pressure pass by way of the medial division of the dorsal root into the posterior funiculus and run with the proprioceptive fibers there. As these fibers ascend they give off collaterals to the gray matter of the successive levels of the spinal cord through which they pass. The tactile impulses from a given root, therefore, do not enter the gray matter all at once, but filter forward through the collaterals and terminals of these dorsal root fibers to reach the posterior gray column in a considerable number of segments above that at which the root enters the cord. Within the posterior gray column at these successive levels the terminals and collaterals of the tactile fibers establish synaptic connections with neurons of the second order, the axons of which cross the midline and form the *ventral spinothalamic tract* of the opposite side (Fig. 144). If the tactile fibers of the second order are destroyed in the anterior commissure at one level, as in syringomyelia, they are likely to be intact at another level so that tactile impulses can get past the lesion. Muscle sensibility is not involved by destruction of commissural fibers because the fibers concerned extend up the posterior funiculus without crossing.

It is in this path in the posterior funiculus, along with the fibers conveying muscle sense impressions to conscious areas, that the more critical types of tactile sensibility, tactile localization and discrimination, are conveyed.

To the ventral spinothalamic tract is assigned crude touch and pressure sense. The uncrossed path in the posterior funiculus for tactile impulses, entering the cord through any given dorsal root, overlaps by many segments the crossed path in the ventral funiculus (Fig. 264), and many uncrossed fibers reach the nuclei of the funiculus gracilis and funiculus cuneatus in the medulla oblongata. This extensive overlapping of the crossed by the uncrossed path accounts for the fact that lateral hemisection of the human spinal cord rarely causes marked disturbance of tactile sensibility as detected by ordinary methods of testing.

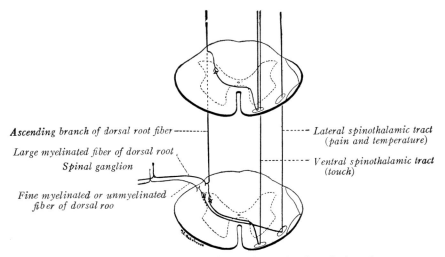

Ascending branch of dorsal root fiber- - - - - - - - - - - - - - - - - *Lateral spinothalamic tract*
                                                                        (pain and temperature)

Large myelinated fiber of dorsal root
  Spinal ganglion   - - - - - - *Ventral spinothalamic tract*
                                                                        (touch)

Fine myelinated or unmyelinated
  fiber of dorsal roo

FIGURE 144.   Exteroceptive pathways in the spinal cord.

The **ventral spinothalamic tract** is an ascending bundle of fibers found in the anterior funiculus. It *mediates tactile sensibility and consists of fibers which take origin from cells in the posterior column of the opposite side, cross the median plane in the anterior white commissure, and ascend in the ventral funiculus to end within the thalamus* (Figs. 144, 264). It is possible that many of the fibers do not reach the thalamus directly, but terminate in the gray matter of the cord and medulla oblongata in relation to other neurons, whose axons continue the course to the thalamus. If this be so, the path consists in part of relays of shorter neurons (Dejerine, 1914).

The Conduction of Sensations of Pain, of Heat, and of Cold.   The small myelinated fibers, which convey thermal sensibility, and the fine myelinated and unmyelinated fibers, which convey pain, enter the spinal cord through the lateral division of the dorsal root and end in the substantia gelatinosa Rolandi within one or two segments of the point of entrance. Here they synapse with cells the axons of which cross the midline in the ventral white commissure and ascend on the opposite side of the cord in the lateral spinothalamic tract. The sensory dissociation characteristic of syringomyelia gives information concerning the course of the sensory pathways within the spinal cord. In this disease, cavity formation begins in the region of the central canal and soon destroys the adjacent commissures. Since the fibers forming the lateral spinothalamic tracts start their course by crossing in the commissures near the level of entrance of the primary afferent fibers, while the tactile fibers give off collaterals at many levels to synapse with commissural neurons forming the ventral spinothalamic tract, there results a loss of pain and temperature sensations in corresponding segments of the body, but with unimpaired tactile sensibility.

It is well established on the basis of clinical observations that the paths for sensations of heat and cold follow closely those for pain. They pass through the gray matter within two segments after entering the cord, cross to the opposite side, and ascend in the lateral spinothalamic tract. According to May (1906), "It is clear that there are distinct and separate paths for the impulses of pain, of heat, or of cold in the spinal cord, and that these different and specific qualities of sensation may be dissociated in an affection of the spinal cord." That is, one of these forms of sensibility may be lost, although the other two are retained. "But as these paths are anatomically very closely associated from origin to termination these three forms of sensation are usually affected to a like degree."

Section of the lateral spinothalamic tract for the relief of intractable pain is now a well recognized surgical procedure. When the section is made on one side only, there is analgesia of the opposite side of the body up to the caudal level of the first segment below the lesion. This analgesia involves the skin, muscles, fasciae, tendons, and bones but not the viscera. Bilateral section is required to abolish visceral pain. A careful study of patients on whom this operation has been performed has shown that in the lateral spinothalamic tract the fibers mediating temperature sensation lie dorsal to those for pain. There is also a lamination of the fibers according to their segmental origin. As it ascends in the spinal cord the tract increases in size by the addition of fibers to its ventromedial border. The fibers from the sacral segments continue to occupy a relatively superficial position. Superficial involvement of the lateral funiculus at any level of the cord is, therefore, likely to produce sensory disturbances limited to the regions supplied by the sacral nerves, deeper injury producing more disturbance of higher spinal levels up to the level of injury (Foerster and Gagel, 1932).

Not all of the fibers of the lateral spinothalamic tract reach the thalamus. According to May (1906), "Some of these fibers certainly pass directly to the thalamus, while others terminate in the intermediate gray matter, and thus, by means of a series of short chains, afford secondary paths to the same end station, which may supplement the direct path, or be made available after interruption of the direct path." It has been shown in many cases in man and animals that, after a complete hemisection of the spinal cord, the loss of sensibility to pain on the opposite side of the body below the lesion was only temporary. In time there may occur a more or less perfect restoration of pain conduction, showing that the homolateral side of the cord is able to supplement or replace the heterolateral path. These short chains, which are of secondary importance in man, are much better developed in the cat. In this animal pain conduction through the spinal cord is bilateral and is effected to a large extent through a series of short relays. (Karplus and Kreidl, 1914; Ranson and Billingsley, 1916.) An excellent account of sensation in patients with spinal cord lesions is given by Foerster (1936).

Evidence has been presented which points toward the fine myelinated and unmyelinated fibers of the spinal nerves and dorsal roots as the pain fibers (Ranson, 1931). Space does not permit a detailed presentation of the evidence here. It should be noted, however, that the delicate fibers of the lateral division of the dorsal root terminate in the gray matter soon after their entrance into the spinal cord, and in this respect correspond to the known course of the fibers carrying painful impulses. The problem can be approached from the experimental standpoint. The seventh lumbar dorsal root of the cat was found to be especially adapted for such a test. This root as it approaches the cord breaks up into a number of filaments which spread out in a longitudinal direction and enter the cord along the posterolateral sulcus. Within each root filament, as it approaches this sulcus, the unmyelinated separate out from among the myelinated fibers and take up a position around the circumference of the filament and along septa that divide it into smaller bundles. As the root enters the cord, these unmyelinated fibers turn laterally into the dorsolateral fasciculus, constituting together with some fine myelinated fibers the lateral division of the root (Fig. 145). A slight cut in

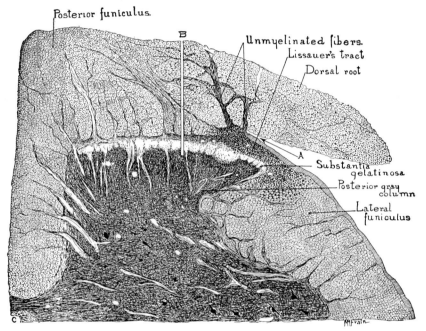

FIGURE 145. From a section of the seventh lumbar segment of the spinal cord of the cat, showing the unmyelinated fibers of the dorsal root entering the tract of Lissauer.

the direction of the arrow, which as shown by subsequent microscopic examination divided the lateral without injury to the medial division of the root, at once eliminated the pain reflexes obtainable from this root in the anesthetized cat, such as struggling, acceleration of respiration, and rise of blood pressure. On the other hand, a long deep cut in the plane indicated by *B*, Fig. 145, which severed the medial division of the root as it entered the cord, had little or no effect on the pain reflexes. This series of experiments, the details of which are given elsewhere (Ranson and Billingsley, 1916), furnishes strong evidence that painful afferent impulses are carried by the fibers of the lateral division of the dorsal root. Convincing physiologic evidence that pain is mediated by unmyelinated as well as fine myelinated fibers of the spinal nerves has been furnished.

The **exteroceptive fibers** under consideration carry afferent impulses from the skin to the spinal cord, in addition to making connection with local reflex mechanisms and with neurons forming the long paths to conscious levels make other connections. Many of the impulses which enter the cord over these fibers expend themselves at various levels of the spinal cord and brain stem in unconscious regulation of muscular activity, for example, those impulses which ascend in the spinotectal tract.

The **spinotectal tract** consists of fibers which arise from cells in the posterior gray column, and which, after crossing, ascend in the lateral funiculus in company with those of the lateral spinothalamic tract to end in the roof (tectum) of the mesencephalon (Fig. 149). Since here are located reflex connections with other afferent impulses, as auditory and visual, it is to be supposed that some integration of the motor responses to stimuli from various sources may take place here.

The **spino-olivary tract** is composed of ascending fibers running from the spinal cord to the inferior olivary nucleus of the medulla oblongata. They are intermingled with the olivospinal or bulbospinal fibers which run in the opposite direction. From the inferior olivary nucleus many fibers pass across the midline to reach the cerebellum.

From animal experiments it appears that impulses carried by spino-olivary fibers are relayed to the same zones of the cerebellum to which the dorsal spinocerebellar tracts are distributed, that is, largely the medial (vermal) portion of the anterior lobe, and to a less extent to the more posterior portions of the vermis (Brodal et al., 1950).

Spinoreticular fibers run in the lateral funiculus of the cord to the medulla oblongata and terminate in the lateral reticular nucleus, especially its caudal and more superficial portions which are the parts of the nucleus sending fibers to the vermis of the cerebellum. This may represent a route of exteroceptive impulses to the cerebellum (Brodal, 1949). There are also **spino-pontine** fibers which ascend in the region between the ventral and lateral corticospinal tracts to terminate on cells of the nuclei pontis. These fibers are both crossed and uncrossed (Walberg and Brodal, 1953).

Interoceptive fibers are known to be present in the thoracic and upper lumbar spinal nerves, and there accompany the thoracicolumbar preganglionic autonomic outflow. There is also evidence that they occur in certain sacral nerves, but they are absent or not discovered in cervical nerves, and the course of the fiber tracts in the spinal cord in mammals is not well known. If visceral pain is taken as an example, the fibers probably pass up the cord in short relays.

In the cat, afferent impulses from splanchnic nerves have been traced by electrical means by two routes to higher centers. One path goes through the homolateral fasciculus gracilis and the opposite medial lemniscus to the nucleus ventralis posterolateralis of the thalamus; another extends bilaterally upward in the region of the spinothalamic tracts reaching the posterior hypothalamus and caudal part of thalamus on both sides. The bilateral character of the path may explain the failure of some unilateral operations on the cord for intractable pain (Aidar, Geohegan, and Ungewitter, 1951).

Summary of the Sensory Pathways.   From what has been said above, it will be apparent that the paths mediating pain and temperature sensibility cross promptly to the opposite side of the cord and ascend in the lateral spinothalamic tract. The path for touch crosses more gradually into the ventral spinothalamic tract of the opposite side, the uncrossed path in the posterior funiculus overlapping by many segments the crossed path in the ventral funiculus. The sensory impulses from the muscles, joints, and tendons, as well as some elements of tactile sensibility, are carried upward on the same side of the cord by the long ascending branches of the dorsal root fibers, which terminate in the nuclei of the funiculus gracilis and the funiculus cuneatus. From here a second neuron conveys the impulses to the thalamus by way of the medial lemniscus of the opposite side.

Referred Pain. The term "referred pain" has no exact limitation and is used to describe pains of more than one type. Pain caused by visceral disease is often felt on the surface of the body. The surface area to which the pain is referred usually lies within the dermatomes associated with the cord segments which receive sensory fibers from the diseased viscus. The outlines of such painful areas resemble the arrangement of the dermatomes and not the distribution of the peripheral nerves. The receptive mechanisms within the spinal cord for visceral and somatic pain are closely associated. The surface area to which the pain is referred may be tender and painful when touched. It seems probable that the spinal receptive mechanism within the segment or segments, corresponding to the dermatomes involved, is activated by the stream of painful impulses from the viscera and for this reason has a lower threshold for impulses from the skin. This involves the assumption "that both somatic and visceral afferent fibers carry impulses which affect a common pool of secondary neurons" (Hinsey and Phillips, 1940).

Experiments by Kellgren (Lewis, 1942) demonstrated that pain experimentally produced by injecting salt solution in muscles or interspinous ligaments of the vertebral column is distributed in a segmental pattern like that from viscera. This segmental distribution is similar to the pattern of dermatomes except that in the extremities some segments are not represented as far distalward.

Lewis points out that pain is localized well in the skin and closely related mucous membranes, fairly well in deep fasciae, and poorly in viscera. He suggests that pain fibers are not as numerous in the viscera as in superficial structures (witness the apparent insensitivity to cutting and burning) and that the production of pain from a viscus involves spatial summation; this could underlie inability to localize visceral pain and at the same time offer explanation of its diffuse quality.

ASCENDING AND DESCENDING DEGENERATION OF SPINAL CORD

When as a result of an injury a nerve fiber is divided, that part which is severed from its cell of origin degenerates, while the part still connected with that cell usually remains intact. This is known as Wallerian degeneration, and,

Table Showing the Location of the Chief Fiber Tracts of the Spinal Cord and the Direction in which They Degenerate

	ASCENDING DEGENERATION	DESCENDING DEGENERATION
Anterior funiculus	Ventral spinothalamic tract	Ventral corticospinal tract Vestibulospinal tract Tectospinal tract
Lateral funiculus	Dorsal spinocerebellar tract Ventral spinocerebellar tract Lateral spinothalamic tract Spinotectal tract	Lateral corticospinal tract Rubrospinal tract Bulbospinal tract
Posterior funiculus	Ascending branches of the dorsal root fibers	Fasciculus interfascicularis Septomarginal tract

as will be readily understood, gives valuable information concerning the course of the fiber tracts. In case of a complete transection of the spinal cord, all the ascending fibers whose cells are located below the cut will degenerate in the segments above, while those descending fibers whose cells of origin are located above will degenerate below the lesion (Fig. 146). Injury to the dorsal roots

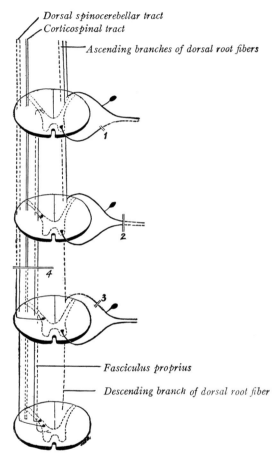

FIGURE 146.   Diagram of the spinal cord to illustrate the principle of Wallerian degeneration. The broken lines represent the degeneration resulting from: 1, Section of the ventral root; 2, section of the spinal nerve distal to the spinal ganglion; 3, section of the dorsal root proximal to the spinal ganglion, and 4, a lesion in the lateral funiculus.

proximal to the spinal ganglia causes a degeneration of the dorsal root fibers throughout their length in the spinal cord. Brain injuries may, according to their location, result in the degeneration of one or more of the tracts which descend into the spinal cord from above.

By the study of a great many cases of injury to the central nervous system in man and of experimentally produced lesions in animals a very considerable amount of information has been obtained concerning the fiber tracts of the spinal cord. This has been supplemented by a study of developmental stages which allows the tracing of tracts since the myelin sheaths of the fibers of separate tracts are acquired at different times. This is summarized in the table (p. 194) and in Fig. 149.

The **fasciculi proprii** or ground bundles are composed of short ascending and descending fibers, which arise and terminate within the gray matter of the spinal cord and link together its various segments. These fascicles, one of which

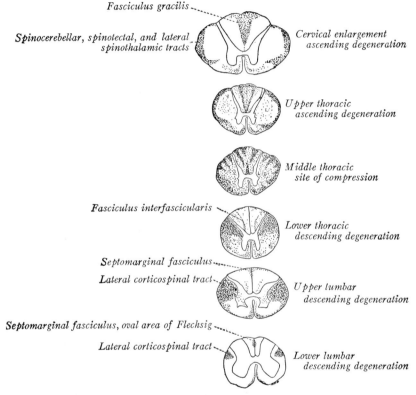

FIGURE 147. Ascending and descending degeneration resulting from a compression of the thoracic spinal cord in man. Marchi method. (Hoche.)

is present in each of the three funiculi, immediately surround the gray columns. After a transection of the spinal cord the fasciculi proprii undergo an incomplete degeneration for some distance both above and below the lesion (Figs. 146, 147). In cross-section the ground bundle of the *posterior funiculus* has the form of a narrow band upon the surface of the posterior column and posterior commissure, and was once called the cornucommissural bundle (Fig. 149). In addition to this fascicle there are in the posterior funiculus two other tracts which in part belong to the same system—the *septomarginal tract* and the *fasciculus interfascicularis,* or comma tract of Schultze. These are both composed of descending fibers, in part of intraspinal origin and in part representing the descending branches of the dorsal root fibers. The septomarginal tract is situated along the dorsal periphery of the posterior funiculus in the thoracic region; it takes up a position along the septum in the lumbar segments (oval area of Flechsig); and in the sacral region it forms a triangular field at the dorsomedial angle of the posterior funiculus (triangle of Gombault and Philippe) (Fig. 147). The fasciculus interfascicularis is best developed in the thoracic segments, where it occupies a position near the center of the posterior funiculus.

In the *anterior funiculus*, in addition to the *fasciculus proprius* which immediately surrounds the gray matter, there is a thin layer of similar fibers spread out along the border of the anterior fissure and known as the *sulcomarginal fasciculus*. This contains also fibers which descend into the cord from the medial longitudinal bundle of the medulla oblongata.

As a general rule, the short fibers of the fasciculus proprius lie nearer the gray substance than the fibers of greater length, and the long tracts, which connect the spinal cord with the brain, occupy the most peripheral position. But the fact must not be overlooked that many fibers of the fasciculus proprius are intermingled with those of the long tracts.

LONG DESCENDING TRACTS OF THE SPINAL CORD

Fibers which arise from cells in various parts of the brain descend into the spinal cord, where they form several well defined tracts. The most important

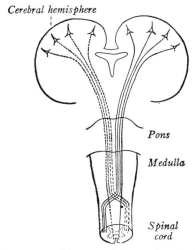

Cerebral hemisphere

Pons

Medulla

Spinal cord

FIGURE 148. Diagram of the corticospinal tracts.

and most conspicuous of these are the cerebrospinal fasciculi, which are more properly called the *corticospinal tracts*. Their constituent fibers take origin from pyramidal cells of the precentral gyrus or motor region of the cerebral cortex (and probably some other regions) and pass through the subjacent levels of the brain to reach the spinal cord (Fig. 148). Just before they enter the spinal cord they undergo an incomplete decussation in the medulla oblongata, giving rise to a ventral and a lateral corticospinal tract in each lateral half of the cord.

The Lateral Corticospinal Tract (Crossed Pyramidal Tract, Fasciculus Cerebrospinalis Lateralis).   The majority of the pyramidal fibers, after crossing the median plane in the decussation of the pyramids, enter the lateral funiculus of the spinal cord as the lateral corticospinal tract, which occupies a position between the dorsal spinocerebellar tract and the lateral fasciculus proprius (Fig. 149). In the lumbar and sacral regions, below the origin of the dorsal spinocerebellar tract, the lateral corticospinal tract is more superficial. It can be traced as a distinct strand as far as the fourth sacral segment, and as it descends in the spinal cord it gradually decreases in size. Throughout its course in the spinal cord it gives off collateral and terminal fibers which end in the gray matter in synapses with the primary motor neurons or with neurons intercalated between

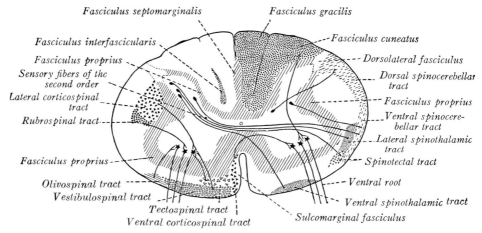

FIGURE 149.   Diagram showing the location of the principal fiber tracts in the spinal cord of man. Ascending tracts on the right side, descending tracts on the left.

the pyramidal endings and the motor neurons. A few fibers from the pyramid run without crossing into the lateral corticospinal tract of the same side (Fulton and Sheehan, 1935).

Approximately half the corticospinal fibers are distributed to cervical segments of the spinal cord, a fifth to the thoracic, and nearly a third to the lumbar and sacral segments. But the cervical segments supply only a third (by weight) of the muscle of the body, and the thoracic segments a tenth while over half of the muscle is supplied by the lumbosacral segments. (Weil and Lassek, 1929.)

The fibers of the corticospinal tract that supply the cervical segments of the cord lie in its medial portion, those supplying lumbar segments lie laterally with fibers to thoracic segments between (Walker, 1940).

The **ventral corticospinal tract** (fasciculus cerebrospinalis anterior or direct pyramidal tract) is formed by those corticospinal fibers, which do not cross in the medulla but pass directly into the ventral funiculus of the same side of the cord. They form a tract of small size, which lies near the anterior median fissure and which can be traced as a distinct strand as far as the middle of the thoracic region of the spinal cord. Just before terminating, these fibers cross in the anterior white commissure. They end like those of the lateral corticospinal tract, either directly or through an intercalated neuron, in relation to the motor cells in the anterior column. Although the crossing of these fibers is delayed, it will be apparent that the fibers of the ventral as well as of the lateral corticospinal tract arising in the right cerebral hemisphere terminate in the anterior column of the left side of the cord, and conversely, those from the left hemisphere end on the right side. It is along these fibers that impulses from the motor portion of the cerebral cortex reach the cord and bring the spinal motor apparatus under voluntary control.

It is not certain that all the fibers of the ventral corticospinal tract cross in the anterior white commissure (Lewandowsky, 1907). Some of them may end in the anterior gray column of the same side. Moreover there are some uncrossed fibers in the lateral corticospinal tract. This may explain the part which the homolateral hemisphere plays in the slight recovery of motor function which occurs in a paralyzed limb long after destruction of the opposite motor area. Hoff (1932) believes that corticospinal fibers terminate in both the anterior and the posterior columns. Evidence that corticospinal tract fibers in the cat end in the dorsal and intermediate gray matter, including the nucleus dorsalis and nuclei of gracilis and cuneatus, has been presented by Chambers and Liu (1957), who furthermore found no signs of such endings in the ventral horn. The corticospinal path is from the standpoint of phylogenesis a relatively new system and varies a great deal in different mammals. It is found in the ventral funiculus in the mole, while in the sheep and rat it occupies the posterior funiculus. In the mole it is almost completely unmyelinated, in the rat largely so. It contains many unmyelinated fibers in the cat, fewer in the monkey. In man it does not become fully myelinated before the second year.

After complete removal of the cortex of one cerebral hemisphere the homolateral pyramid loses practically all its fibers, but in the spinal cord the regions occupied by lateral and ventral corticospinal tracts show many scattered fibers, emphasizing the overlap of tracts in the cord by the entrance of fibers from other sources (Lassek and Evans, 1946).

The **rubrospinal tract** (tract of Monakow) is situated near the center of the lateral funiculus just ventral to the lateral corticospinal tract (Fig. 149). Its fibers come from the red nucleus of the mesencephalon, cross the median plane, and descend into the spinal cord. While in most mammals it is one of the most conspicuous tracts in the cord, it is small in man, and its course in the human spinal cord has never been accurately traced (André-Thomas, 1936). Probably it ends, either directly or through an intercalated neuron, in relation to the primary motor cells of the anterior gray column. In the cat it has been shown to extend as a completely crossed path all the way to the lumbosacral cord (Pompeiano and Brodal, 1957).

Other Descending Tracts. The *olivospinal tract* is a small bundle of fibers found in the cervical region near the surface of the lateral funiculus opposite the anterior column. The fibers arise from cells in the medulla oblongata, possibly in the inferior olivary nucleus, and end somewhere in the gray matter of the spinal cord. The exact origin and termination of the tract is unknown. The *tectospinal tract* is composed of fibers which take origin in the roof (tectum) of the mesencephalon, cross the median plane and descend into the anterior funiculus of the spinal cord, and end in the gray matter of the anterior column. The tract is concerned with optic and auditory reflexes. The *vestibulospinal tract*, also located in the anterior funiculus, arises from the lateral nucleus of the vestibular nerve in the medulla oblongata and conveys impulses concerned in the maintenance of tonus and equilibrium. Some of its fibers can be traced as far as the lower lumbar segments. They end in the gray matter of the anterior column. Fibers have been traced into the spinal cord from large cells of the reticular formation of the pons and medulla oblongata constituting the *reticulospinal tracts* (Papez, 1926). The work of Magoun has emphasized the importance of the facilitating and inhibitory mechanisms found in the reticular formation which are related to the control of activity of skeletal muscle. Reticulospinal fibers must be involved here.

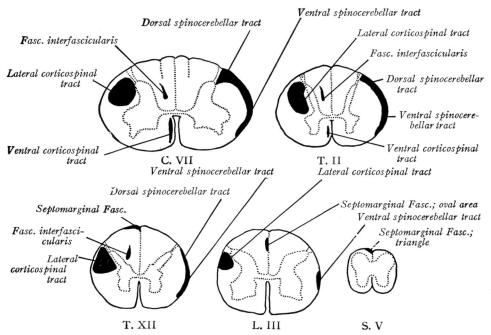

FIGURE 150.   Diagrams showing the shape and location of certain fiber tracts at several levels of the human spinal cord. Ascending tracts on the right side, descending tracts on the left.

Descending fibers carrying facilitating influences to spinal motor mechanisms arise throughout the brain stem while those carrying inhibitory influences to the cord arise in the medulla oblongata. The influence of the centers giving rise to these fibers is exerted bilaterally, the facilitatory fibers crossing in brain stem and cord, the inhibitory fibers crossing only in the cord. The reticulospinal fibers run in the lateral and ventral funiculi widely scattered and overlapping, although there is some concentration of facilitatory fibers dorsally and inhibitory fibers ventrally in this region (Niemer and Magoun, 1947).

Since the medulla has within it reflex centers concerned with respiration, heart rate, and other visceral mechanisms, the pathways carrying such influences must in part take origin there.

Descending paths concerned with visceral control have been obscure. In the monkey, Beaton and Leininger (1943) found paths concerned with sweating in the lateral and anterolateral region of the spinal cord which crossed, probably completely, just before reaching the level of their appropriate preganglionic outflow.

The **outlines of the various tracts** given in Fig. 149 should not be taken too seriously. The spinotectal and the ventral and lateral spinothalamic tracts do not form well defined bundles. On the contrary, their fibers are widely scattered and intermingled with those of the fasciculus proprius. Exact information is not available about the rubrospinal, vestibulospinal, and tectospinal tracts in man. Information obtained from experiments on animals cannot always be safely applied. A large and compact rubrospinal tract has been traced through the spinal cord in cats and other mammals; there is good reason to believe that rubrospinal fibers are present in man (Stern, 1938). It is known that some of the fascicles and tracts undergo changes in size, shape, and location at various levels of the human spinal cord as indicated in Fig. 150. The ventral corticospinal tract diminishes rapidly in size and usually ends in the midthoracic region. Since the dorsal spinocerebellar tract arises chiefly in the thoracic region, it is not present in the lumbar or sacral cord and here the lateral corticospinal tract occupies a superficial position.

Hemisection of the spinal cord in man produces a characteristic symptom complex known as Brown-Séquard's syndrome, which can be studied to advantage at this time since analysis of the symptoms requires consideration of details of the connections and functions of the tracts of the spinal cord. Below the level of the lesion and on the same side, there is found a paralysis of the muscles with a loss of sensation from the muscles, joints, and tendons; while on the opposite side of the body, beginning as a rule about one segment below the level of the lesion, there is loss of sensations of pain and temperature. Tactile sensibility is normal or only slightly impaired.

CHAPTER X

The Structure of
the Medulla Oblongata

The primitive animal meets the environment head on, so to speak, and its developed special sense organs, the nose, eyes, ears and tongue, accumulate information about objects more or less distant from it, and record alterations of equilibrium. Furthermore, the feeding and respiratory mechanisms develop at the head end, and in air breathing forms there commonly develops a mechanism for vocalization. The innervation required for these various features is supplied through cranial nerves that attach to the brain and pass through foramina of the skull. These specializations are related to appropriate changes in form of the brain stem, as compared with the spinal cord with its simpler segmental pattern.

In addition to the connections of rather specialized cranial nerves, the form of the brain stem is modified by the presence of suprasegmental structures, such as the cerebellum, tectum and cerebral hemispheres with their heavy bundles of connections. Among these various new masses of nerve cells and fibers, the long tracts from and to the spinal cord pass, with some modification of their positions and relations.

The **central connections of the cranial nerves,** except those of the first two pairs, are located in the medulla oblongata and in the tegmental portions of the pons and mesencephalon. In many respects they resemble the connections of the spinal nerves within the spinal cord. The following general statements on this topic, most of which are illustrated in Fig. 151, will help to elucidate the structure of the brain stem.

1. The *cells of origin of the sensory fibers* of the cranial nerves (Fig. 151, 1) are found in ganglia which lie outside the cerebrospinal axis and are homologous with the spinal ganglia. These are the semilunar ganglion of the trigeminal, the geniculate ganglion of the facial, the superior and petrous ganglia of the glossopharyngeal, the jugular and nodose ganglia of the vagus, the spiral ganglion of the cochlear, and the vestibular ganglion of the vestibular nerve.

2. All of these sensory ganglia except the last two, the cells of which are

bipolar, are formed by unipolar cells, the axons of which divide dichotomously into peripheral and central branches. The latter (or in the case of the acoustic nerve the central processes of the bipolar cells) form the sensory nerve roots and enter the brain stem, within which they form longitudinal fiber tracts. The fibers from the trigeminal and vestibular nerves divide into short ascending and long descending branches. It is the *descending branches* of the sensory fibers of the *trigeminal nerve* which form the *spinal tract* of that nerve illustrated in Figs. 151, 154, 155, 157. But the ascending branches may be entirely wanting, as in the case of the *sensory fibers of the seventh, ninth, and tenth nerves,* all of which bend caudally and form a descending tract in the medulla oblongata, known as the *tractus solitarius* (Figs. 151, 157, 160).

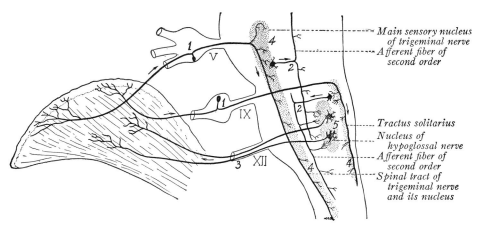

FIGURE 151. Diagram of the tongue and rhombencephalon to illustrate the central connections and functional relationships of certain of the cranial nerves: 1, Sensory neurons of the first order of the trigeminal and glossopharyngeal nerves; 2, sensory neurons of the second order; 3, motor fibers of the hypoglossal nerve; 4, sensory nuclei; 5, motor nucleus of hypoglossal nerve. (Cajal.)

3. These ascending and descending sensory fibers and the collaterals derived from them end in gray masses known as *sensory nuclei* or *nuclei of termination.*

4. The *sensory nuclei* (Fig. 151, 4) within which the afferent fibers terminate contain the cells of origin of the *sensory fibers of the second order* (Fig. 151, 2). Some of these are short; others are long, and these may be either direct or crossed. Many of them divide into ascending and descending branches. They run in the reticular formation and some of the ascending fibers reach the thalamus.

5. These sensory fibers of the second order give off *collaterals to the motor nuclei.* Direct collaterals from the sensory fibers of the cranial nerves to the motor nuclei are few in number or entirely wanting.

6. The motor nuclei (Fig. 151, 5) are aggregations of multipolar cells which give origin to the motor fibers of the cranial nerves (Fig. 151, 3). These are of two types which are segregated in different nuclei. One type is comparable to the anterior horn cells of the spinal cord and includes the neurons innervating skeletal muscle of the head region. The second type is comparable to the cells

of the intermediolateral cell column of the spinal cord and includes only the preganglionic neurons to the ganglia of the cranial division of the autonomic nervous system. To the cranial nerve nuclei supplying skeletal muscle run descending fibers of the corticobulbar path, which cross the midline just before terminating in the nuclei in somewhat the same manner as fibers of the ventral corticospinal tract reach anterior horn cells in the spinal cord. It has also been shown that descending fibers from the cortex reach sensory nuclei, for example, the trigeminal sensory nuclei and the nucleus solitarius (Brodal, Szabo, and

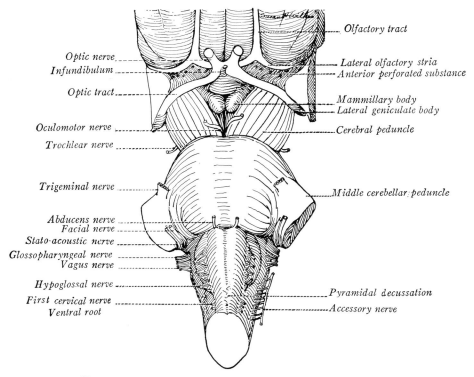

FIGURE 152. Ventral view of brain stem showing cranial nerves.

Torvik, 1956). The function of these is not clear, but it has been suggested they relate to inhibition of afferent messages.

The Rearrangement Within the Medulla Oblongata of the Structures Continued Upward from the Spinal Cord.   At the level of the rostral border of the first cervical nerve the spinal cord goes over without a sharp line of demarcation into the medulla oblongata. The transition is gradual both as to external form and internal structure, but in the caudal part of the medulla there occurs a gradual rearrangement of the fiber tracts and alterations in the shape of the gray matter, until at the level of the olive, a section of the medulla bears no resemblance to one through the spinal cord.

The realignment of the corticospinal tracts and the termination of the fibers of the posterior funiculi of the spinal cord are two of the most important factors responsible for this gradual transformation. Traced rostrally from the spinal cord, the *ventral corticospinal tracts* are seen to enter the pyramids within the ventral area of the medulla oblongata, that is to say, they enter the medulla without realignment. The fibers of the *lateral corticospinal tracts* traced rostrally into the medulla swing ventromedially in coarse bundles, which run through the anterior gray columns and cut them off from the gray matter surrounding

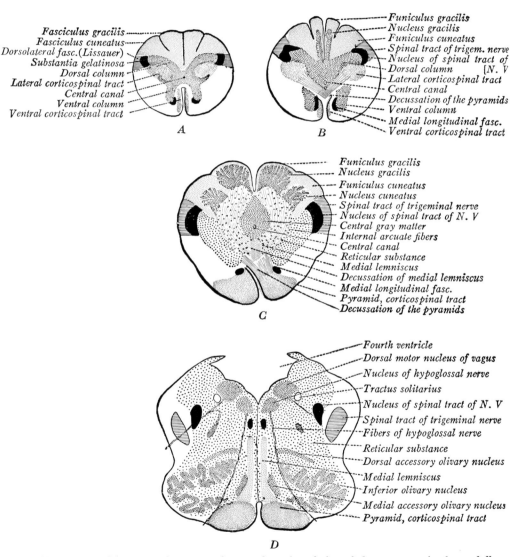

FIGURE 153. Diagrammatic cross-sections to show the relation of the structures in the medulla oblongata to those in the spinal cord: *A*, First cervical segment of spinal cord; *B*, medulla oblongata, level of decussation of pyramids; *C*, medulla oblongata, level of decussation of medial lemniscus; *D*, medulla oblongata, level of olive.

the central canal (Figs. 152, 153). After crossing the median plane in the decussation of the pyramids these fibers join those of the opposite ventral corticospinal tracts and form the pyramids (Fig. 153). Thus fibers from the lateral funiculus come to lie ventral to the central canal and displace this dorsally, and at the same time a start is made toward breaking up the **H**-shaped gray figure characteristic of the spinal cord.

Shortly after entering the medulla oblongata, the *fibers of the posterior funiculi* end in nuclear masses which invade the funiculus gracilis and funiculus cuneatus as expansions from the posterior gray columns and central mass of gray substance (Fig. 153). These are known as the *nucleus gracilis* and *nucleus cuneatus*. They cause a considerable increase in the size of the posterior funiculi and a corresponding ventrolateral displacement of the posterior columns of gray matter. The fibers of the posterior funiculi end in these nuclei about cells, the axons of which run ventromedially as the *internal arcuate fibers*. These sweep in broad curves through the gray substance, and decussate ventral to the central canal in what is known as the *decussation of the medial lemniscus*. After crossing the median plane, they turn rostrally between the pyramids and the central gray matter to form on either side of the median plane a broad band of fibers known as the *medial lemniscus* (Fig. 153). At the level of the middle of the olive most of the fibers of the funiculus cuneatus and funiculus gracilis have terminated in their respective nuclei, and the nuclei also disappear a short distance farther rostrally (Fig. 153). With the disappearance of these fibers and nuclei there ceases to be any nervous substance dorsal to the *central canal*, and this, which has been displaced dorsally by the pyramid and medial lemniscus, opens out as *the fourth ventricle*. The floor of the ventricle is the whole dorsal surface of the medulla while the roof is thinned to an ependymal layer into which a plexus of vessels is invaginated to form the chorioid plexus.

The *outline of the gray matter* in the most caudal portions of the medulla oblongata closely resembles that of the spinal cord. The anterior columns are first cut off by the decussation of the pyramids. Then the posterior columns are displaced ventrolaterally because of the increased size of the posterior funiculi and the disappearance of the lateral corticospinal tracts from their ventral aspects. This rotation of the posterior column causes the apex of that column with its *spinal tract* and *nucleus of the trigeminal nerve*, which are continuous with the fasciculus dorsolateralis and substantia gelatinosa of the spinal cord (Fig. 153), to lie almost directly lateralward from the central canal. The shape of the gray figure is still further altered by the development of special nuclear masses, many of which are very conspicuous. These include the *nucleus gracilis, nucleus cuneatus, inferior olivary nucleus,* and the *nuclei of the cranial nerves*. The greater part of the gray substance now becomes broken up by nerve fibers crossing in every direction, but especially by the internal arcuate fibers. This mixture of gray and white matter is known as the *reticular substance*. The *central gray matter* is pushed dorsad first by the pyramids and later by the medial lemniscus until it finally spreads out to form a thin gray covering for the floor of the fourth ventricle.

The Pyramids and Their Decussation. The pyramids are large, somewhat rounded fascicles of longitudinal fibers, which lie on either side of the anterior median fissure of the medulla oblongata (Fig. 29). The constituent fibers take origin from the pyramidal cells of the anterior central gyrus or motor cerebral cortex and certain other portions of the cortex (see p. 363). The *decussation of the pyramids* or motor decussation occurs near the caudal extremity of the medulla oblongata (Fig. 152). Something more than three fourths of the cortico-spinal tract passes through the decussation into the lateral funiculus of the opposite side of the spinal cord, as the *lateral corticospinal tract* (fasciculus cerebrospinalis lateralis or lateral pyramidal tract); while the remainder is continued without crossing into the ventral funiculus of the same side as the *ventral corticospinal tract* (fasciculus cerebrospinalis anterior or anterior pyramidal tract—Figs. 153, 154). The decussating fibers are grouped into relatively

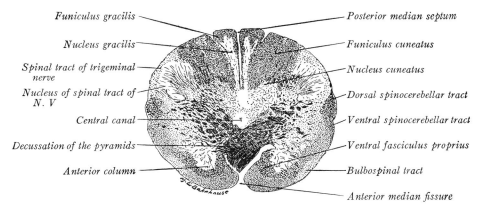

Funiculus gracilis — Posterior median septum

Nucleus gracilis — Funiculus cuneatus

Spinal tract of trigeminal nerve — Nucleus cuneatus

Nucleus of spinal tract of N. V — Dorsal spinocerebellar tract

Central canal — Ventral spinocerebellar tract

Decussation of the pyramids — Ventral fasciculus proprius

Anterior column — Bulbospinal tract

Anterior median fissure

FIGURE 154. Section through the medulla oblongata of a child at the level of the decussation of the pyramids. Pal-Weigert method. (×6.)

large bundles as they cross the median plane, the bundles from one side alternating with similar bundles from the other, and largely obliterating the anterior median fissure at this level (Figs. 272, 307). There is great individual variation as to the relative size of the ventral and lateral corticospinal tracts, and there may even be marked asymmetry due to a difference in the proportion of the decussating fibers on the two sides.

The fibers of the pyramidal tracts supplying the region of the cervical enlargement, and so the arm musculature, cross in the cranial portion of the decussation, those to the lumbar enlargement cross in the caudal portion. A lesion on one side in this region may therefore result in paralysis of an arm and a leg on opposite sides of the body if the lesion damages fibers which supply the arm after they have crossed, and fibers supplying the leg before crossing.

There is evidence that some corticospinal fibers are uncrossed, and so influence movement homolaterally.

The **nucleus gracilis** and **nucleus cuneatus** (nucleus funiculi gracilis and nucleus funiculi cuneati) are large masses of gray matter located in the posterior funiculi of the caudal portion of the medulla oblongata (Figs. 308–320, grac and cun). They are surrounded by the fibers of these funiculi except on their ventral aspects, where they are continuous with the remainder of the gray substance (Fig. 155). The fibers of the gracile and cuneate fasciculi terminate in the corresponding nuclei, and their terminal arborizations are synaptically related to the neurons, whose cell bodies and dendrites are located there. Accordingly, in sections through successive levels we see the fibers decreasing in number as the nuclei grow larger (Figs. 154, 155). It is because of the presence of these nuclei that the funiculi become swollen to form the club-shaped prominences with which we are already familiar under the names *clava* and *cuneate tubercle.* At the level of the pyramidal decussation, the gracile nucleus has the form of a rather thin and ill defined plate, while the cuneate nucleus is represented by a

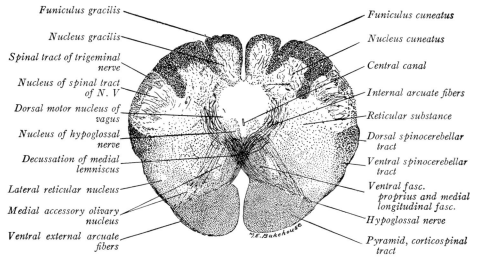

FIGURE 155. Section through the medulla oblongata of a child at the level of the decussation of the medial lemniscus. Pal-Weigert method. (×6.)

slight projection from the dorsal surface of the posterior gray column (Fig. 154). At the level of the decussation of the lemniscus, both have enlarged and the gracile nucleus has become sharply outlined (Fig. 155). As the central canal opens out into the fourth ventricle, the nuclei are displaced laterally and gradually come to an end as the restiform body becomes clearly defined (Fig. 157).

The lateral or accessory cuneate nucleus lies lateral to the rostral part of the main cuneate nucleus between this and the restiform body (Figs. 319–322). It is composed of large cells similar to those in the nucleus dorsalis of the spinal cord. This serves to differentiate it from the other nuclei of the posterior funiculi which contain much smaller cells. The fibers, which arise in the lateral cuneate nucleus, run by way of the dorsal external arcuate fibers and the restiform body of the same side to the cerebellum (Brun, 1925; Ferraro and Barrera, 1935).

The Medial Lemniscus and Its Decussation. The great majority of fibers which arise from the cells in the nucleus gracilis and nucleus cuneatus sweep ventromedially in broad concentric curves around the central gray substance toward the median raphe (Fig. 155). As has been stated on a preceding page, these are known as *internal arcuate fibers*, and as they cross those from the opposite side in the raphe they form the *decussation of the lemniscus* (decussatio lemniscorum, sensory decussation). After crossing the median plane they turn rostrally in the medial lemniscus (fillet), and end in the thalamus (Fig. 269). These longitudinal fibers constitute a broad band which lies close to the median raphe, medial to the inferior olivary nucleus, and dorsal to the pyramids (Fig. 153). By the accession of additional internal arcuate fibers this band increases in size and spreads out dorsally until, at the level of the middle of the olive, it

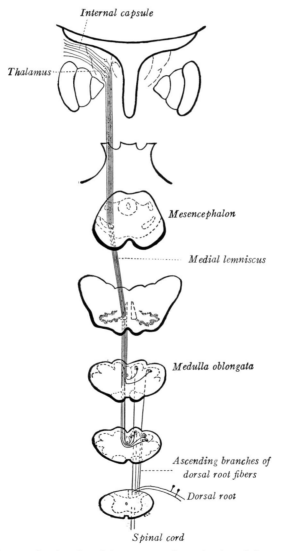

FIGURE 156.   Diagram showing the origin, course, and termination of the medial lemniscus.

is separated from the gray matter of the ventricular floor only by the fibers of the fasciculus longitudinalis medialis and the tectospinal tract (Fig. 157). The decussation of the lemniscus begins at the upper border of the decussation of the pyramids, where the sensory fibers are grouped into course bundles arching around the central gray matter (Fig. 155), and extends as far rostrally as do the gracile and cuneate nuclei, that is, to about the middle of the olive. In sections through the lower half of the olive the internal arcuate fibers describe broad curves through the reticular formation and their decussation occupies a considerable ventrodorsal extent of the raphe (Fig. 319).

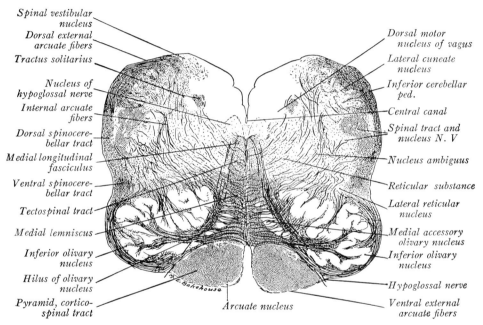

Spinal vestibular nucleus
Dorsal external arcuate fibers
Tractus solitarius
Nucleus of hypoglossal nerve
Internal arcuate fibers
Dorsal spinocerebellar tract
Medial longitudinal fasciculus
Ventral spinocerebellar tract
Tectospinal tract
Medial lemniscus
Inferior olivary nucleus
Hilus of olivary nucleus
Pyramid, corticospinal tract

Dorsal motor nucleus of vagus
Lateral cuneate nucleus
Inferior cerebellar ped.
Central canal
Spinal tract and nucleus N. V
Nucleus ambiguus
Reticular substance
Lateral reticular nucleus
Medial accessory olivary nucleus
Inferior olivary nucleus
Hypoglossal nerve
Ventral external arcuate fibers

Arcuate nucleus

FIGURE 157. Section through the medulla oblongata of a child at the level of the olive. Pal-Weigert method. (×6.)

The **arcuate fibers** of the medulla oblongata may be separated into two groups: those which run through the reticular formation constitute the internal arcuate fibers, and those which run over the surface of the medulla, the external arcuate fibers. The *internal arcuate fibers* are of at least three kinds: (1) those described in the preceding paragraph, which arise in the gracile and cuneate nuclei and form the medial lemniscus; (2) sensory fibers of the second order, arising in the sensory nuclei of the cranial nerves, and (3) olivocerebellar fibers, which will be considered in another paragraph. *Dorsal external arcuate fibers* arise from the large cells of the lateral cuneate nucleus and run laterally to the inferior cerebellar peduncle and through it to the cerebellum. Some of the *ventral external arcuate fibers* take origin from cells in the reticular formation, cross the raphe, emerge from the anterior median fissure, traverse the arcuate nuclei (Figs. 157, 159), and circumvent the pyramid and inferior olivary nucleus to reach the inferior cerebellar peduncle. These are joined by a considerable number from the lateral reticular and arcuate nuclei. Some fibers from the striae medullares which have passed ventrad in the raphe and decussated mingle with the ventral external arcuate fibers. The arcuate nuclei are small irregular patches of gray matter situated on the ventromedial aspect of the pyramids.

It was formerly supposed that some of the internal arcuate fibers from the nuclei gracilis and cuneatus emerged from the anterior median fissure and became ventral external arcuate fibers of the opposite side but no such fibers are mentioned by Brun (1925) or by Ferraro and Barrera (1935, 1936). The latter authors state that, "The axons of the cells of the nucleus gracilis and nucleus cuneatus are sent into the medial lemniscus; whereas the axons of the cells of the external cuneate nucleus are sent to the cerebellum via the inferior cerebellar peduncle of the same side."

Olivary Nuclei. The oval prominence in the lateral area of the medulla, known as the olive, is produced by the presence just beneath the surface of a

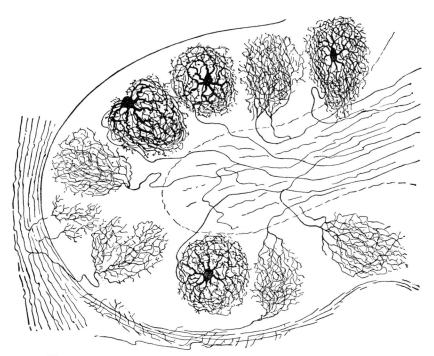

FIGURE 158. Diagram to illustrate the structure of the inferior olivary nucleus. (Cajal, Edinger.)

large gray mass, the inferior olivary nucleus, with which there are associated two accessory olivary nuclei. The *inferior olivary nucleus* is very conspicuous in the sections of this part of the medulla (Fig. 157). It appears as a broad, irregularly folded band of gray matter, curved in such a way as to enclose a white core, which extends into the nucleus from the medial side through an opening, known as the hilus. Considered as a whole this nucleus resembles a crumpled leather purse, with an opening, the hilus, directed medially. Sections at either end of the nucleus do not include this opening, and at these points the central core of white matter is completely surrounded by the gray lamina. The fibers which stream in and out of the hilus constitute the olivary peduncle. The two accessory olives are plates of gray substance, which in transverse section appear as rods. The *medial accessory olivary nucleus* is placed between the hilus of the inferior olive and the medial lemniscus, while the *dorsal accessory olivary nucleus* is located close to the dorsal aspect of the chief nuclear mass (Figs. 317–328).

STRUCTURE AND CONNECTIONS. The gray lamina of the inferior olivary nucleus consists of neuroglia and many rounded nerve cells beset with numerous short frequently branching dendrites, the axons of which run through the white core of the nucleus and out at the hilus as *olivocerebellar fibers*. About these cells there ramify the end branches of several varieties of afferent fibers. Though a thalamo-olivary tract is often labelled, Walberg (1956) found no evidence in the cat of fibers to the olivary nucleus from the thalamus; but he did observe them descending to it from the sensorimotor cerebral cortex, caudate nucleus, globus pallidus and especially from the red nucleus and periaqueductal gray matter. According to Bebin (1956), the most rostral component of these descending fibers which are included in the term, *central tegmental bundle*, came from the pallidum and zona incerta. On the way to the olive additional fibers from the red nucleus and descending branches of the brachium conjunctivum are added. The bundle terminates also in the region adjacent to the olive in the central reticular substance. Another group of fibers, consisting chiefly of collaterals, comes from the ventral funiculus of the spinal cord and may be regarded as ascending sensory fibers (Cajal, 1909). These belong to the so-called spino-olivary fasciculus. Connections have been demonstrated with the zona incerta and associated structures, the gray matter about the cerebral aqueduct, and some other nearby areas (Snider and Barnard, 1949).

Olivocerebellar Fibers. The axons from the cells of the inferior olivary nucleus stream out of the hilus, cross the median plane, and either pass through or around the opposite nucleus. Here they are joined by some uncrossed fibers from the olivary nucleus of the same side (Brun, 1925). Thence they curve dorsally toward the inferior cerebellar peduncle, passing through the spinal tract of the trigeminal nerve which becomes split up into several bundles (Fig. 159). They form an important group of internal arcuate fibers, which run through the inferior peduncle to the cerebellum and constitute the olivocerebellar tract.

Cells of the inferior olivary nuclei are connected to the cerebellar cortex in orderly topographic sequence, and functionally the olive and cerebellum are closely related. Destruction of an olivary nucleus produces signs of cerebellar deficit in the limbs, largely contralaterally, but sectioning the olivary decussation in the monkey did not produce cerebellar signs (Orioli and Mettler, 1956). It has been suggested that the inferior olivary nucleus stands in the same relation to a subcortical motor controlling system as the pontine nuclei do to the corticopontocerebellar connections (Wilson and Magoun, 1945; King, 1948).

The **inferior cerebellar peduncle** is a large and prominent strand of fibers which gradually accumulate along the lateral border of the caudal part of the fourth ventricle. It forms the floor of the lateral recess of that cavity and then turns dorsally into the cerebellum (Figs. 32, 33, 159, 326). It is composed for the most part of two large and important fascicles: (1) the *olivocerebellar fibers*, both direct and crossed, but chiefly from the inferior olivary nucleus of the opposite side; and (2) the *dorsal spinocerebellar tract*, from the nucleus dorsalis of the spinal cord. In addition, there are fibers in smaller number from other sources: (3) the *dorsal external arcuate fibers* from the lateral cuneate nuclei of the same side; and *fibers* (4) *from the arcuate nucleus*, (5) *from the lateral reticular nucleus*, and possibly also from other cells scattered through the reticular formation (Van Gehuchten, 1904).

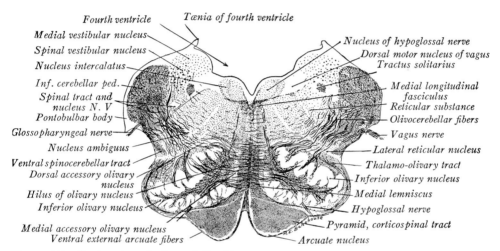

FIGURE 159. Section through the medulla oblongata of a child at the level of the restiform body. Pal-Weigert method. (×4.)

The **dorsal spinocerebellar tract** can readily be traced in serial sections of the medulla because the large, heavily myelinated fibers of which it is composed cause it to be deeply stained by the Weigert technique. It can be followed from the spinal cord along the periphery of the medulla oblongata near the posterior lateral sulcus. At first it lies ventral to the spinal tract of the trigeminal nerve (Figs. 154, 155). But at the level of the lower part of the olive it inclines dorsally, passing over the surface of the spinal tract of this nerve to reach the inferior cerebellar peduncle (Fig. 157). Between this tract and the olive we find the *ventral spinocerebellar tract* also in a superficial position.

The **spinal tract of the trigeminal nerve** is formed by the descending branches of the sensory fibers of that nerve. They give off collateral and terminal branches to a column of gray matter, resembling the substantia gelatinosa Rolandi, with which it is directly continuous, and designated as the *nucleus of the spinal tract of the trigeminal nerve* (Figs. 151, 154, 155, 157, 159, 308–328, sp. V). The tract lies along the lateral side of the nucleus and is superficial except in so far as it is covered by the external arcuate fibers, the dorsal spinocerebellar tract, and the restiform body. It forms an elongated elevation, the tuberculum cinereum, on the surface of the medulla oblongata (Fig. 32).

The **formatio reticularis** fills the interspaces among the larger fiber tracts and nuclei. It is composed of small islands of gray matter, separated by fine bundles of nerve fibers which run in every direction, but which are for the most part either longitudinal or transverse. It is subdivided into two parts. The *formatio reticularis alba* is located dorsal to the pyramid and medial to the root filaments of the hypoglossal nerve and is composed in large part of longitudinal nerve fibers belonging to the *medial lemniscus, tectospinal tract,* and the *medial longitudinal fasciculus* (Fig. 160). The latter is closely associated with the vestibular nerve and can best be described with the central connections of that nerve. The *formatio reticularis grisea* is found dorsal to the olive and lateral to the hypoglossal nerve. In it the nerve cells predominate and the horizontally coursing internal arcuate fibers form a conspicuous feature. Its longitudinal fibers, though less prominent, are of great importance. The

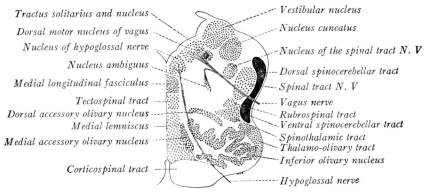

Figure 160.   Diagram showing the location of the nuclei and fiber tracts of the medulla oblongata at the level of the olive.

descending fibers include those of the *rubrospinal tract*, which can be followed into the lateral funiculus of the spinal cord, and the *thalamo-olivary fasciculus,* or tegmento-olivary tract, the fibers of which can be seen surrounding the lateral aspect of the inferior olivary nucleus in which it ends. Among the *ascending fibers* are those of the *ventral* and *dorsal spinocerebellar,* the *spino-thalamic,* and *spinotectal tracts.*

The term **reticular formation,** formerly applied to the mingled gray and white matter adjacent to the gray matter of the spinal cord and filling in areas between the larger named paths and nuclei of the medulla and pons, has acquired a somewhat more specific meaning as the understanding of its connections and functions has increased. Brodal (1956), who has contributed to knowledge of the anatomy of the system, has summarized much of what is known of it and his work should be consulted for further details.

The reticular formation consists of paths and nuclei. The cell groups described are similar in man and lower mammals, though certain giant cells in the nuclei that are common in the cat and rabbit are less conspicuous in man. The lateral reticular nucleus is large in the bat and relatively small in the porpoise (Walberg, 1952).

The more conspicuous nuclei are as follows: (1) the *lateral reticular nucleus* lying dorsolateral to the olive; (2) the reticular nucleus of the pontine tegmentum lying dorsal to the pontine nuclei; (3) the paramedian reticular nucleus, which lies near the midline dorsal to the olive; (4) the large-celled reticular nucleus (gigantocellularis), extending from the middle of the olive to the level of the facial nucleus occupying the medial two thirds of the reticular formation; (5) the caudal reticular nucleus of the pons extending cranialward from the large-celled nucleus, and (6) the oral reticular nucleus of the pons extending up to the mesencephalon.

Other less conspicuous nuclei include the small-celled reticular nucleus medial to the spinal nucleus of the 5th nerve; the ventral reticular nucleus extending caudalward from the large-celled nucleus; and some other small groups.

Connections of the reticular formation include intrinsic interconnecting systems of fibers, and long efferent connections to the spinal cord, the cerebellum and to higher centers, as well as cortico-reticular connections. Reticulospinal fibers extend from both pontine and medullary reticular nuclei and are widely scattered in the ventrolateral part of the white matter, ending, presumably, in the anterior horns of gray matter. Some such fibers extend from the mesencephalon and mingle in their passage with rubrospinal and vestibulospinal paths. Torvik and Brodal (1957) found that the reticulospinal fibers from the pontine region are entirely homolateral and those from the medulla are mainly homolateral in distribution, and that neither type extended so far as lumbosacral segments. There is no evidence of somatotropic localization in the cord.

Reticulocerebellar fibers extend from the lateral reticular nuclei, the paramedian and the reticular nuclei of the pontine tegmentum. Fibers from the lateral reticular nucleus reach the paramedian lobule of the cerebellum in the area of somatotropic representation of afferent spinal paths, and Brodal believes this nucleus to be in the route taken by tactile impulses from the spinal sources. The vermis of the cerebellum receives fibers from the small-celled reticular nucleus and adjacent portions of the large-celled nucleus; the hemispheres and paraflocculus from the remaining portion of the large-celled nucleus; the flocculonodular lobe from the small subtrigeminal portion.

Both facilitatory and inhibitory effects have been produced on stimulation of the reticular formation (Suda et al., 1958), and in some areas at least there is good evidence that the responsible neurons are intermingled, e.g., areas affecting respiratory movements (Fig. 282). Much has been made of the ascending reticular activating system in the brain stem which on stimulation results in activation of cerebral mechanisms affecting the electroencephalogram. There is yet no adequate explanation for the phenomenon, but it is noteworthy that afferent impulses from many sources act similarly. The reticular formation supplies basic patterns available in lower forms and in higher forms, but made less conspicuous by the appearance of the newer more elaborate pathways accompanying the development of higher brain mechanisms.

The **nuclei of the cranial nerves** can best be considered in a separate chapter. At this point it will only be necessary to enumerate and locate the nuclei of those nerves which take origin from the medulla oblongata.

The **nucleus of the hypoglossal nerve** contains the cells of origin of the motor fibers which compose that nerve. It forms a long column of nerve cells on either side of the median plane in the ventral part of the gray matter surrounding the central canal and in the floor of the fourth ventricle (Figs. 155, 157, 160, 180, 317, 328). In the latter region it lies immediately beneath that part of the floor which was described in the preceding chapter under the name of the trigonum hypoglossi (Fig. 33). In reality, it corresponds only to the medial part of this eminence, for on its lateral side there is found another group of cells known as the nucleus intercalatus, the connections and functions of which have not been satisfactorily determined (Fig. 159). From their cells of origin the fibers of the hypoglossal nerve stream forward through the reticular formation to emerge at the lateral border of the pyramid.

The **nucleus ambiguus** is a long column of nerve cells which give origin to the motor fibers that run through the *glossopharyngeal, vagus,* and *accessory nerves* to supply the striated musculature of the pharynx and larynx. It is located in the reticular formation of both the open and the closed portions of the medulla, ventromedial to the nucleus of the spinal tract of the trigeminal nerve (Figs. 157, 160, 308–332).

The **dorsal motor nucleus of the vagus** lies along the lateral side of the nucleus of the hypoglossal. It occupies the ala cinerea of the rhomboid fossa and extends into the closed part of the medulla oblongata along the lateral side of the central canal (Figs. 33, 155, 157, 159, 180, 311–332). From the cells of this nucleus arise the efferent fibers of the vagus nerve which innervate smooth muscle and glandular tissue.

The *afferent fibers of the vagus and glossopharyngeal nerves* bend caudally and run within the tractus solitarius. This tract can be traced throughout almost the entire length of the medulla. It decreases in size as the descending fibers terminate in the gray matter which surrounds it (Figs. 151, 157, 160, 180, 319, 326).

The **nucleus of the tractus solitarius** is the nucleus of reception of the afferent fibers of the facial, glossopharyngeal, and vagus nerves, i. e., it contains the cells about which these afferent fibers terminate. It surrounds the tractus solitarius, and that part of it which lies dorsal to this tract is sometimes called the dorsal sensory nucleus of the glossopharyngeal and vagus nerves. The caudal end of the nucleus joins that of the opposite side, forming the commissural nucleus (Fig. 317), which is associated with the most caudal fibers of the tractus solitarius that cross the midline at this level.

CHAPTER XI

Internal Structure of the Pons

The pons consists of two portions which differ greatly in structure and significance. The *dorsal* or *tegmental part* resembles the medulla oblongata, of which it is the direct continuation. The *ventral* or *basilar portion* contains the longitudinal fibers which go to form the pyramids, but except for these it is composed of structures which are peculiar to this level. It forms a prominent feature of the brain only in those mammals which have relatively large cerebral and cerebellar hemispheres, as might be expected from the fact that it forms part of a conduction path uniting these structures. There is however a pontine homologue in birds (Brodal, Kristiansen and Jansen, 1950).

THE BASILAR PART OF THE PONS

The basilar portion of the pons is the larger of the two divisions. It is made up of fascicles of longitudinal and transverse fibers and of irregular masses of gray substance, which occupy the spaces left among the bundles of nerve fibers and which are known as the nuclei pontis.

The **longitudinal fasciculi** of the pons consists of two kinds of fibers: (1) those of the *corticospinal tract,* which are continued through the pons into the pyramids of the medulla oblongata; and (2) those which end in the nuclei of the pons and are known as *corticopontile or corticopontine fibers* (Fig. 161). As they pass through the pons the corticospinal fibers give off collaterals which also end in these nuclei. The longitudinal fibers enter the pons at its rostral border from the basis pedunculi. At first they form on either side a single compact bundle, but this soon becomes broken up into many smaller fascicles, which are separated from each other by the transverse fibers and nuclei of the pons (Fig. 163). At the caudal border these bundles again become assembled into a compact strand which is continued as the pyramid of the medulla oblongata (Fig. 162). It is evident, however, that the volume of the bundles is much greater at the rostral than at the caudal border. This is to be explained by the fact that the corticopontile fibers have left these bundles during their passage through the pons and have come to an end by arborization within the nuclei pontis.

The **transverse fibers** are designated as *fibrae pontis* and are divisible into

217

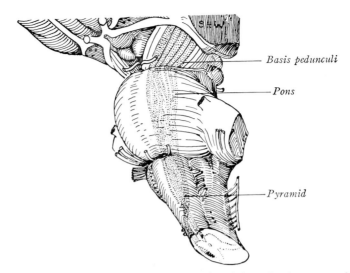

Basis pedunculi

Pons

Pyramid

FIGURE 161. Corticospinal pathway shown in dotted path in peduncle, pons, and pyramid. The decussation at the lower end of the pyramid is shown with separate courses for ventral and lateral tracts in the cord.

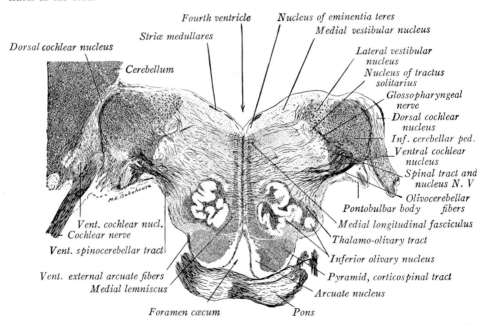

Fourth ventricle

Nucleus of eminentia teres
Medial vestibular nucleus

Striæ medullares

Dorsal cochlear nucleus

Lateral vestibular nucleus
Nucleus of tractus solitarius
Glossopharyngeal nerve
Dorsal cochlear nucleus
Inf. cerebellar ped.
Ventral cochlear nucleus
Spinal tract and nucleus N. V
Olivocerebellar fibers
Pontobulbar body
Medial longitudinal fasciculus
Thalamo-olivary tract
Inferior olivary nucleus
Pyramid, corticospinal tract
Arcuate nucleus

Cerebellum

Vent. cochlear nucl.
Cochlear nerve
Vent. spinocerebellar tract

Vent. external arcuate fibers
Medial lemniscus

Foramen cæcum   Pons

FIGURE 162. Section through caudal border of the pons and the cochlear nuclei of a child. Pal-Weigert method. (×4.)

a superficial and a deep group (fibrae pontis superficiales and fibrae pontis profundae). Those of the superficial group lie ventral to the longitudinal fasciculi, while the deep transverse bundles interlace with the longitudinal ones or lie dorsal to them. The majority of the fibrae pontis cross the median plane. These are joined by some uncrossed fibers and gathered together on either side of the pons to form a compact and massive strand, known as the *middle cerebellar peduncle,* which curves dorsally to enter the white center of the cerebellum (Figs. 32, 162).

Along the rostral border of the pons and brachium pontis one or two fiber bundles are some-times found which run an isolated course to the cerebellum. These are known as the *fila lateralia pontis* or *taenia pontis* (Fig. 32). According to Horsley (1906) the constituent fibers arise from a ganglion situated caudal to the interpeduncular ganglion, decussate at once, and end in the cere-bellum in the neighborhood of the dentate nucleus. Perhaps they represent slightly displaced fibrae pontis. It also seems likely that the striae medullares and the ventral external arcuate fibers

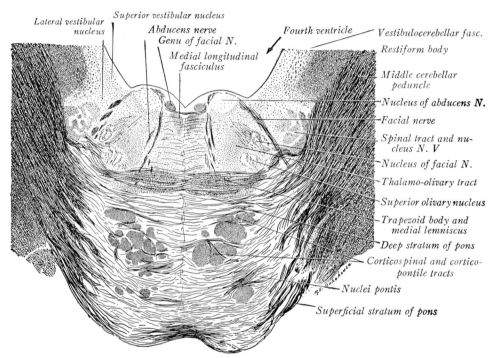

FIGURE 163. Section through the pons of a child at the level of the facial colliculus. Pal-Weigert method. (×4.)

belong to the same system and are also displaced pontine fibers (Rasmussen and Peyton, 1946). Some of the transverse fibers on reaching the median plane bend at right angles and run as fibrae rectae toward the pars dorsalis pontis (Fig. 345). According to Edinger (1911) these belong in part to the tractus cerebellotegmentalis pontis, which arises in the nuclei of the cerebellum and runs through the brachium to end in the reticular formation of the opposite side. Others are fibers joining cells in the tegmentum with the cerebellum (Kappers, Huber and Crosby, 1936).

The **nuclei pontis,** which are continuous with the arcuate nuclei of the medulla oblongata, contain medium-sized rounded or polygonal cells, the axons of which are continuous with the fibrae pontis (Figs. 336–357). There are also some small nerve cells of Golgi's Type II, the short axons of which end in adjacent gray matter. Within these nuclei terminate the fibers of the cortico-pontile tracts and some collaterals from the corticospinal fibers. Collaterals from the medial lemniscus are also found arborizing in those nuclei of the pons which lie immediately ventral to that bundle.

The pons serves to establish an important and for the most part crossed connection between the cerebral hemispheres and the cerebellum, a *cortico-pontocerebellar path*. The corticopontile fibers take origin from pyramidal cells in the frontal and temporal lobes and end in the nuclei pontis. Arising from the cells in these nuclei, most of the transverse fibers cross the median plane and reach the opposite cerebellar hemisphere through the middle cerebellar peduncle (Fig. 161).

THE DORSAL OR TEGMENTAL PART OF THE PONS

The dorsal or tegmental part of the pons (pars dorsalis pontis) resembles in structure the medulla oblongata (Fig. 163). On its dorsal surface there is a thick layer of gray matter which lines the rhomboid fossa. Between this layer and the basilar portion of the pons is the *reticular formation* divided by the median raphe into two symmetric halves. This has essentially the same structure here as in the medulla oblongata, and contains the continuation of many longitudinal tracts with which we are already familiar, as well as groups of neurons not belonging to the cranial nerve nuclei The inferior cerebellar peduncle (restiform body) at first occupies a position similar to that which it has in the medulla, along the lateral border of the rhomboid fossa, but it soon bends dorsally into the cerebellum.

The Cochlear Nuclei. At the point of transition between the medulla and pons, the inferior cerebellar peduncle is partly encircled on its lateral aspect by a mass of gray matter formed by the *terminal nuclei of the cochlear division of the stato-acoustic nerve* (Figs. 162, 330, 334, 331–335). There may be distinguished a *dorsal* and a *ventral cochlear nucleus* at the dorsal and ventral borders of the restiform body. Within these nuclei the fibers of the cochlear nerve end, while those of the vestibular nerve plunge into the substance of the pons ventromedially to the restiform body to reach the floor of the fourth ventricle (Figs. 187, 189). Fibers from the dorsal cochlear nucleus run medially beneath the floor of the fourth ventricle and, sinking into the tegmentum, join the fibers from the ventral cochlear nucleus in the trapezoid body.

The **trapezoid body** (corpus trapezoideum) is covered by the pars basalis pontis. In sections through the more caudal portions of the pons, the trapezoid body forms a conspicuous bundle of transverse fibers in the ventral portion of the reticular formation (Fig. 163). The fibers are associated with the terminal nuclei of the cochlear nerve, especially the ventral one, and with the superior olivary nucleus, around the ventral border of which they swing in such a way as to form a bay for its reception. Farther medialward they pass through the medial lemniscus at right angles to its constituent fibers and decussate in the median raphe. The trapezoid body describes a curve with convexity directed rostrally as well as ventrally, and as a result its lateral portions are seen best in sections through the lower border of the pons, while the rest of it is in evidence in sections at a higher level. Arising from the ventral nucleus of the cochlear nerve (Fig. 162) these fibers pass, with or without interruption in the superior olivary nucleus, across the median plane. (Fig. 163), and, on reaching the lateral border of the opposite superior olivary nucleus, they turn rostrally to form a longitudinal band of fibers known as the lateral lemniscus (Fig. 164). This is a part of the central auditory pathway, the connections of which are represented diagrammatically in Fig. 187.

The **superior olivary nucleus** is a small mass of gray matter located in the ventrolateral portion of the reticular formation of the pons in close relation to the trapezoid body and not far from the rostral pole of the inferior olivary nucleus (Figs. 163, 164, 340). It consists of two or three separate but closely associated nuclear masses, within which there ramify collaterals from the fibers of the trapezoid body. From the dorsal aspect of this nucleus, a bundle of fibers, known as the peduncle of the superior olive, makes its way toward the nucleus of the abducens nerve (Fig. 177). In the cat they have been shown to arise from cell bodies dorsal to the nucleus of the trapezoid body. Some fibers of the peduncle have been seen to cross the midline and emerge between the nervus intermedius and the vestibular division of the eighth nerve, with which they course as far as the vestibular ganglion, and then pass to the cochlear where they are distributed as spiral fibers in all turns of the organ of Corti (Rasmussen, 1953). Other fibers descend in the medial longitudinal fasciculus, and still others are contributed from the superior olive to the lateral lemniscus on both sides (Rasmussen, 1946).

The **nuclei of the vestibular nerve** lie in the floor of the fourth ventricle, where they occupy a field with which we are already familiar, namely the *area acustica* (Fig. 33). The vestibular fibers on approaching the rhomboid fossa divide into ascending and descending branches, and terminate in four nuclear masses: (1) the *medial* (dorsal or principal) *vestibular nucleus* (Figs. 159, 162); (2) the *lateral vestibular nucleus* of Deiters; (3) *the superior vestibular nucleus* of Bechterew (Fig. 163), and (4) the *spinal* or *descending vestibular nucleus*. These are represented diagrammatically in Fig. 189.

The Vestibulocerebellar Fasciculus. Ascending branches from some of the vestibular nerve fibers, accompanied by fibers from the lateral and superior vestibular nuclei, run to the cerebellum along the medial side of the inferior cerebellar peduncle. These fibers constitute the vestibulocerebellar fasciculus (Fig. 163). They end in the vestibular parts of the cerebellum (nodulus, uvula, lingula, and the fastigial nuclei).

The **medial longitudinal fasciculus** is an important bundle which extends from near the floor of the third ventricle to the spinal cord, and is especially concerned with the reflex control of the movements of the head and eyes. A large proportion of its fibers are derived from the vestibular nuclei. From this origin the fibers pass through the reticular formation to the medial longitudinal fasciculus of the same or the opposite side. Some of the fibers bifurcate, but a majority of them turn either up or down to become ascending or descending fibers within the fasciculus (Fig. 189). The former terminate in the nuclei of the oculomotor, trochlear, and abducens nerves, the latter in the nucleus of the spinal accessory nerve and in the columna anterior of the cervical portion of the spinal cord. In this way there is established a path for the reflex control of the movement of the head, neck, and eyes, in response to stimulation of the nerve endings in the semicircular canals of the ears. Another important group of fibers within this fasciculus takes origin from the *interstitial nucleus* situated in the zone of transition between the hypothalamus and mesencephalon medial to the rostral end of the red nucleus (Fig. 374). The nucleus of Darkschewitsch, often called the nucleus of the posterior commissure, is said to contribute fibers to the medial longitudinal fasciculus. Still other fibers serve to connect the nuclei of the third, fourth, and sixth cranial nerves with each other, with the motor nuclei of the seventh and eleventh cranial nerves and with the motor cells of the cervical spinal cord. Details concerning the origin of the vestibular fibers of the medial longitudinal fasciculus are given on page 264 and in Fig. 189.

The *medial longitudinal fasciculus* contains fibers which are continued upward from the *ventral funiculus* of the spinal cord. These fibers are displaced dorsolaterally by the decussation of the pyramids (Fig. 154) and then still farther dorsally by the decussation of the lemniscus (Fig. 155) until they come to lie in the most dorsal part of the substantia reticularis alba (Fig. 157), which position they occupy throughout the remainder of their course. The fasciculus is found ventral to the nucleus of the hypoglossal nerve (Fig. 159) and in close apposition to the nuclei of the three motor nerves of the eye (Figs. 163, 168, 170).

The **medial lemniscus** can also be traced within the reticular formation from the medulla into and through the pons. But this broad band of longitudinal fibers, which was spread out along the median raphe in the medulla, shifts ventrally in the pons, assuming first a somewhat triangular outline and a ventromedian position (Fig. 162); then by shifting farther lateralward it takes again the form of a flat band (Figs. 163, 164). But now it is compressed ventrodorsally and occupies the ventral part of the reticular formation, its fibers crossing those of the trapezoid body at right angles. It must not be forgotten that the medial lemniscus is composed of longitudinal fibers, and it is by the gradual shifting of these that the bundle as a whole changes shape and position. As it is displaced ventrally it separates from the medial longitudinal bundle, which retains its dorsal position.

The **motor nucleus of the facial nerve** occupies a position in the reticular formation dorsal to the superior olive (Figs. 163, 335–340). It is an oval mass of gray matter, which extends from the lower border of the pons to the level of the facial colliculus, and contains the cells of origin of the fibers which innervate the platysma and muscles of the face. These fibers emerge from the dorsal surface of the nucleus and run dorsomedially toward the floor of the fourth ventricle. Somewhat widely separated at first, they become united on the medial side of the abducens nucleus into a compact strand, which as the *genu of the facial nerve* partly encircles this nucleus, and which then runs ventrolaterally between the spinal tract of the trigeminal nerve and its own nucleus toward its exit from the brain (Figs. 163–177).

The **nucleus of the abducens nerve** along with the genu of the facial produces a rounded elevation in the rhomboid fossa, known as the *facial colliculus* (Figs. 33, 163, 340). It is a spheric mass of gray matter containing the cells of origin of the fibers which innervate the lateral rectus. These emerge from the dorsal and medial surfaces of the nucleus and run ventrally more or less parallel to the median raphe toward their exit at the lower border of the pons.

The Nuclei of the Trigeminal Nerve. In transverse section through approximately the middle of the pons we encounter the fibers of the trigeminal nerve and two associated masses of gray matter, the *motor* and *main sensory nuclei* of that nerve (Fig. 164). These are located close together in the dorsolateral part of the reticular formation near the groove between the middle and superior

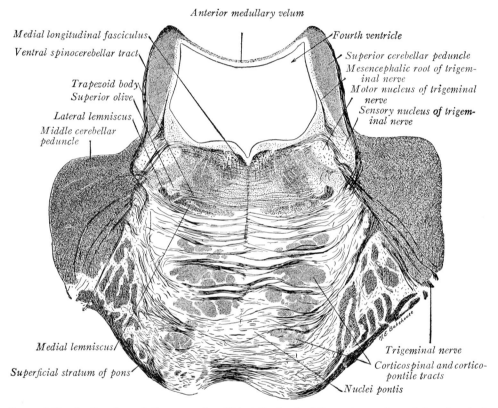

FIGURE 164. Section through the pons of a child at the level of the motor nucleus of the trigeminal nerve. Pal-Weigert method. (×4.)

cerebellar peduncles. Of the two, the *sensory nucleus* is the more superficial. It is, in reality, not a new structure, but rather the enlarged rostral extremity of the column of gray matter which we have followed upward from the substantia gelatinosa Rolandi of the spinal cord and have designated as the *nucleus of the spinal tract* of the trigeminal nerve (Figs. 154, 157). On the medial side of the main sensory nucleus is found the *motor nucleus,* a large oval mass of gray matter from the cells of which arise the motor fibers for the muscles of mastication. Some of the fibers of the trigeminal nerve, passing between these two nuclei, are continued as the *mesencephalic root of the trigeminal nerve*

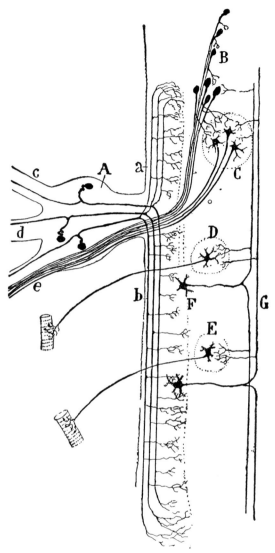

FIGURE 165. Diagram of the nuclei and central connections of the trigeminal nerve: *A*, Semilunar ganglion; *B*, mesencephalic nucleus, N. V; *C*, motor nucleus, N. V; *D*, motor nucleus N. VII; *E*, motor nucleus, N. XII; *F*, nucleus of the spinal tract of N. V; *G*, sensory fibers of the second order of the trigeminal path; *a*, ascending and *b*, descending branches of the sensory fibers, N. V; *c*, ophthalmic nerve; *d*, maxillary nerve; *e*, mandibular nerve. (Cajal.)

(Figs. 164, 165). Reaching the gray matter in the lateral wall of the rostral part of the fourth ventricle, this bundle of fibers turns rostrally along the medial side of the superior cerebellar peduncle (Fig. 166). It extends into the mesencephalon in the lateral part of the gray matter which surrounds the cerebral aqueduct (Fig. 168). The fibers of this root take origin from large unipolar cells scattered along its course and constituting the *mesencephalic nucleus* of the trigeminal nerve.

It will be apparent from this description that there are four nuclear masses associated with the trigeminal nerve, namely, the nucleus of the spinal tract, the main sensory, the motor, and mesencephalic nuclei. The relations which each of these groups of cells bears to the fibers of the trigeminal nerve are illustrated in Fig. 165. Note that those fibers which arise from cells in the semilunar ganglion divide into short ascending and long descending branches. The former end in the main sensory nucleus, while the latter run in the spinal tract of the trigeminal nerve and end in the nucleus which accompanies it.

The **superior cerebellar peduncle** (Fig. 33) is seen in sections through the rostral half of the pons, where it enters into the lateral boundary of the fourth

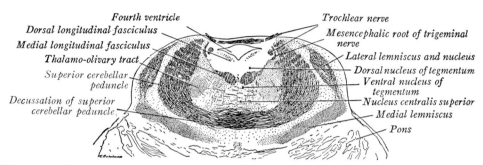

FIGURE 166. Dorsal half of a section through the rostral part of the human pons. Pal-Weigert method.

ventricle (Fig. 164). It is a large strand of fibers which runs from the dentate nucleus of the cerebellum to the red nucleus of the mesencephalon (Fig. 169). As it emerges from the white center of the cerebellum this peduncle is superficially placed, with its ventral border resting on the tegmental portion of the pons (Fig. 164). To its dorsal border is attached a thin plate of white matter, the *anterior medullary velum,* which roofs in the rostral part of the fourth ventricle. As the superior peduncle ascends toward the mesencephalon it sinks deeper and deeper into the dorsal part of the pons (Fig. 351) until it is entirely submerged (Fig. 166). Near the rostral border of the pons it assumes a crescentic outline and lies in the lateral part of the reticular formation. From its ventral border fibers stream across the median plane, decussating with similar fibers from the opposite side. This is the most caudal portion of the *decussation of the superior cerebellar peduncle,* which increases in volume as it is followed rostrally, reaching its maximum in the mesencephalon at the level of the inferior colliculi (Fig. 168). In this decussation the fibers of the peduncle undergo a complete crossing.

The **ventral spinocerebellar tract,** which has made its way through the reticular formation of the pons, turns dorsolaterally near the rostral end of the pons, winds around the superior peduncle, and enters the anterior medullary velum, in which it passes to the vermis of the cerebellum (Figs. 164, 198).

The **lateral lemniscus** is an important tract of fibers which we have already traced from the cochlear nuclei. It first takes definite shape about the middle of the pons, where it is situated lateral to the medial lemniscus (Fig. 164). As it ascends it becomes displaced dorsolaterally until it occupies a position on the lateral aspect of the superior peduncle (Fig. 166). In this position there is developed in connection with it a collection of nerve cells, the *nucleus of the lateral lemniscus*, to which its fibers give off collaterals.

CHAPTER XII

The Internal Structure
of the Mesencephalon

A diagram of a transverse section through the rostral part of the mesencephalon will make clear the relation of the various parts of the midbrain to each other (Fig. 167). The *cerebral aqueduct* is surrounded by a thick lamina of gray matter, the central gray stratum (stratum griseum centrale). The aqueduct varies in diameter in different portions of its course. Its area in cross section has been found to vary from about one-half square millimeter to around ten (Flyger and Hjelmquist, 1957). Dorsal to this lies the *lamina quadrigemina*, a plate of mingled gray and white matter which bears four rounded elevations, the corpora quadrigemina. The ventral part of the midbrain is formed by the *cerebral peduncles*, each of which is separated into two parts by a lamina of pigmented gray substance, known as the *substantia nigra*. Dorsal to this the peduncle consists of reticular formation continuous with that of the pons and known as the *tegmentum*. Ventral to the substantia nigra is a thick plate of longitudinal fibers, called the *basis pedunculi*, composed of fibers which are continuous with the longitudinal fasciculi of the pons.

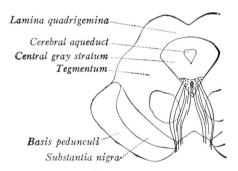

FIGURE 167. Diagrammatic cross-section through the human mesencephalon.

The Tegmentum. The dorsal portion of the pons is directly continuous with the tegmentum of the mesencephalon. Both are composed of reticular formation, consisting of interlacing longitudinal and transverse fibers grouped in fine bundles and separated by minute masses of gray substance, in which are embedded important nuclei and fiber tracts. In the caudal part of the midbrain and the rostral part of the pons are five cellular masses the locations of which are indicated in Figs. 166, 346–356. They are the *dorsal nucleus of the*

227

raphe, the *superior central nucleus*, the *ventral tegmental nucleus*, the *dorsal tegmental nucleus*, and the *reticulotegmental nucleus*. Both the ventral and dorsal tegmental nuclei receive fibers from the mammillary body (tractus mammillotegmentalis), and within the dorsal one there also terminate fibers from the interpeduncular ganglion. The tegmentum contains many *longitudinal fiber tracts* which are continued into it from the dorsal part of the pons. The most conspicuous of these is the superior cerebellar peduncle.

The Decussation of the Superior Cerebellar Peduncles. In the sections of the pons we saw that, as the superior peduncles ascend toward the me-

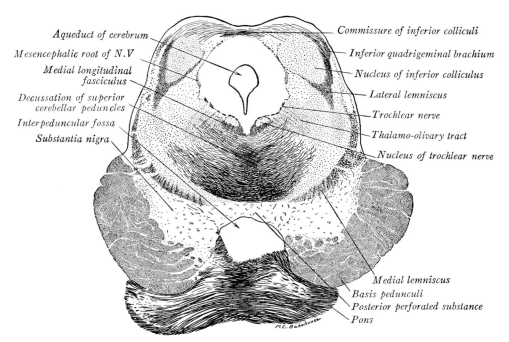

FIGURE 168. Section through the mesencephalon of a child at the level of the inferior colliculus. Pal-Weigert method. (×4.)

sencephalon, they sink deeper and deeper into the pars dorsalis pontis (Fig. 166). When they reach the level of the inferior colliculi of the corpora quadrigemina they are deeply placed in the tegmentum; and here they cross the median plane in the *decussation* (Fig. 168). After crossing, each peduncle turns rostrally and forms a rounded bundle of ascending fibers, which almost at once come into relation with the *red nucleus* (Fig. 170). Many of the fibers enter this nucleus directly, while others are prolonged over its surface to form a capsule that is best developed on its medial surface. While the majority of these fibers ultimately end in the red nucleus, some reach and end within the ventral part of the thalamus (Fig. 169).

According to Cajal (1911), the fibers of the superior cerebellar peduncle give off two sets of descending branches, which he has seen in Golgi preparations of the mouse, rabbit and cat. The

CHAPTER XIII

The Cranial Nerves and Their Nuclei

When the embryonic neural tube closes and the cells of the ependymal layer have proliferated to form mantle and marginal layers, there is left a groove in each lateral wall which separates dorsal and ventral portions. These are known respectively as the alar and basal laminae. Within the alar laminae throughout the neural tube sensory cell clusters develop, while in the basal laminae motor cells develop. This is exemplified in the mature spinal cord by the origin of the motor fibers of ventral roots of the spinal nerves from cells of the ventral horn of gray matter, and the connections which sensory fibers of the dorsal roots establish with cells of the dorsal horn of gray matter. There is in the basal laminae in the region of the spinal cord evidence of a further longitudinal segregation of functional groups of cells. Not only is subdivision of longitudinal columns of somatic motor cells evident, but dorsolateral to the somatic motor columns appears the visceral motor column, that is, the preganglionic visceral efferent group of cells in the intermediolateral cell column of gray matter.

The spinal cord remains tubular in form and its segmental arrangement presents no marked variation in plan at different levels. The size of the cord varies with the amount of tissue to be supplied in the region; witness the quantitative increase in the region of the lumbar and cervical enlargements where the limbs attach. In the head end of the animal, where specialized sense organs occur and special mechanisms for feeding, respiration, and vocalization are formed, there is an accompanying specialization of the nerves supplying various parts and of the cranial portion of the neural tube with which these nerves are connected. During development the simple tubular pattern of the nervous system is distorted and becomes less evident owing to the flexures which occur, the thinning of the roof of the fourth ventricle, the suprasegmental accumulations of nervous tissue, and the mushroom growth of nerve cell groups associated with some cranial nerves.

There is, however, evidence of the original tubular structure, especially well retained in the mesencephalon; and a study of the nerve cell groups related to the cranial nerves reveals a more or less clear columnar arrangement of nuclear masses associated with functional types of fibers. The line of division between the alar and basal laminae, the sulcus limitans, is visible in the floor of the

237

fourth ventricle though somewhat effaced in the caudal portion. Between this sulcus and the midline may be found the nuclei of origin of the motor fibers of the cranial nerves, while beneath the floor lateral to the sulcus limitans lie the nuclei of reception of sensory fibers of the cranial nerves (except nerves I and II).

Functional Components. The functional components of a typical spinal nerve are four: general somatic and visceral, each subdivided into afferent and efferent. The same components occur in cranial nerves (not all in each nerve), but there are also *special* groups of fibers so that if each of these four components could be subdivided into *special* and *general* subdivisions, eight functional types of components would result. Actually, only seven types are listed since somatic efferent fibers are not considered as divided into special and general groups.

The following diagram will illustrate the classification of fibers of cranial nerves into seven components:

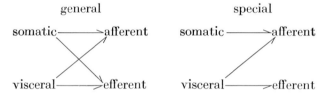

A few conflicts arise in the functional classification of cranial nerve fibers because either of two separate criteria has been used to make the classification. This is in reality a logical error, but at the head end of the animal where the "visceral" entodermal canal joins the superficial ectoderm of the head covering, a "somatic" area, such conflicts are unavoidable. As long as the student is aware of the dilemma and can see the reasonableness of either classification no misunderstanding need arise.

Nerves supplying sensory fibers to ectodermally derived structures, as the skin, the eye, and the internal ear, are classed as somatic, those to the skin are termed general, those to the eye and ear as special. An exception occurs in the case of the first cranial nerve, which, though derived from cells in an ectodermal structure, the nasal pit, is classed as visceral because of its association with feeding, a dominantly visceral function. It is at least distinguished by being called special visceral as are also the fibers from taste buds.

On the motor side nerve fibers to smooth muscle, cardiac muscle, and glands are classed as general visceral efferent, and those which supply skeletal muscles derived from the mesoderm of the somites are classed as somatic efferent. About the mouth and face a set of muscles identical histologically with those derived from segmental mesoderm are formed out of the diffuse mesoderm of the branchial arches which develop in intimate relation to the anterior end of the alimentary canal. These are striated and in every way resemble the somatic muscle but are termed visceral muscles. However, because they are very different from the smooth visceral musculature of the gut, the motor nerve fibers to them are classed as special visceral. (These nerve fibers do *not* belong to the autonomic system.) A third conflict arises out of this situation. The proprioceptive fibers

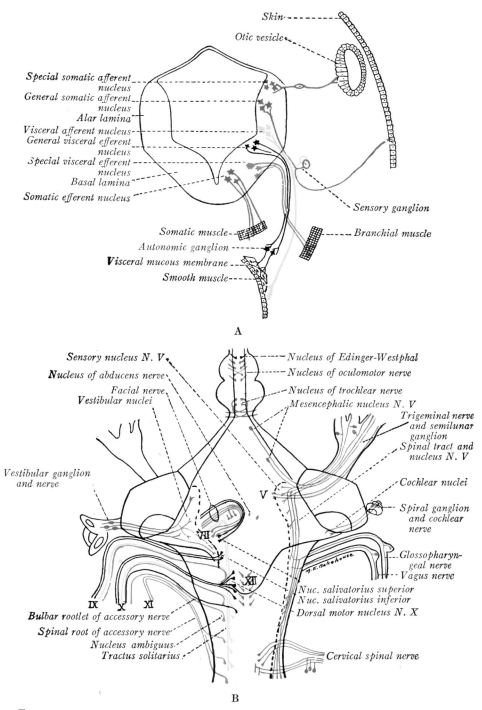

FIGURE 173. Diagrams showing the origin, course, and termination of the functional components of the cranial nerves. Somatic afferent and efferent, red; visceral afferent, yellow; general visceral
efferent, black; special visceral efferent, blue. A, shows the locations of the several functional cell
columns in a section through the medulla oblongata of a human embryo and the peripheral terminations of the several varieties of fibers. B, dorsal view of the human brain stem, showing the
location of the nuclei and the intramedullary course of the fibers of the cranial nerves.

throughout the body have been grouped with the general somatic afferent fibers. Since the proprioceptive neurons related to somatic muscle and those to the branchiomeric muscle are histologically alike, they have been left in the same classification, giving rise to the peculiar situation in which a set of muscles receiving motor fibers classed as special visceral are supplied with sensory fibers classed as general somatic. Again, in the facial nerve are fibers conveying deep

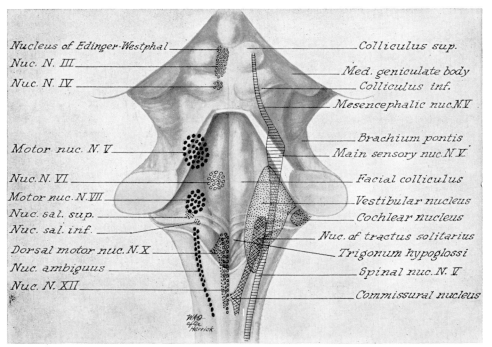

FIGURE 174. Dorsal view of the human brain stem with the positions of the cranial nerve nuclei projected upon the surface. Sensory nuclei on the right side, motor nuclei on the left. Circles indicate somatic efferent nuclei; small dots, general visceral efferent nuclei; large dots, special visceral efferent nuclei; horizontal lines, general somatic sensory nuclei; cross-hatching, visceral sensory nuclei; stipple, special somatic sensory nuclei. (Herrick.)

sensibility from the face. Whether these fibers are identical with the proprioceptive fibers from facial muscles is not known, but they have been classified as general visceral afferent.

From what has been said it will be evident that there are seven distinct *functional components* in the cranial nerves, namely, somatic efferent, general somatic afferent, special somatic afferent, general visceral efferent, special visceral efferent, general visceral afferent, and special visceral afferent components (Figs. 173, 174). No single nerve contains all seven types of fibers and the individual cranial nerves vary greatly in their functional composition. On entering the brain a nerve breaks up into its several components, which separate from each other and pass to their respective nuclei, enumerated below. These nuclei may be widely separated in the brain stem. Fibers having the same function tend to be associated together within the brain irrespective of the nerves to which they belong. For example, all the visceral afferent fibers of the facial, glossopharyngeal, and vagus nerves are grouped in the tractus solitarius (Fig. 173, yellow). The analysis of the cranial nerves into their functional components has involved a great amount of labor which has been carried through for the most part by American investigators. Among those who have made important contribution to this subject may be mentioned the following: Gaskell (1886), Strong (1895), Herrick (1899), Johnson (1901), Coghill (1902), Norris (1908), and Willard (1915). The nerve cells, with which the fibers of the several functional varieties are associated within the brain stem, are arranged in *longitudinal nuclear columns*, which incidentally show more conspicuously in the selachian than in the higher vertebrate brain.

Longitudinal Nuclear Columns. As stated above, the sensory nuclei of the cranial nerves develop within the alar plate and the motor nuclei within the basal plate of the neural tube. In the rhombencephalon both plates come to lie in the floor of the fourth ventricle, the alar occupying the more lateral position. In spite of the changes of position which occur during development, the sensory nuclei retain, on the whole, a lateral, and the motor nuclei a more medial, location. From the basal plate there differentiate a somatic and a visceral column of efferent nuclei, and from the alar plate a visceral and a somatic column of afferent nuclei.

The *somatic efferent column* includes the nuclei of those motor nerves which supply the extrinsic muscles of the eye and the musculature of the tongue (Fig. 175, 176).

The *visceral efferent* cells lie in two columns: (1) a ventrolateral column of nuclei, from which arise the *special visceral efferent* fibers to the striated visceral or branchial musculature, and which includes the nucleus ambiguous and the motor nuclei of the fifth and seventh nerves, and (2) a more dorsally placed group for the innervation of involuntary musculature and glandular tissue, of which the dorsal motor nucleus of the vagus is the chief example. The former may be called the *special visceral efferent* and the latter the *general visceral efferent column*.

The *visceral afferent column* is represented by the nucleus of the tractus solitarius, within which end the visceral afferent fibers, both general and special, of the facial, glossopharyngeal, and vagus nerves. The somatic afferent nuclei may be separated into two groups: a *general somatic afferent column,* within which terminate the sensory fibers from the skin; and a *special somatic* group of nuclei for the reception of the fibers of the acoustic nerve and, in aquatic vertebrates, of the lateral line nerves also.

While the classification of cranial nerve components is analytically useful, it is often too arbitrary for the actual details. In the specialization that occurred, certain cranial nerves usurped, as it were, functions which in the spinal nerves are shared by successive segmental nerves. For example, the trigeminal has taken over the job of supplying general sensibility to the head and face, but the vagus and probably the glossopharyngeal and the facial supply a small cutaneous area in the neighborhood of the external auditory meatus and ear.

The fibers from this area on entering the medulla join the spinal nucleus of the trigeminal. Such contributions are not commonly listed in an analysis of cranial nerve components, and there are other exceptions to the general rule. For example, some fibers from the trigeminal nerve enter the nucleus solitarius (Torvik, 1956).

THE SOMATIC EFFERENT COLUMN

As can be seen by reference to Figs. 157, 163, 168, and 170, the nuclei of the hypoglossal, abducens, trochlear, and oculomotor nerves are arranged in linear order in the central gray matter near the median plane. They represent the continuation into the medulla oblongata of the large cells of the anterior column of the spinal cord. The cells of these nuclei are large and multipolar with well developed Nissl bodies (Fig. 169), and from them arise large myelinated fibers. This group of nuclei is indicated in red in Fig. 173 and by small circles in Figs. 174 and 176.

The muscles supplied by this column of cells do not come from myotomes as do those supplied by the spinal nerves. The extrinsic eye muscles develop from premandibular and maxillomandibular condensations of mesoderm that lie anterior to the notochord (Gilbert, 1947). The tongue musculature apparently arises from the mesoderm of the branchial arches forming the floor of the mouth.

The **nucleus of the oculomotor nerve** is an elongated mass of cells in the central gray matter ventral to the cerebral aqueduct at the level of the superior colliculus (Figs. 174, 176). Even a superficial examination shows that it is divided into a lateral paired and a medial unpaired portion (Fig. 170). The lateral group of cells spreads out upon the surface of the medial longitudinal bundle, and extends throughout the entire length of the nucleus (Fig. 175). The medial portions of the two nuclei are fused into an unpaired median nucleus, which at its caudal end is rather ill defined, but in sections through the middle third of the oculomotor complex forms a well defined spindle-shaped mass, the medial nucleus of Perlia (Fig. 175, *M* and *MP*). The paired lateral nuclei form plates of cells lying upon and infiltrating the medial longitudinal fasciculi. Each of these plates is divided rather indistinctly into a larger ventral and a small dorsal portion. These lateral nuclei are composed of large multipolar cells of the type supplying skeletal muscle. The medial nucleus, including the medial nucleus of Perlia, is composed of cells, which although smaller than those of the lateral nucleus, have the discrete Nissl bodies characteristic of motor neurons.

Some of the fibers from the medial nucleus enter the right and the others enter the left oculomotor nerve. Some from the lateral nucleus cross the median plane and enter the nerve of the opposite side, but the majority remain uncrossed. After sweeping in broad curves through the tegmentum and red nucleus the fibers emerge through the oculomotor sulcus (Fig. 170). They supply all of the extrinsic muscles of the eye except the lateral rectus and superior oblique.

As one might expect from the fact that the oculomotor nerve supplies several distinct muscles, its nucleus seems to be made up of a number of more or less distinct groups of cells. Szentágothai (1942), Bender and Weinstein (1943), and Danis (1948) found the pattern of representation the reverse of that formerly described. From the cranial end caudalward according to Danis the cell groups supply nerve fibers to the extrinsic eye muscles in the following order: rectus inferior, rectus medialis, obliquus inferior, rectus superior, and levator palpebrae superioris, the last three over-

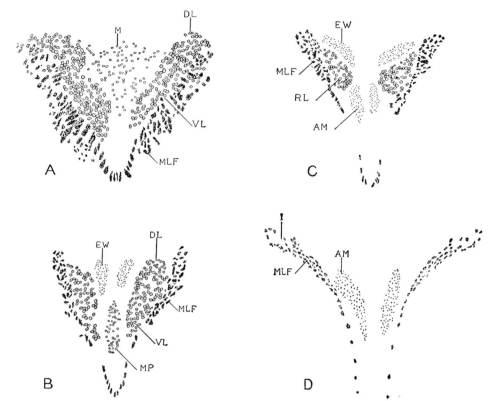

FIGURE 175. Diagrams showing the changes in topography of the several divisions of the oculomotor nucleus seen in following a series of sections from below upward through the mesencephalon: *A*, From near the caudal end of the oculomotor nucleus; *B*, middle portion; *C*, rostral end; *D*, just rostral to the lateral large-celled portion of the nucleus. *AM*, Anterior medial nucleus; *DL*, dorsal portion of lateral nucleus; *EW*, Edinger-Westphal nucleus; *I*, interstitial nucleus; *M*, diffuse portion of medial nucleus; *MLF*, medial longitudinal fasciculus; *MP*, medial nucleus of Perlia; *RL*, rostral end of lateral nucleus; *VL*, ventral portion of lateral nucleus.

lapping. The fibers leaving these subdivisions and passing to the rectus inferior, rectus medialis, and obliquus inferior muscles were observed to be uncrossed, while those passing to rectus superior and levator palpebrae were largely, but not entirely, crossed. Warwick (1953) confirmed these observations except that he found the fibers to the levator palpebrae superiores wholly crossed in the monkey.

The **nucleus of the trochlear nerve** has already been located in the central gray matter ventral to the cerebral aqueduct at the level of the inferior colliculus, close to the caudal extremity of the oculomotor nucleus (Figs. 168, 174, 176). The fibers of the trochlear nerve emerge from the dorsal and lateral aspects of this nucleus, and, encircling the central gray matter along an angular course which carries them also caudally, enter the anterior medullary velum, decussate within it, and make their exit from its dorsal surface (Fig. 166). They supply the superior oblique muscle.

The **nucleus of the abducens nerve** was encountered in the dorsal portion of the pons as a spheric gray mass, which with the genu of the facial nerve forms the facial colliculus of the rhomboid fossa (Figs. 163, 174, 176). The fibers of the abducens nerve leave the nucleus chiefly on its dorsal and medial surfaces and become assembled into several root bundles, which are directed ventrally toward their exit from the lower border of the pons near the pyramid of the medulla oblongata. It supplies the lateral rectus muscle.

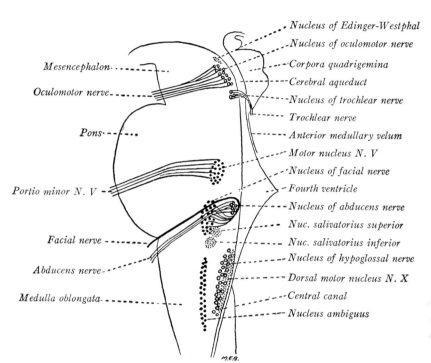

FIGURE 176. Motor nuclei of the cranial nerves projected on a medial sagittal section of the human brain stem. Circles indicate somatic efferent nuclei; small dots, general visceral efferent nuclei; large dots, special visceral efferent nuclei.

A diagram of the representation of the craniocaudal sequence of the ocular muscles within the brain stem alongside the pattern of movements of the bulbus oculi shows some correlation of topography.

Cranio-caudal Position in Brain Stem	Nerve Fibers from Nucleus to Muscle	Movements of Right Eye in Direction of Arrows. (Initials indicate eye muscles responsible for movements)
Nuc. N. III		
Rectus Inferior Rectus Medialis Obliquus Inferior	homolateral	O.I. ↖ ↗ R.S.
Rectus Superior Levator Palpebrae Superioris	largely contralateral	R.L. ← X → R.M. O.S. ↙ ↘ R.I.
Nuc. N. IV		
Obliquus Superior - contralateral		
Nuc. N. VI		
Rectus Lateralis - homolateral		

overlapping

The *axons,* which ramify within the three nuclei for the motor nerves of the eye, are derived from many sources. The most important of these sources are the corticobulbar tract, the medial longitudinal bundle, and the tectobulbar tract. These various fibers provide for voluntary movements of the eyes, and for reflex ocular movements in response to vestibulbar, visual, and auditory impulses. The nuclei probably also receive branches from the central sensory path of the fifth nerve.

The **nucleus of the hypoglossal nerve** is a slender cylindric mass of gray matter nearly 2 cm. in length, extending between the levels of the lower borders of the olive and of the cochlear nuclei. We have already identified it in both the open and the closed portions of the medulla oblongata. In the floor of the fourth ventricle it lies beneath the trigonum hypoglossi, while more caudally it lies ventral to the central canal (Figs. 155, 159, 174, 176, 317–327). The root fibers are assembled into bundles which run ventrally toward their exit along the lateral border of the pyramid.

A conspicuous plexus of myelinated fibers gives the hypoglossal nucleus a characteristic appearance in Weigert preparations. Fibers from many sources reach the nucleus and ramify within it. These include some from the corticobulbar tract and others from the sensory nuclei of the fifth nerve and from the nucleus of the tractus solitarius. The part which such fibers may play in reflex movements of the tongue is illustrated in Fig. 151.

THE SPECIAL VISCERAL EFFERENT COLUMN

The special visceral efferent column of nuclei contains the cells of origin of the motor fibers for the striated musculature derived from the branchial arches, as distinguished from the general skeletal musculature that develops from the myotomes. The branchial musculature includes the following groups of muscles: the *muscles of mastication,* derived from the mesoderm of the first branchial arch and innervated by the trigeminal nerve; the *muscles of expression,* derived from the second or hyoid arch and innervated by the facial nerve; the *musculature of the pharynx and larynx,* derived from the third and fourth arches and innervated by the glossopharyngeal, vagus, and the bulbar portion of the accessory nerve; and probably also the *sternocleidomastoid* and *trapezius muscles,* innervated through the spinal root of the accessory nerve. Some authors prefer to call this column, which includes the *motor nuclei of the fifth and seventh nerves* and the *nucleus ambiguus,* the lateral somatic column, because the cells of these nuclei and the fibers which arise from them possess the characteristics of somatic motor cells and fibers. The nuclei are composed of large multipolar cells with well developed Nissl bodies. These cells give origin to large myelinated fibers which run through the corresponding nerve and terminate in neuromuscular endings in one or another of the muscles indicated above.

The motor nuclei of the fifth and seventh nerves and the nucleus ambiguus of the ninth, tenth, and eleventh nerves form a broken column of gray matter, located in the ventrolateral part of the reticular formation of the pons and medulla oblongata some distance beneath the floor of the fourth ventricle (Figs.

174, 176). The cells of this column and the special visceral efferent fibers which arise from them have been colored blue in Fig. 173.

The **motor nucleus of the trigeminal nerve** lies on the medial side of the main sensory nucleus of that nerve, and is located at the level of the middle of the pons in the lateral part of the reticular formation some distance from the ventricular floor (Figs. 164, 174, 176, 346–352). The fibers, which take their origin here, are collected in the motor root or portio minor of the fifth nerve and run with its mandibular division to the muscles of mastication. Within the nucleus there terminate fibers from the corticobulbar tract and many fibers, chiefly collaterals, from the central sensory tract of the trigeminal nerve. It also receives collaterals from the mesencephalic root of the trigeminal and from other sources (Fig. 184).

Within the motor nucleus of the trigeminal nerve muscles are represented by groups of cells that supply them: the more dorsally placed muscles in the ventral part of the nucleus, the more ventral muscles in the dorsal part. Muscles more oral in position are represented more anteriorly in the nucleus than those posterior in position (Szentágothai, 1949).

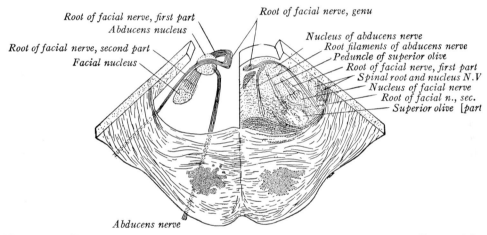

FIGURE 177. Diagram of the root of the facial nerve, shown from the rostral side as if exposed by dissection in a thick section of the pons.

The **motor nucleus of the facial nerve** is located in the ventrolateral part of the reticular formation of the pons near its caudal border (Figs. 162, 174, 176, 335–340). Its constituent cells are arranged so as to form a varying number of subgroups which may possibly be concerned with the innervation of individual facial muscles.

From the dorsal aspect of this nucleus there emerges a large number of fine bundles of fibers, directed dorsomedially through the reticular formation. These rather widely separated bundles constitute the *first part of the root of the facial nerve* (Fig. 177). Beneath the floor of the fourth ventricle the fibers turn sharply rostrad and are assembled into a compact strand of longitudinal fibers, often called the ascending part of the facial nerve. This ascends along the medial side of the abducens nucleus dorsal to the medial longitudinal bundle for a considerable distance (5 mm.). The nerve then turns sharply lateralward over the dorsal surface of the nucleus of the abducens nerve, and helps to form the elevation in the rhomboid fossa, known as the *facial colliculus*. This bend around the abducens nucleus, including the ascending part of the facial nerve, is known as the *genu*. The *second part of the root of the facial nerve* is directed ventro-laterally and at the same time somewhat caudally, passing close to the lateral side of its own nucleus, to make its exit from the lateral part of the caudal border of the pons (Fig. 163).

Fibers from many sources terminate in the facial nucleus in synaptic relation with its constituent cells. Those from the corticobulbar tract place the facial muscles under voluntary control. Others are collaterals from the secondary sensory paths in the reticular formation and are concerned with bulbar reflexes. Some of these collaterals are given off by fibers arising in the trapezoid body and carry auditory impulses. Others are collaterals of fibers arising in the nucleus of the spinal tract of the fifth nerve; and still others are given off by ascending sensory fibers from the spinal cord (Cajal, 1909).

A type of topographic localization of cell groups supplying the various facial muscles similar to that shown in the trigeminal motor nucleus has been demonstrated in the cat. Muscles in concentric zones beginning about the mouth and extending posteriorly are represented in the nucleus in similar order anteroposteriorly. Muscles in the upper part of the face are represented in the more ventral part of the nucleus, those in the lower part of the face in the more dorsal part of the nucleus. The platysma was represented medially in the nucleus, the orbicularis oculi laterally (Szentágothai, 1948).

The **nucleus ambiguus** is a long slender column of nerve cells, extending through the length of the medulla oblongata in the ventrolateral part of the reticular formation (Figs. 158, 174, 176, 308–332). Its constituent cells give rise to the *special visceral efferent fibers* that run through the glossopharyngeal, vagus, and accessory nerves to supply the musculature of the pharynx and larynx. It reaches from the border of the pons to the end of the medulla, but is most evident in transverse sections through the caudal part of the rhomboid fossa. Here it can be found in the reticular formation ventral to the nucleus of the spinal root of the trigeminal nerve. The fibers arising from its cells are at first directed dorsally; then curving laterally and ventrally they join the root bundles of the ninth, tenth, and eleventh nerves with which they emerge from the brain (Fig. 160). A few of the fibers cross the median plane and join the corresponding root bundles of the opposite side.

The **sensory collaterals** which arborize among the cells of the nucleus ambiguus are derived from the central tracts of the trigeminal, glossopharyngeal, and vagus nerves, from ascending sensory fibers of spinal origin, and from other longitudinal fibers in the reticular formation. Other fibers reach this nucleus from the corticobulbar tract.

The accessory nerve consists of a bulbar and a spinal portion. The fibers of the *spinal root* take origin from a linear group of cells in the lateral part of the anterior gray column in the upper cervical segments of the spinal cord. This root ascends along the side of the spinal cord, passes through the foramen magnum, and is joined by the bulbar rootlets of the accessory (Fig. 178). The nerve then divides into an internal and an external branch. In the latter run all the fibers of spinal origin and these are distributed to the trapezius and sternocleidomastoid muscles. If, as seems probable, these muscles are derived from the branchial arches (Lewis, 1910), the fibers which supply them may be regarded as special visceral efferent fibers, and the spinal nucleus of the accessory nerve may be considered as homologous to the nucleus ambiguus. The *bulbar rootlets* of the accessory nerve, which contain both general and special visceral efferent fibers, form a well defined fascicle, readily distinguished from the spinal portion of the nerve, and which, as the internal ramus, *joins the vagus nerve and is distributed through its branches* (Fig. 173; Chase and Ranson, 1914).

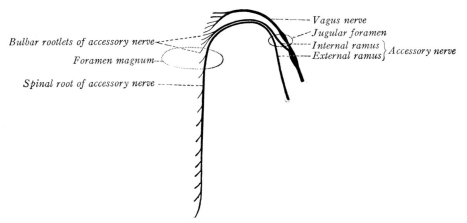

Bulbar rootlets of accessory nerve

Foramen magnum

Spinal root of accessory nerve

Vagus nerve
Jugular foramen
Internal ramus }
External ramus } *Accessory nerve*

FIGURE 178.   Diagram of the roots of the vagus and accessory nerves.

The afferent and efferent fibers of the vagus become segregated into separate rootlets before entering the medulla. The motor rootlets are small and are in vertical alignment with the bulbar rootlets of the accessory. Like the latter they are composed of fibers from the nucleus ambiguus and from the dorsal motor nucleus. The fibers from the jugular as well as those from the nodose ganglion form sensory rootlets which join the tractus solitarius (Ranson, Foley and Alpert, 1933; Foley and DuBois, 1934; Tarlov, 1940).

THE GENERAL VISCERAL EFFERENT COLUMN

The general visceral efferent column of nuclei is composed of the cells from which arise the efferent fibers innervating cardiac and smooth muscle and glandular tissue. The cells of these nuclei are relatively small and their Nissl bodies are not well developed (Fig. 179, *B*). They give rise to the *general visceral efferent fibers* of the cranial nerves. These are small myelinated fibers, which end in autonomic ganglia, where they arborize about autonomic cells, the axons of which terminate in smooth or cardiac muscle or in glandular tissue. The neurons of this series are, therefore, characterized by the fact that the impulses which they transmit must be relayed by neurons of a second order before reaching the innervated tissue (Fig. 173). This group of nuclei is indicated by black in Fig. 173 and by fine stipple in Figs. 174, 176.

The **dorsal motor nucleus of the vagus** (nucleus vagi dorsalis medialis) has been noted in the transverse section through the medulla oblongata (Figs. 155, 159). It lies along the dorsolateral side of the hypoglossal nucleus, subjacent to the ala cinerea of the rhomboid fossa, and lateral to the central canal in the closed part of the medulla oblongata (Figs. 182, 311–332). The *general visceral efferent fibers* which arise from the cells in this nucleus, leave the medulla oblongata through the roots of the vagus and accessory nerves; but those entering the accessory nerve leave that nerve by its internal ramus and join the vagus (Fig. 173). Hence all of the fibers from this nucleus are distributed through the branches of the vagus to the vagal autonomic plexuses of the thorax and abdomen for the innervation of the involuntary musculature of the heart, respiratory passages, esophagus, stomach, and small intestines (Van Gehuchten and Molhant, 1912), and for the innervation of the pancreas, liver, and other glands.

There is some topographic representation in the nucleus: abdominal organs are represented throughout the nucleus except at its caudal end; the oral part is also related to lungs; the caudal part is related to trachea, bronchi, and esophagus; the central part of the nucleus is related to heart and abdominal organs (Getz and Sirnes, 1949).

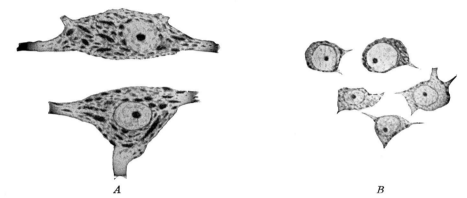

A   B

FIGURE 179.   Two types of motor nerve cells from medulla oblongata of lemur: *A*, Cells of the somatic motor type from the hypoglossal nucleus; *B*, cells of the visceral efferent type from the rostral part of the dorsal motor nucleus of the vagus. Toluidine blue stain. (Malone.)

There are relatively few myelinated sensory collaterals reaching the dorsal motor nucleus, and these come in large part from sensory fibers of the second order, arising in the receptive nuclei of the trigeminal, glossopharyngeal, and vagus nerves.

The **nucleus salivatorius** is located in the reticular formation at the junction of the pons and medulla oblongata. The exact location of this nucleus is unknown and its representation in Figs. 174 and 176 is to be regarded as purely diagrammatic. The more caudal portion, or *nucleus salivatorius inferior*, sends general visceral efferent fibers by way of the *glossopharyngeal nerve* to the otic ganglion for the innervation of the *parotid gland*. The rostral part, or *nucleus salivatorius superior*, sends general visceral efferent fibers to the facial nerve. These run from the facial nerve through the *chorda tympani* to the submaxillary ganglion for the innervation of the *submaxillary* and *sublingual salivary glands*.

The **Edinger-Westphal nucleus** is a group of relatively small nerve cells located in the rostral part of the nucleus of the oculomotor nerve. Here it is placed dorsolateral to the median unpaired portion of that nucleus (Figs. 174–176). This group of small cells has been said to give origin to the general visceral efferent fibers of the *oculomotor nerve* which run to the ciliary ganglion for the innervation of the *intrinsic muscles of the eye*. The Edinger-Westphal nucleus begins at about the middle of the oculomotor complex and is situated medial to the dorsal border of the lateral nucleus (Fig. 175, *EW*). It can be traced rostrally in this position and then ventrally around the rostral end of the lateral nucleus to form a ventrodorsally directed column of cells which has been called the anterior medial nucleus (*AM*). This has the same structure as the Edinger-Westphal nucleus proper and is considered to be a part of the latter (Brouwer, 1918). The two nuclei are continuous one with the other and both are com-

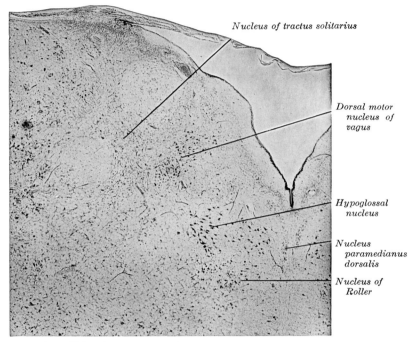

FIGURE 180.   Nuclei in the floor of the fourth ventricle. Cresyl violet.

posed of oval or fusiform cells of the general visceral efferent type. It has been suggested that the preganglionic outflow to the ciliary ganglion does not arise from the Edinger-Westphal nucleus but from some other cell group in that neighborhood. (Benjamin, 1939; White and Smithwick, 1941).

Szentágothai suggested that the preganglionic neurons are within the oculomotor nucleus and that the midline nuclei are not the visceral efferent ones. But Bender and Weinstein found definite pupillary constriction from stimulation of cells at the rostral end of the oculomotor nucleus corresponding to the general position of the nucleus of Edinger-Westphal.

Neurobiotaxis. The position of the motor nuclei of the brain stem varies greatly in different orders of vertebrates, and is determined by the source of the principal afferent impulses which reach them. The cell bodies of neurons are said to migrate in the direction of the chief fiber tracts from which they receive impulses (Ariëns Kappers, 1914, 1917; Black, 1917). This orientation

longitudinal bundles from which collaterals are given off to the motor nuclei of the brain stem (Fig. 184). There are at least two such longitudinal bundles in each lateral half of the brain. The *ventral secondary afferent path of the trigeminal nerve* consists for the most part of crossed fibers and is located in the ventral part of the reticular formation, close to the spinothalamic tract in the medulla, and dorsal to the medial lemniscus in the pons and mesencephalon (Fig. 185). It is composed in large part of long fibers which reach the thalamus. The *dorsal secondary afferent path of the trigeminal nerve* consists chiefly of uncrossed fibers and lies not far from the floor of the fourth ventricle and the central gray matter of the cerebral aqueduct. It consists in considerable part of short fibers (Cajal, 1911; Wallenberg, 1905; Economo, 1911;

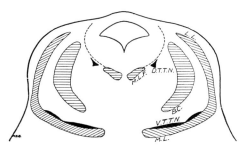

FIGURE 185.   Diagram to show the location of the secondary sensory tracts of the trigeminal nerve (solid black) in the tegmental portion of the rostral part of the pons: *B.C.*, Brachium conjunctivum; *D.T.T.N.*, dorsal secondary sensory tract of the trigeminal nerve; *L.L.*, lateral lemniscus; *M.L.*, medial lemniscus; *M.L.F.*, medial longitudinal fasciculus; *V.T.T.N.*, ventral secondary sensory tract of trigeminal nerve.

Déjerine, 1914). The uncrossed trigeminothalamic pathway has been found to arise from cells in the dorsomedial portions of the main sensory trigeminal nucleus in the cat (Torvik, 1957).

The **proprioceptive nuclei** of the cranial nerves have to do with afferent impulses arising in the muscles of mastication and in the extrinsic muscles of the eye. The *mesencephalic nucleus* of the fifth nerve contains large unipolar cells of the sensory type (Fig. 82, *C*). Fibers arising from this nucleus run through the mesencephalic root to join the motor root of the trigeminal nerve (Fig. 184) and are distributed chiefly to the muscles of mastication. Some also go to the teeth and palate. They are afferent fibers concerned in the reflex control of mastication (Corbin, 1940; Corbin and Harrison, 1940). The mesencephalic nucleus presents an exception to the rule that the afferent fibers of the cerebrospinal nerves take origin from cells located outside the cerebrospinal axis. This nucleus lies in the lateral wall of the rostral portion of the fourth ventricle and in the lateral part of the gray matter surrounding the cerebral aqueduct (Figs. 174, 183, 346–360). Cells of the mesencephalic nucleus become mingled with fibers of the trochlear nerve at its decussation, and fibers of the mesencephalic root which extend into the cerebellum have a few of the mesencephalic cells among them, a situation reminiscent of lower forms. Cells of the mesencephalic nucleus of the fifth nerve may have other than proprioceptive function. They vary in size and appearance (Sheinin, 1930; Pearson, 1949).

The origin of the afferent fibers for the extrinsic muscles of the eye is unknown, although we know that such afferent fibers are present in the oculomotor, trochlear, and abducens nerves.

If, as Corbin suggests, the cells of origin are mingled with the cells of the motor nuclei this would form an interesting exception to the usual pattern of distribution of sensory and motor cells in parts derived from alar and basal laminae. Tozer and Sherrington found that the sensory fibers supplying the extrinsic ocular muscles degenerate along with their neuromuscular and neuro-tendinous endings after section of the oculomotor, trochlear, and abducens nerves. Clumps of ganglion cells have been found along the course of these nerves, but their number is inconstant and it is not certain that they give origin to proprioceptive fibers. Perhaps these come from the mesencephalic nucleus of the fifth nerve or some other similar nucleus in the brain stem. The cells in the mesencephalic nucleus of the trigeminal have in Nissl preparations an appearance very similar to that of the cells of the spinal ganglia, but the cells found scattered along the third, fourth, and sixth nerves have quite a different arrangement of Nissl granules (Clark, 1926). On the other hand the proprioceptive terminations within the extrinsic muscles of the eye are much simpler than the usual muscle spindle, though they are distributed more widely through the muscles.

SPECIAL SOMATIC AFFERENT NUCLEI

The special somatic afferent nuclei are associated with the stato-acoustic nerve, which is composed of two divisions. One part, the *cochlear nerve,* conveys impulses aroused by sound waves reaching the cochlea through the outer ear and tympanic cavity. Since it responds to stimuli from without, the cochlear apparatus subserves *exteroceptive* functions. The *vestibular nerve,* on the other hand, conveys impulses from the semicircular canals of the ear. These are important *proprioceptive* sense organs and give information concerning the movements and posture of the head. Though termed proprioceptive, the receptors of vestibular apparatus resemble in fundamental histology those of the auditory division of the ear and the lateral line system of lower forms; that is, each of these receptors has a specialized epithelium with hair cells in contact with a fluid through which pressure waves are transmitted. The range of sensitivity in these is of interest. The vestibular apparatus responds to gross movements of the head. The lateral line organs respond to frequencies as low as 6 per second, and so respond to waves caused by movement of the fish itself, thus aiding it when these are reflected from other objects to find its way around in the dark. The cochlea is not sensitive to frequencies as low as these but in man audible sounds range from around 14 to 20,000 cycles per second. However, in the bat much higher frequencies are perceived and utilized to guide the nocturnal animal, which emits supersonic squeaks that are reflected from nearby objects. The ear and lateral line organs were successful forerunners of radar.

The **cochlear nuclei** are the terminal nuclei of the cochlear nerve, the fibers of which take origin in the *spiral ganglion of the cochlea.* This is composed of bipolar cells, each having a short peripheral and a longer central process (Fig. 186). The peripheral process terminates in the *spiral organ* of Corti. The central process is directed toward the brain in the cochlear nerve. These central fibers terminate in two masses of gray matter, located on the restiform body near the point where the latter turns dorsally into the cerebellum (Figs. 162, 183, 328–336). One of these masses, the *dorsal cochlear nucleus,* is placed on the dorsolateral aspect of the restiform body and produces a prominent elevation on the surface of the brain (Fig. 32). The other, known as the *ventral cochlear nucleus,* is in contact with the ventrolateral aspect of the restiform body.

Within the spiral organ of Corti a definite gradation of sensitivity to different frequencies of sound occurs, the higher pitched sounds being received in the more basal turns of the cochlear duct, the lower tones in that portion nearer the apex. Specific frequencies are detected by localized parts of the organ

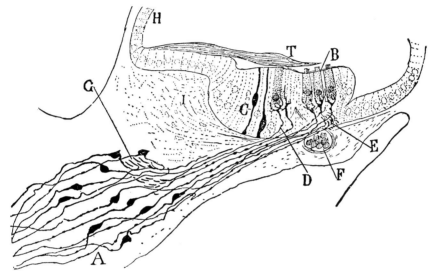

FIGURE 186. Section of the spiral ganglion and organ of Corti of the mouse: *A,* Bipolar cells of the spiral ganglion; *B,* outer hair cells; *C,* sustentacular cells; *D,* terminal arborization of the peripheral branch of a bipolar cell about an inner hair cell; *T,* tectorial membrane. Golgi method. (Cajal.)

of Corti, and so transmitted by different groups of axons. When electrical recording is done from the eighth nerve or the auditory paths in the brain, the sounds introduced in the ear can be reproduced within limits by amplification of the nerve impulses detected in the neural paths. It can be readily seen, however, that since it requires at least half a thousandth of a second for a nerve fiber to recover from the passage of one impulse sufficiently to be ready to transmit another, frequencies much greater than a thousand per second cannot be transmitted by a single nerve fiber. It is supposed that groups of nerve fibers take part in the transmission of sounds of high frequency, successive vibrations activating members of the group in rotation, thus allowing time for recovery. The center receiving the impulses has the responsibility for interpretation. Rasmussen (1950, 1953) has traced efferent fibers from the superior olivary nucleus of the opposite side to cochlear ganglion and organ of Corti, where they run as internal spiral fibers. Their function is unknown, but it was suggested by Herrick (1948) that these may be involved in efferent discharge to a receptor that has been excited by peripheral stimulus.

Secondary Auditory Path.   Experimental studies of the auditory pathway in the monkey show that three bundles of fibers extend from the cochlear nuclei toward the opposite side. From the dorsal cochlear nucleus a dorsally placed stria runs beneath the floor of the fourth ventricle below the level of the medial longitudinal fasciculus. From cells of the ventral cochlear nucleus an intermediate stria extends over the restiform body and transversely through the reticular formation, and a more conspicuous bundle known as the *trapezoid*

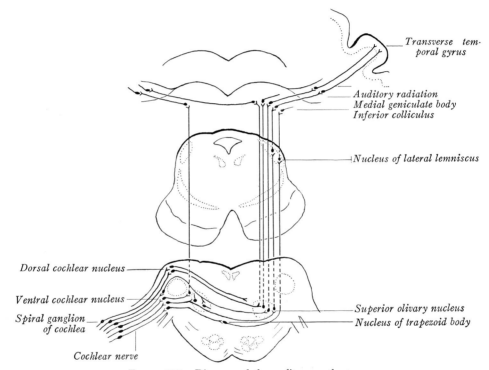

FIGURE 187.   Diagram of the auditory pathway.

body runs ventral to the restiform body and medialward in the ventral part of the pars dorsalis pontis (Figs. 163, 187). On reaching the lateral border of the opposite superior olivary nucleus, the fibers turn rostrally as a compact bundle known as the *lateral lemniscus* (Figs. 164, 166, 168).

Mingled with the fibers of the trapezoid body are nerve cells constituting nuclei, which receive fibers from the contralateral cochlear nuclei that end in synapses formed like a calyx. Many fibers from the cochlear nuclei of each side reach each *superior olivary nucleus.* The lateral part of each superior olive sends fibers upward by way of the lateral lemniscus of both sides, the medial part projects upward homolaterally, but the cells of this part receive impulses from both ears (Stotler, 1953). On reaching the mesencephalon many fibers of the lateral lemniscus terminate in the inferior colliculus; others extend to the medial geniculate body, a few of which were contributed by the homolateral superior olivary nucleus. From the medial geniculate body fibers arise which pass to the cerebral cortex. A homolateral acoustic pathway is provided by connection of fibers from the cochlear nuclei to the homolateral superior olivary nuclei and thence to the homolateral inferior colliculus. While there are fibers crossing at the inferior colliculus, these are probably for integration of activity at this level (Barnes, Magoun, and Ranson, 1943; Ades and Brookhart, 1950).

The **vestibular apparatus** consists of the three semicircular canals, the sacculus and the utriculus. At each end the canals join the utriculus. The sacculus is also connected with the utriculus and with the auditory portion of the membranous labyrinth of the internal ear, the cochlear duct. Within the ampulla on each semicircular canal is a small patch of hair cells (crista acustica) related to peripheral endings of divisions of the vestibular nerve. A similar but larger patch of hair cells (macula acustica) occurs in the utricle and in the saccule.

Stimulation of one of these specialized endings by alteration of the position of the head (or by mechanical direct stimuli) results in changes in the tone of muscles of the body and limbs in such a way as to adjust the body position, the general pattern of adjustment being such that it would tend to restore the body to proper orientation with the force of gravity. Similar shifts in the tension of muscles occur when the body of an animal is pushed out of its normal position, or rotated in some plane. The movements altering the posture in response to the changed position are termed compensatory.

When an animal is rotated slowly, the eyes tend to maintain their fixation on the original field and so deviate in the direction opposite to that of rotation. When their limit of deviation is reached, the eyes quickly move back to the other extreme, fix on an object in the field of vision and deviate again in the slow movement. This is termed nystagmus. If the body is rotated more rapidly the eyes may stay fixed in extreme deviation during rotation, but, when rotation ceases, there follows a series of eye movements (after-nystagmus) opposite in character to the original ones. That is, the eyes behave as if the body were slowly rotating in the opposite direction from that just experienced. Though not the primary movement, the nystagmus receives its name (right, left, up, or down) from the direction of the quick component.

Impulses apparently pass constantly along the vestibular nerve from individual semicircular canals, even in the resting condition. Canals on opposite sides reinforce the activity of each other. When an animal is rotated in the plane of the horizontal canal, there is a facilitation of the impulses discharged when rotation is toward the side from which the recording is made, and inhibition of impulses when rotation is in the opposite direction. According to Szentágothai (1950), there appears to be a functional relation between a given crista and two of the extraocular muscles. The crista of the superior canal is especially related to the superior rectus muscle of the homolateral eye and the inferior oblique of the contralateral eye; the crista of the posterior canal is related to the homolateral superior oblique and the contralateral inferior rectus; the crista of the horizontal canal to the homolateral medial rectus and the contralateral lateral rectus. The reflex pathway between the crista and the primary motor neuron to the eye muscle is said to be made of three neurons, and involves the medial longitudinal fasciculus.

The Vestibular Nuclei. The fibers of the vestibular nerve take origin from the bipolar cells of the *vestibular ganglion* located in the internal auditory

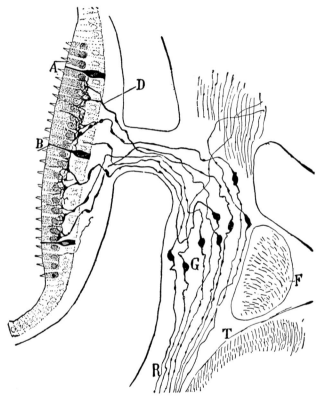

FIGURE 188. The vestibular ganglion and the termination of the peripheral branches of its bipolar cells in a macula acustica: *A*, Hair cells and *B*, sustentacular cells of the macula; *D*, terminal arborization of the peripheral branches of the bipolar cells of the vestibular ganglion (*G*) about the hair cells of the macula; *F*, facial nerve; *R*, central branches of the bipolar cells directed toward the medulla oblongata, *T*. Mouse. Golgi method. (Cajal.)

meatus (Fig. 188). The cochlear and vestibular divisions of the acoustic nerve separate at the ventral border of the restiform body. Here the vestibular nerve penetrates into the brain, passing between the restiform body and the spinal tract of the trigeminal nerve toward the vestibular area of the rhomboid fossa. Under cover of the vestibular area the fibers divide into short ascending and longer descending branches (Fig. 189). There may be enumerated five cellular masses within which these fibers terminate, namely: (1) the *medial* or *principal nucleus*, (2) the *descending* or *spinal nucleus*, (3) the *superior nucleus* of Bechterew, (4) the *lateral nucleus* of Deiters, and (5) the *cerebellum* (Figs. 183, 189).

The *medial, principal,* or dorsal *vestibular nucleus* is very large. It lies subjacent to the major portion of the vestibular area and belongs, therefore, to both the pons and the medulla oblongata (Figs. 33, 159, 162, 324–335). It can be followed in serial sections as far as the rostral extremity of the nucleus gracilis. The gray matter, associated with the descending branches from the vestibular nerve, lies on the medial side of the inferior cerebellar peduncle, and constitutes the *spinal* or descending *vestibular nucleus* (Figs. 308, 311, 332). The *lateral*

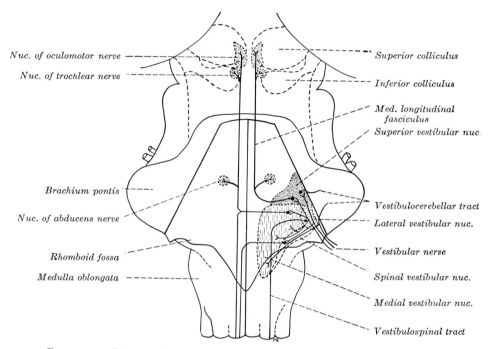

Nuc. of oculomotor nerve

Nuc. of trochlear nerve

Brachium pontis

Nuc. of abducens nerve

Rhomboid fossa

Medulla oblongata

Superior colliculus

Inferior colliculus

Med. longitudinal fasciculus

Superior vestibular nuc.

Vestibulocerebellar tract

Lateral vestibular nuc.

Vestibular nerve

Spinal vestibular nuc.

Medial vestibular nuc.

Vestibulospinal tract

FIGURE 189.   Diagram of the nuclei and central connections of the vestibular nerve.

vestibular nucleus of Deiters is situated along the course of the vestibular nerve within the pons and also at the point where the vestibular nerve fibers begin to branch close to the inferior cerebellar peduncle (Figs. 162, 335–340). It is composed of large multipolar cells. Directly continuous with the medial and lateral nuclei is a mass of medium-sized cells, the *superior vestibular nucleus* of Bechterew, located in the floor and lateral wall of the fourth ventricle at the level of the abducens nucleus and extending rostrally as far as the caudal border of the main sensory nucleus of the trigeminal nerve (Figs. 163, 339–346) (Weed, 1914).

Some of the ascending branches of the vestibular nerve run to the cerebellum. These are joined by cerebellipetal fibers arising in the superior vestibular nucleus and probably also by some from the lateral vestibular nucleus. Together these ascending fibers form the *vestibulocerebellar fasciculus* which lies on the medial side of the inferior cerebellar peduncle ((Figs. 163, 189).

Secondary Vestibular Paths. Besides the fibers to the cerebellum mentioned in the preceding paragraph two important tracts of fibers take origin in the vestibular nuclei. One of these was encountered in the study of the *medial longitudinal bundle.* Cells in the superior, spinal, and medial vestibular nuclei give rise to fibers which run to the medial longitudinal fascicle, and through it reach the motor nuclei of the ocular muscles (Fig. 189). In this way there is established an arc, which makes possible the reflex response of the eye muscles to afferent impulses arising in the vestibule and semicircular canals of the ear. The other bundle was considered in connection with the spinal cord as the *vestibulospinal tract,* the fibers of which take origin from the cells of the lateral nucleus and descend into the anterior funiculus of the same side of the cord. These fibers serve to place the primary motor neurons of the spinal cord under the reflex control of the vestibular apparatus. No tract to the thalamus is known. However, Aronson precipitated seizures in animals by whirling after painting the cerebral cortex with strychnine in an area near the lateral fissure which by other evidence received vestibular impulses, and cortical representation of the vestibular apparatus has been demonstrated in the cat.

The course of the secondary vestibular fibers in the medial longitudinal fasciculus has been investigated by Gray (1926), Rasmussen (1932), and Buchanan (1937) with results which are on the whole concordant. Figure 189 presents the origin and course of those fibers concerning which at least two of these authors are in agreement. From the superior vestibular nucleus fibers ascend in the fasciculus of the same side. From the medial nucleus fibers cross the midline and divide into ascending and descending branches in the fasciculus of the opposite side. From the descending nucleus, fibers cross and run downward in the opposite fasciculus.

THE VISUAL APPARATUS

While the eye develops as an evagination of the diencephalon and the optic nerve has the same embryonic origin and mature histologic structure as a pathway of the central nervous system, it is customary to refer to the optic nerve as a cranial nerve. It, however, contains the axons of the third neuron in the visual path counting the receptive elements, the rod and cones, as the primary afferent neurons. According to Bruesch and Arey (1942), 38 per cent of all the fibers entering or leaving the central nervous system are in the optic nerve. In man the optic nerve contains a million fibers which are all myelinated, though unmyelinated fibers are numerous in the optic nerve of lower forms and even of some mammals. The ratio of ganglion cells of the retina to optic nerve fibers is one to one.

The **retina** presents for consideration three layers of superimposed nervous elements: (1) the visual cells, (2) the bipolar cells, and (3) the ganglion cells (Fig. 190). These, with some horizontally arranged association neurons and supporting elements, form the nervous portion of the retina and are derived from the inner layer of the optic cup. The pigmented stratum of the retina is derived from the outer layer of the cup.

The *visual cells* are bipolar elements, whose perikarya are located in the *outer nuclear layer* (Fig. 190). Each presents an external process in the form of a *rod* or *cone,* so differentiated as to respond to photic stimulation and thus to serve as a visual receptor. The other process terminates in the *outer molecular layer* in relation to processes from the *bipolar cells.* These latter elements have their perikarya in the *inner nuclear layer* and branches in the inner and outer molecular layers. The *ganglion cells* send their denrites into the *inner molecular layer,* where they are related to the inner branches of the bipolar cells, while the axons form the innermost stratum of the retina, the *stratum opticum,* through which they enter the optic nerve. The nerve also contains some efferent fibers which terminate in the retina (Arey, 1916). It will be apparent from Fig. 190 that the visual cells are the receptors and neurons of the first order in the optic path. The impulses are transmitted through the bipolar cells to the ganglion cells, whose axons, in turn, carry them by way of the optic nerves to the superior colliculus, pretectal region, and lateral geniculate body. The

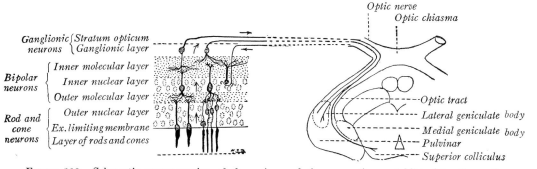

FIGURE 190.   Schematic representation of the retina and the connections established by the optic nerve fibers.

rods are more sensitive to low intensities of light and serve in twilight vision. When the light is adequate the cones are the more efficient receptors. They are responsible for sharp vision and for color discrimination. The cones alone are present in the fovea where vision is the sharpest and sensibility to color at the maximum. The part of the retina responsible for central vision is the macula lutea. It is located a little to the temporal side of the posterior pole.

Within the retina the details of connections of neurons, as worked out minutely by Polyak (1941), show a variety of relationship of the rod and cone receptor units to the bipolar cells and the latter to the ganglion cells. While there are single synaptic relations between some cones and bipolar units, several rods may synapse with one bipolar cell, and in some instances both rods and cones synapse with the same bipolar cell. The original work should be consulted for details. The significant point is made that the connections allow means of intensifying the original stimuli, as well as minute accuracy in the visual patterns.

Numerical relationships of rods and cones to fibers of the optic nerve become interesting in relation to the way the retina functions. In the human optic nerve there are about one million nerve fibers, the processes of the ganglion cells of the retina, which must carry all the visual information to the brain. But there are a million cones and about 37 million rods which supply them with stimuli.

By careful measurements and appropriate calculations, Hecht (1944) has been able to state that as few as five to eight quanta of light can activate the retina, with this amount acting over an area containing as many as 500 rods. It appears probable from the photochemical equivalent theory that one quantum acts upon one rod, and the necessity for 5 to 8 rods being activated must lie in central interpretation, that many impulses being received from a small area being more than the brain might accept as random phenomena without retinal stimulation.

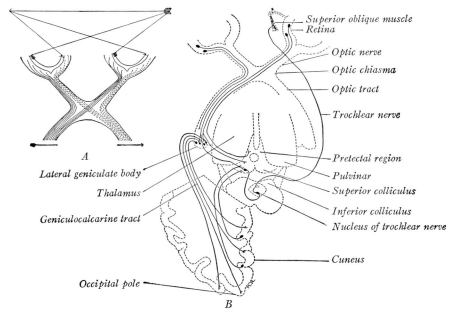

FIGURE 191.   *A*, Diagram showing why destruction of one optic tract causes blindness in both eyes for the opposite lateral half of the field of vision. *B*, Schematic representation of the optic pathways.

The Optic Chiasma and Optic Tracts.   The optic nerve emerges from the bulbus oculi at the nasal side of the posterior pole and, after entering the cranium through the optic foramen, unites with its fellow of the opposite side to form the optic chiasma, in which a partial decussation of the fibers takes place (Fig. 191). Beyond the decussation fibers from both retinae are continued in each of the optic tracts. In the chiasma the fibers from the two optic nerves are so distributed that each tract receives the fibers from the lateral half of the retina of its own side and those from the medial half of the opposite retina. The optic tract partially encircles the cerebral peduncle and runs to the *lateral geniculate body,* the *pretectal region,* and to the *superior colliculus* of the corpora quadrigemina (Barris, Ingram, and Ranson, 1935).

The ventral and dorsal supraoptic decussations are bundles of fibers which ascend from the brain stem and which cross the midline in close relation to the dorsal border of the optic chiasma to reach various parts of the forebrain and midbrain of the opposite side. It is now well established that the commissure of Gudden, which was supposed to unite the two medial geniculate bodies, does not exist (Magoun and Ranson, 1942).

Bishop and O'Leary (1940) point out that the larger fibers in the optic nerve go to the lateral geniculate body relaying impulses to the cortex; and that because of the difference in size, and so the speed of transmission of impulses, there would be time for visual impulses to reach the cortex and be relayed to midbrain centers by corticotectal fibers before the slower travelling impulses over smaller fibers reach the midbrain directly from the retina.

The *pretectal region* is the zone of transition between the thalamus and tectum. It is situated lateral to the posterior commissure and rostral to the superior colliculus. The optic fibers which subserve the pupillary light reflex enter it and bilateral lesions of this part of the brain abolish the reflex (Ranson and Magoun, 1933; Magoun and Ranson, 1935). The *superior colliculus* is not concerned with pupillary reactions but is responsible for somatic optic reflexes, such as movements of the head and eyes in response to visual, auditory, and exteroceptive stimuli. Here, however, visual connections are dominant.

Certain topographic relationships are of interest in the optic connections. The more rostral and medial parts of the superior colliculi are concerned with impulses arising from objects in the upper part of the visual fields, the caudal and caudolateral portions with impulses from the lower part of the visual fields. Clinical cases of pineal tumor give evidence that the rostral portions of the superior colliculi are involved with upward conjugate movements of the eyes, a movement characteristic of response to stimuli in the upper fields of vision. Parts of the oculomotor nuclei are related rostrocaudally with corresponding regions of the superior colliculi.

The Geniculocalcarine Tract.   The lateral geniculate body receives impulses from the retina by way of the optic nerve and relays them to the cerebral cortex where they give rise to visual sensation. It is connected with the striate area or visual cortex (Fig. 259) by the geniculocalcarine tract. Many of the fibers of this bundle are at first directed forward and lateralward from the lateral geniculate body above the inferior horn of the lateral ventricle, and then, bending lateralward through the sublenticular part of the internal capsule and finally backward, they run through the external sagittal stratum of the temporal and occipital lobes to the striate area of the occipital cortex (Figs. 192, 399-401). The internal sagittal stratum was formerly thought to contain visual fibers and was often designated as the optic radiation, but it is now known that the geniculocalcarine fasciculus contains all of the visual fibers and that this bundle occupies the external sagittal stratum (Poliak, 1932; Barris, Ingram, and Ranson, 1935).

Hemianopsia.   The significance of the partial decussation in the chiasma is made clear by Figs. 191, 193. The properties of the refracting media of the eyes are such that images of objects to the right of the axis of vision are produced on the nasal side of the right retina and the temporal side of the left retina. And, because of the manner of decussation of the optic nerve fibers, impulses from both these sources reach the visual area of the left cortex. In the same way the visual cortex of the right side receives impressions from objects to the left of the axis of vision. That is to say, the sensory representation of the outer world in the cerebral cortex is contralateral in the case of sight just as it is in the case of cutaneous sensations. Furthermore, it will be evident that, while destruction of one optic nerve causes total blindness in the corresponding eye, destruction of one optic tract, lateral geniculate body, or geniculocalcarine fasciculus, or the visual cortex of one hemisphere, will produce blindness in both eyes for the opposite lateral half of the field of vision.

The course of impulses from the retinal quadrants to the visual cortex and their distribution within it is shown in Fig. 193. The left lateral geniculate

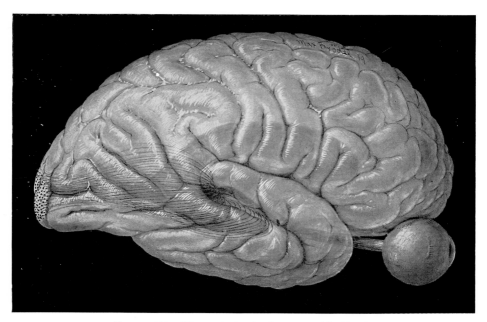

FIGURE 192.   The geniculocalcarine tract.   (Cushing.)

body is illustrated receiving fibers from the left sides of both retinae and sending fibers to the visual cortex of the left hemisphere. From the upper nasal quadrant of the right retina and the upper temporal quadrant of the left retina, fibers go to the medial part of the left lateral geniculate body and from there fibers go to the upper part of the left visual cortex. From the lower nasal quadrant of the right retina and the lower temporal quardrant of the left retina, fibers go to the lateral part of the left lateral genciculate body and from there fibers go to the lower part of the left visual cortex. These statements hold for the macular as well as the peripheral portions of the retinal quadrants. The fibers from the upper quadrants occupy the upper part of the cross-section of the optic nerve, but in passing through the optic chiasma they undergo a partial rotation so that within the optic tract they lie medially and inferiorly.

In the visual cortex and in the geniculocalcarine tract, as the fibers pass back through the temporal lobe and into the occipital lobe, the representation of the upper quadrants lies above that for the lower quadrants. The fibers from the maculae occupy central positions within the optic nerves and optic tracts. They end in the superior and posterior part of the lateral geniculate body, whence the impulses from the maculae are relayed to the posterior part of the visual cortex.

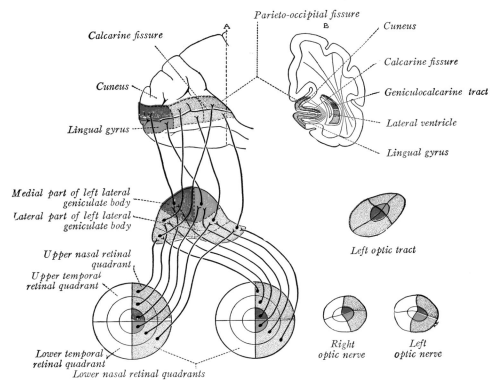

Figure 193.   Diagram of the optic pathway showing the course of visual impulses from the left halves of both retinae through the left lateral geniculate body to the visual cortex of the left hemisphere. *A,* Line representing plane along which section *B* was cut. (Redrawn after Rasmussen: The Principal Nervous Pathways. The Macmillan Company.)

SUMMARY OF THE ORIGIN, COMPOSITION, AND CONNECTIONS OF THE CRANIAL NERVES

The olfactory nerve, the nervus terminalis, and the vomeronasal nerve, which have not yet been considered in detail, have been included in this summary for the sake of completeness.

The **nervus terminalis** is a nerve which arises from the cerebral hemisphere in the region of the medial olfactory tract or stria. It is closely associated with the olfactory nerve and its fibers run to the nasal septum (Fig. 7). The origin, termination, and function of its component fibers are not yet understood (McKibben, 1911; Huber and Guild, 1913; McCotter, 1913; Johnston, 1914; Brookover, 1914, 1917; Larsell, 1918, 1919). Since it was unknown at the time the cranial nerves were first enumerated, it bears no numerical designation. The nervus terminalis has scattered ganglion cells along it and is considered to be related to vasomotor control in the region of the nasal septum supplied by it.

The nerve to the vomeronasal organ (Jacobson) is connected with the accessory olfactory bulb centrally, which in turn connects with the amygdaloid nucleus. Sinclair (1951) has described a ganglion of some size lying on the dura at the edge of the cribriform plate. The function of this is not known.

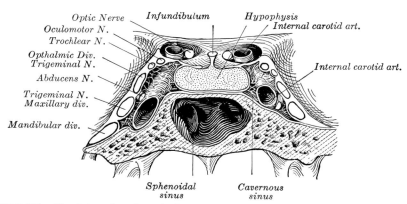

FIGURE 194. Frontal section through the hypophysis and cavernous sinus showing the relationships of five cranial nerves and the internal carotid artery to these structures. The carotid artery is surrounded in this part of its course by the cavernous sinus. (After Cunningham-Robinson.)

I. Olfactory Nerve. Superficial origin from the olfactory bulb in the form of a number of fine fila which separately pass through the openings in the cribriform plate. It is composed of special visceral afferent fibers with cells of origin in the olfactory mucous membrane. The fibers terminate in the glomeruli of the olfactory bulb.

II. Optic Nerve. Not a true nerve, but from the standpoint of both its structure and development, a fiber tract of the brain. Superficial origin, from the optic chiasma, or after partial decussation, from the lateral geniculate body, and superior colliculus. Component fibers; special somatic afferent— exteroceptive; origin, ganglion cells of the retina; terminations in the lateral geniculate body, and superior colliculus. The fibers from the nasal half of each retina cross in the optic chiasma.

It has been demonstrated by Arey that there are also efferent fibers in the optic nerves of fishes which control the movement of the retinal elements in response to light.

III. Oculomotor Nerve. Superficial origin from the oculomotor sulcus on the medial aspect of the cerebral peduncle. Composition:

1. SOMATIC EFFERENT FIBERS. Cells of origin in the oculomotor nucleus of the same and to a less extent of the opposite side (Fig. 173). Termination in the extrinsic muscles of the eye except the superior oblique and the lateral rectus.

2. GENERAL VISCERAL EFFERENT FIBERS. Cells of origin in the Edinger-Westphal nucleus. Termination in the ciliary ganglion, from the cells of which postganglionic fibers run to the intrinsic muscles of the eye.

3. GENERAL SOMATIC AFFERENT FIBERS. Proprioceptive fibers for the eye muscles.

IV. **Trochlear Nerve.** Superficial origin, from the anterior medullary velum. Composition (Fig. 173):

1. SOMATIC EFFERENT FIBERS. Cells of origin in the trochlear nucleus; decussation in the anterior medullary velum; termination in the superior oblique muscle of the eye.

2. GENERAL SOMATIC AFFERENT FIBERS. Proprioceptive fibers for the superior oblique muscle.

V. **Trigeminal Nerve.** Superficial origin from the lateral aspect of the middle of the pons by two roots: the portio major or sensory root and the portio minor or motor root. Composition (Fig. 173):

1. GENERAL SOMATIC AFFERENT FIBERS. A, Exteroceptive: Cells of origin in the semilunar ganglion (Gasserii), chiefly unipolar with T-shaped axons, peripheral branches to skin and mucous membrane of the head, central branches by way of the portio major to the brain. Termination in the main sensory nucleus and nucleus of the spinal tract of the trigeminal nerve.

2. GENERAL SOMATIC AFFERENT FIBERS. B, Proprioceptive: Cells of origin probably located in the mesencephalic nucleus of the fifth nerve. Fibers by way of the portio minor, distributed as sensory fibers to the muscles of mastication.

3. SPECIAL VISCERAL EFFERENT FIBERS. Cells of origin in the motor nucleus of the fifth nerve. Fibers by way of the portio minor and the mandibular nerve to the muscles of mastication.

VI. **Abducens Nerve.** Superficial origin from the lower border of the pons just rostral to the pyramid. Composition:

1. SOMATIC EFFERENT FIBERS. Cells of origin in the abducens nucleus; termination in the lateral rectus muscle of the eye.

2. GENERAL SOMATIC AFFERENT FIBERS. Proprioceptive fibers for the lateral rectus muscle.

VII. **Facial Nerve and Nervus Intermedius.** Superficial origin from the lateral part of the lower border of the pons separated from the flocculus by the eighth nerve. Composition (Fig. 173):

1. GENERAL VISCERAL AFFERENT FIBERS. Cells of origin in the ganglion geniculi. The peripheral branches run through the branches of the facial nerve, supplying deep sensibility to the face. The central branches run by way of the nervus intermedius to the tractus solitarius and end in the nucleus of that tract, or perhaps they enter the spinal tract of the trigeminal and end in its nucleus. In the latter case it would be proper to question their classification as visceral.

2. SPECIAL VISCERAL AFFERENT FIBERS. Cells of origin in the ganglion geniculi. The peripheral branches run by way of the chorda tympani and lingual nerves to the taste buds of the anterior two-thirds of the tongue. The

central branches run by way of the nervus intermedius to the tractus solitarius and end in the nucleus of that tract. It is probable that the taste fibers terminate in the rostral part of this nucleus.

3. GENERAL VISCERAL EFFERENT FIBERS. Cells of origin in the nucleus salivatorius superior. These fibers run by way of the nervus intermedius, facial nerve, chorda tympani, and lingual nerve to the submaxillary ganglion for the innervation of the submaxillary and sublingual salivary glands.

4. SPECIAL VISCERAL EFFERENT FIBERS. Cells of origin in the motor nucleus of the facial nerve. These fibers run by way of the facial nerve to end in the superficial musculature of the face and scalp, and in the platysma, posterior belly of the digastric, and stylohyoid muscles.

VIII. **Stato-acoustic Nerve.** Superficial origin from the lateral part of the lower border of the pons near the flocculus. Consists of two separate parts known as the vestibular and cochlear nerves.

The Vestibular Nerve. The component fibers belong to the *special somatic afferent* group and are proprioceptive. Cells of origin, in the vestibular ganglion, are bipolar. Their peripheral branches run to the semicircular canals, utricle, and saccule. Their central branches terminate in the medial, lateral, superior, and spinal vestibular nuclei. Some of them run without interruption to the cerebellum.

The Cochlear Nerve. The component fibers belong to the *special somatic afferent* group and are exteroceptive. Cells of origin, in the spiral ganglion of the cochlea, are bipolar. Their peripheral branches end in the spiral organ of Corti. Their central branches terminate in the ventral and dorsal cochlear nuclei.

IX. **The Glossopharyngeal Nerve.** Superficial origin, from the rostral end of the posterior lateral sulcus of the medulla oblongata in line with the tenth and eleventh nerves. Composition (Fig. 173):

1. GENERAL VISCERAL AFFERENT FIBERS. Cells of origin in the ganglion petrosum; peripheral branches form the general sensory fibers to the pharynx and posterior third of the tongue; central branches run to the tractus solitarius and its nucleus.

2. SPECIAL VISCERAL AFFERENT FIBERS. Cells of origin in the ganglion petrosum; peripheral branches to the taste buds of the posterior third of the tongue, central branches to the tractus solitarius and its nucleus.

3. GENERAL VISCERAL EFFERENT FIBERS. Cells of origin in the inferior salivatory nucleus; fibers run to the otic ganglion, from the cells of which post-ganglionic fibers carry the impulses to the parotid gland.

4. SPECIAL VISCERAL EFFERENT FIBERS. Cells of origin in the nucleus ambiguus. Termination in the stylopharyngeus muscle.

X. **Vagus Nerve.** Superficial origin from the rostral part of the posterior lateral sulcus of the medulla oblongata in line with the ninth and eleventh and just caudal to the ninth. Composition (Fig. 173):

1. GENERAL SOMATIC AFFERENT FIBERS. Cells of origin in the ganglion jugulare; peripheral branches to the skin of the external ear by way of the **ramus auricularis**; central branches to the spinal tract of the trigeminal nerve

and its nucleus. According to Herrick, some of the fibers from the external ear run by way of the glossopharyngeal nerve also.

2. GENERAL VISCERAL AFFERENT FIBERS. Cells of origin in the ganglion nodosum; peripheral branches run as sensory fibers to the pharynx, larynx, trachea, esophagus, and the thoracic and abdominal viscera; central branches run to the tractus solitarius and terminate in its nucleus.

3. SPECIAL VISCERAL AFFERENT FIBERS. Cells of origin in the ganglion nodosum; peripheral branches to the taste buds of the epiglottis probably by way of the internal laryngeal nerve; central branches run to the tractus solitarius and terminate in its nucleus.

4. GENERAL VISCERAL EFFERENT FIBERS. Cells of origin in the dorsal motor nucleus of the vagus. Fibers run to the autonomic ganglia of the vagal plexuses for the innervation of the thoracic and abdominal viscera.

5. SPECIAL VISCERAL EFFERENT FIBERS. Cells of origin in the nucleus ambiguus. Termination in the striated musculature of the pharynx and larynx.

It will be noted that the facial, glossopharyngeal, and vagus nerves each contain general and special visceral afferent and general and special visceral efferent fibers.

XI. **Accessory Nerve.** Superficial origin from the posterior lateral sulcus of the medulla oblongata caudal to the ninth and tenth and from the lateral aspect of the first five or six cervical segments of the spinal cord. Composition (Fig. 173):

1. GENERAL VISCERAL EFFERENT FIBERS. Cells of origin in the dorsal motor nucleus of the vagus. Fibers run in the bulbar rootlets and then by way of the internal ramus of the accessory to join the vagus, and end in the autonomic plexuses, associated with the vagus nerve, for the innervation of thoracic and abdominal viscera.

2. SPECIAL VISCERAL EFFERENT FIBERS. These fall into two groups: A, fibers whose cells of origin are located in the nucleus ambiguus, and which run by way of the internal ramus of the accessory to join the vagus and are distributed through it to the striated muscles of the pharynx and larynx; B, fibers whose cells of origin lie in the lateral part of the anterior gray column of the first five or six cervical segments of the spinal cord, and which ascend in the spinal root of the accessory nerve and then run in its external ramus to end in the trapezius and the sternocleidomastoid muscles.

XII. **Hypoglossal Nerve.** Superficial origin from the anterior lateral sulcus of the medulla between the pyramid and the olive. It is composed of somatic efferent fibers, whose cells of origin are located in the hypoglossal nucleus and whose termination is in the musculature of the tongue. According to Langworthy (1924), this nerve also carries the proprioceptive fibers for the tongue. Scattered cells having the shape of sensory neurons occur along the hypoglossal nerve fibers within the medulla, and in the embryo a ganglion (Froriep) lies on a kind of dorsal root to the hypoglossal. This ganglion at times persists in the adult in lower forms, but it is not sufficiently constant to account for all the proprioceptive fibers to the tongue (Pearson, 1945).

CHAPTER XIV

The Cerebellum

The cerebellum, like the other specialized accumulations of neurons, the tectum and the cerebral cortex, is applied to the main axis of the central nervous system as a suprasegmental structure. It receives great bundles of afferent fibers bringing impulses to it from spinal cord, medulla, pons, mesencephalon, and cerebrum, and from its central nuclei pass efferent fibers to each of these regions. Newer knowledge of cerebellar connections in higher vertebrates, which is accumulating rapidly, is emphasizing that many afferent paths other than those from proprioceptive endings and vestibular apparatus reach the cerebellum, a fact long recognized in lower forms. The full significance of its many connections must await further investigation, although like other suprasegmental accumulations, the cerebellum must aid in modifying the response to stimulus at a segmental level based on whatever "information" there is available to it at the time from all sources.

The cerebellum is primarily concerned with synergy in the action of voluntary muscles, which implies widespread action at one time, since the mere shifting of the weight from one foot to the other necessitates adjustment of muscles in all parts of the body. This implies that proprioceptive information from the entire bodily musculature, as well as exteroceptive impulses giving details of the environment both near and at a distance, must be brought into use simultaneously by the cerebellum and that the action of the cerebral motor centers in setting off activity of voluntary muscles must be synchronized with the action of the cerebellum. The structure of the cerebellum should therefore allow for complete connection with sources of proprioceptive and other information throughout the body, equally intimate connection with higher centers in the cerebrum concerned with motion, and an internal mechanism for correlating all incoming influences and sending out properly integrated impulses to the entire bodily musculature at one time if necessary. There is evidence also of cerebellar influence upon certain visceral structures which are controlled by the action of smooth muscle.

Although complete answers to them are not available, the problem set in the study of the cerebellum can be expressed in the following questions, which incidentally arise in relation to most structures in the brain that may be under

274

scrutiny. What tracts bring impulses to the cerebellum from what sources? What tracts carry impulses from the cerebellum to what destinations? What is its internal structure, i. e., the connection of incoming and outgoing fibers? With what functions is the cerebellum concerned? Can local portions of the cerebellum be assigned specific responsibilities in its functioning?

In order to attempt even partial answers to these questions some details of structure are necessary, and as they are examined it is helpful to keep in mind that the key to functional principles is often found in the details of morphology.

Structure of the Cerebellum.   The cerebellum differs from the spinal cord in that the relative position of the gray and white matter is reversed. The gray substance forms a thin superficial layer, the *cerebellar cortex,* which covers a central white *medullary body* (corpus medullare). Originally the cerebellar plate

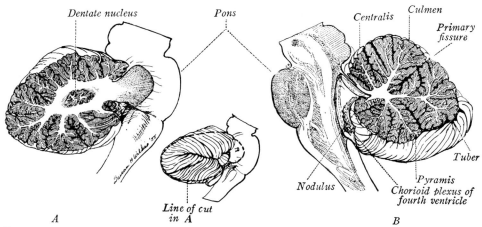

FIGURE 195.   Sagittal sections of the human cerebellum: *A,* Passes through the hemisphere and dentate nucleus; *B,* through the vermis in the median plane.

is formed, like other parts of the neural tube, of an ependymal, a nuclear or mantle, and a cell-free marginal zone. The neuroblasts of the *mantle zone* take only a small part in the formation of the cortex, but become grouped in the internal nuclear masses of the cerebellum. The superficial or *marginal zone* is at first devoid of nuclei; most of the neuroblasts, from which the cerebellar cortex is differentiated, migrate into this zone from the rhombic lip. These developing neurons send their axons inward instead of outward as in the case of the spinal cord. These axons accumulate, along with others which enter the cerebellum from without, in the deep part of the marginal layer and form the central medullary body of the cerebellum, separating the developing cortex from the deep nuclear masses that are differentiated from the mantle layer (Dowd, 1929).

As the mass of the cerebellum is attained in its growth, certain fissures appear which separate portions of the cortex into lobulations having functional significance. The first to appear is not the primary fissure but the *fissura postero-lateralis,* which separates the flocculonodular lobe from the rest of the cerebellum termed *corpus cerebelli.* The *fissura prima* next appears and divides the corpus cerebelli into anterior and posterior lobes. The further details of developmental change have been followed in several species and found to conform to a common pattern (Larsell, 1954).

The white medullary body forms a compact mass in the interior and is continuous from hemisphere to hemisphere through the vermis, within which, however, it is smaller than in the hemispheres (Fig. 195). As is most readily seen in sagittal sections through the cerebellum, the medullary body gives off numerous thick laminae, which project into the lobules of the cerebellum; from these there are given off secondary and tertiary laminae at various angles. Thus, a very irregular white mass is formed, over the surface of which the much folded

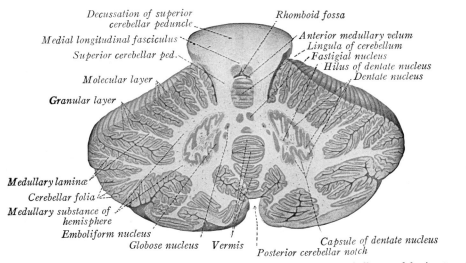

Decussation of superior
cerebellar peduncle
Medial longitudinal fasciculus
Superior cerebellar ped.
Molecular layer
Granular layer

Rhomboid fossa
Anterior medullary velum
Lingula of cerebellum
Fastigial nucleus
Hilus of dentate nucleus
Dentate nucleus

Medullary laminæ
Cerebellar folia
Medullary substance of
    hemisphere
Emboliform nucleus
    Globose nucleus   Vermis

Capsule of dentate nucleus
Posterior cerebellar notch

FIGURE 196. The cerebellar nuclei as seen in a section through the cerebellum and brain stem in a plane corresponding to the long axes of the brachia conjunctiva. (Sobotta-McMurrich.)

cortex is spread in a thin but even layer. Supported by the white laminae, the cortex forms long narrow folds, known as *folia,* which are separated by sulci and which are aggregated into lobules that, in turn, are separated by more or less deep fissures. Sections through the cerebellum at right angles to the long axis of the folia thus present an arborescent appearance to which the name *arbor vitae* has been applied. This is particularly evident in sections through the vermis.

The cerebellum has a thousand square centimeters of surface, only about one-sixth of which is exposed. As a general principle, all of the impulses coming to the cerebellum reach the cortex and the cortex in turn sends impulses to the central nuclei, which send impulses out of the cerebellum to the brain stem. An exception to this occurs in the case of a small part of the vestibular connections, some fibers from the vestibular nuclei are said to end in the fastigial nucleus, and a few fibers from the cortex are believed to reach vestibular nuclei directly.

The Nuclei of the Cerebellum. The *dentate nucleus* is a crumpled, purse-like lamina of gray matter within the massive medullary body of each cerebellar hemisphere (Figs. 196, 197). Like the inferior olivary nucleus, which it closely resembles, it has a white center and a medially placed hilus. In close relation to this hilus lies a plate of gray matter, the *emboliform nucleus,* and medial to this is the small *globose nucleus.* Close to the median plane in the white center of the vermis, where this forms the covering of the fourth ventricle, is the nu-

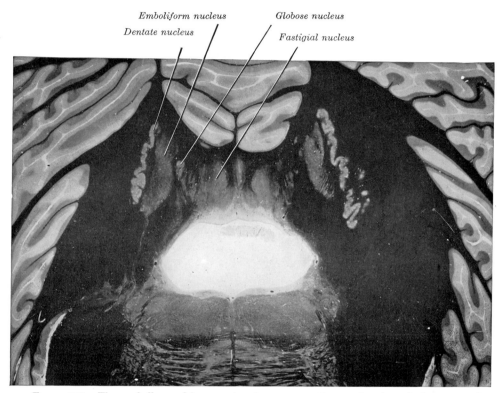

FIGURE 197. The cerebellar nuclei as seen in a transverse section passing through the pons at the level of the motor nucleus of the trigeminal nerve and through the cerebellum rostral to the main mass of the dentate nucleus.

cleus of the roof or *nucleus fastigii.* The fastigial nuclei like the other cerebellar nuclei are paired. They lie close together, one on either side of the midline.

The *dentate nucleus* receives fibers from the cortex of the neocerebellar part of the posterior lobe and also some fibers from the anterior lobe. From its large multipolar cells, fibers arise which run in the superior cerebellar peduncle to the red nucleus and to the lateral ventral nucleus of the thalamus. The *fastigial nucleus* receives fibers from the anterior lobe, pyramis, uvula, nodulus (paleocerebellum) and vestibular nuclei. It gives rise to the fastigiobulbar tract (Fig. 199). The *emboliform nucleus* receives fibers from both the paleocerebellum and the neocerebellum, and sends fibers by way of the brachium conjunctivum to the large-celled portion of the red nucleus. The *globose nucleus* receives fibers from the paleocerebellum and sends fibers by way of the brachium conjunctivum to the large-celled portion of the red nucleus (Fulton, 1938).

Fibers from the cerebellar nuclei reach the central gray matter adjacent to the ventricular lining of medulla, pons and midbrain; the nucleus of Darkschewitsch and the interstitial nucleus of the medial longitudinal fasciculus, and the inferior olivary nuclear complex (Rand, 1954).

The Cerebellar Peduncles. The white core of the cerebellum is formed in part by fibers which run from the cerebellar cortex to the nuclei and in part by fibers which enter and leave the cerebellum through its three peduncles.

The *middle cerebellar peduncle* is formed by the transverse fibers of the pons and carries impulses which come from the cerebral cortex of the opposite side. It enters the cerebellum on the lateral side of the other two peduncles. In man, as might be expected from the large size of the pons and cerebellar hemisphere, the middle is the largest of the three peduncles (Fig. 33).

The *inferior cerebellar peduncle* ascends along the lateral border of the fourth ventricle, and at a point just rostral to the lateral recess, it makes a sharp turn dorsally to enter the cerebellum between the other two peduncles (Figs. 32, 33). It consists of the following bundles of ascending fibers from the spinal cord and medulla oblongata: (1) the *dorsal spinocerebellar tract*, which arises from the cells of the nucleus dorsalis of the spinal cord and whose termination will be discussed in another paragraph; (2) the *olivocerebellar tract*, which consists of fibers from the opposite inferior olivary nucleus and to a less extent from that of the same side and which ends in the cortex of the vermis and of the hemisphere and in the central nuclei; (3) the *dorsal external arcuate fibers*, from the lateral cuneate nucleus of the same side, and (4) the *ventral external arcuate fibers* from the arcuate and lateral reticular nuclei and scattered cells of the reticular formation of the opposite side (Figs. 311–323).

The vestibulocerebellar fasciculus courses along the medial side of the inferior cerebellar peduncle as it turns dorsally into the cerebellum (Fig. 163). Some are secondary trigeminal fibers from the spinal nucleus of the fifth nerve, but most of them arise from the superior and lateral vestibular nuclei or represent the ascending branches of the fibers of the vestibular nerve.

The *superior cerebellar peduncle* (Fig. 32) consists of efferent fibers from the dentate, globose, and emboliform nuclei to the red nucleus and the thalamus of the opposite side. It is the smallest and most medial of the three peduncles. The *ventral spinocerebellar tract* enters the cerebellum in company with the superior peduncle. It ascends through the medulla oblongata and pons, curves over the superior peduncle (Fig. 164), and enters the anterior medullary velum, within which it runs to the cerebellum. A bundle of fibers, the *tectocerebellar tract,* arises in the tectum and descends in the anterior medullary velum alongside of the superior cerebellar peduncle to the cerebellum (Ogawa, 1937).

Afferent Cerebellar Tracts. Fibers from the vestibular nuclei and also direct fibers from the vestibular nerve reach the flocculonodular lobe, uvula, lingula, and the fastigial nuclei (Larsell, 1937; Dow, 1938). Fibers from the ventral spinocerebellar tract pass to a narrow zone near the midplane of each

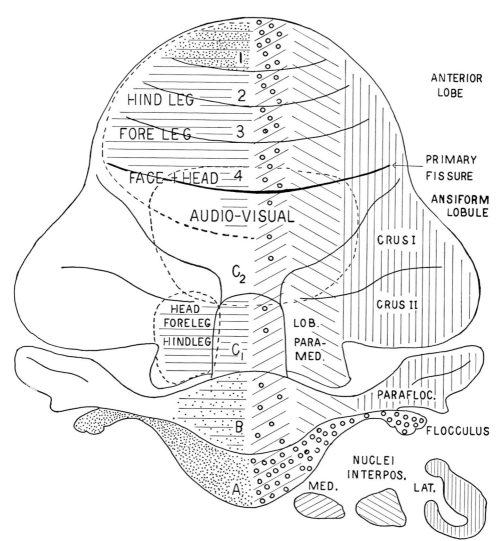

FIGURE 198. Generalized diagram of the cerebellum to show regional specialization as described from the work of various authors. On the right are represented the cerebellonuclear projections: small circles for projection to vestibular nuclei, oblique lines (/), next to midline, for projection to nucleus medialis (fastigii); oblique lines (\) for projection to nucleus interpositus (globose and emboliform); vertical lines for projection to nucleus lateralis (dentate). On the left side afferent connections are indicated: dots for vestibulocerebellar connections; horizontal lines for spinocerebellar connections; blank space for pontocerebellar projections but all other parts of the cortex except the flocculonodular lobe receive these. The lettering and numbering of midline structures is that of Bolk (cf. Figs. 38, 39).

portion of the anterior lobe and to lobulus simplex and pyramis of the posterior lobe. The fibers of the dorsal spinocerebellar tract overlap the distribution of the ventral but are distributed to the lateral parts of the vermis and to the lobulus paramedianus (Anderson, 1943). As determined by following degenerated fibers, each of the spinocerebellar paths carries fibers from both sides of the spinal cord, and those fibers conveying impulses from the region of the legs terminate in the same general region reached by those from head, neck, and arms. Spinocerebellar fibers from caudal segments of the cord which supply the tail in monkeys have been traced not only into the lingula but have been seen on each side of the secondary fissure heading toward paraflocculus (Chang and Ruch, 1949).

Recently the method of electrical recording following stimulation to peripheral receptors or other parts of the nervous system has yielded valuable information regarding connections (Dow, 1939; Adrian, 1944; Snider and Stowell, 1942; Snider and Eldred, 1952). Impulses can be picked up from the cerebellum after peripheral proprioceptive, tactile, auditory, and visual stimuli. The areas responding to cutaneous stimuli did not exactly correspond to the zones of distribution of spinocerebellar fibers (Fig. 198). Separate zones on each side in the anterior and posterior part of the cerebellum duplicated representation of the extremities with distinct overlapping from opposite sides of the body. In the anterior zone the head was represented about the primary fissure and lobulus simplex with foreleg next in sequence anteriorly and forward of that the hindleg areas of representation. In the region of the paramedian lobule, there was representation of face, arm, and leg in that order and in anteroposterior sequence, and bilateral representation was conspicuous. Connection also has been shown between the anterior zones and the paramedian lobule. Auditory and visual impulses were picked up from the vermis and overlapped largely.

In the areas of overlapping representation, diverse types of external and internal (proprioceptive) stimuli pass to the same cerebellar neurons (Bremer and Bonnet, 1951).

Furthermore, by electrical means connection has been shown between the somatosensory and motor, the visual and auditory areas of the cerebrum and the corresponding zones of representation in the cerebellum. The vestibular areas of cerebellar cortex (flocculus, nodulus, uvula, pyramis, and lingula) display by electrical recording connections with the sensorimotor area of the cerebrum and the area to which the vestibular nuclei project (Ruwaldt and Snider, 1956).

There is projection from the pons, and so indirectly from the cerebral cortex, to all parts of the cerebellar cortex except the flocculonodular lobe (Brodal and Jansen, 1946). The pattern is definite with specific zones of the pons projecting to corresponding parts of the cerebellar cortex of the opposite side.

Olivocerebellar fibers reach all parts of the cerebellar cortex (Dow, 1939). The olivocerebellar fibers are not distributed at random. On the contrary each part of the olive projects to a specific part of the cerebellar cortex (Brodal, 1940).

Efferent Cerebellar Tracts.   These arise from the central nuclei, except for some fibers, which come from the cortex of the flocculus, uvula, and nodulus and run to the vestibular nuclei (Dow, 1938).

The *superior cerebellar peduncle* arises from the *dentate nucleus* and, according to Fulton (1938), also from the globose and emboliform nuclei (Figs. 169, 199). It undergoes a complete decussation beneath the inferior colliculus in the tegmentum of the mesencephalon. Some fibers of the superior cerebellar peduncle reach the lateroventral nucleus of the thalamus and the globus pallidus (Carpenter and Stevens, 1957) by way of the ansa lenticularis, but others end in the

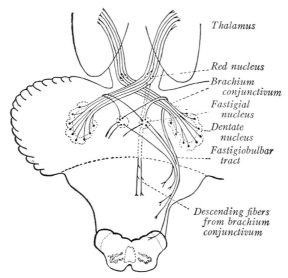

FIGURE 199.   Efferent tracts which arise in the central nuclei of the cerebellum.

red nucleus, whence the impulses they carry are relayed upward to the thalamus or downward along the rubroreticular and rubrospinal tracts to motor neurons in the brain stem and spinal cord (Figs. 169, 199).

According to Kappers, Huber and Crosby (1936), descending fibers are given off in two bundles, one just before and the other just after the peduncular fibers pass through their decussation. These fibers descend in the reticular formation of the pons and medulla (Fig. 169). They enter the medial longitudinal fasciculus and pass to the superior central, reticulotegmental and inferior olivary nuclei and into the spinal cord as far as the cervical enlargement (Carpenter and Stevens, 1957).

Other *efferent tracts arise in the fastigial nuclei* and after a partial crossing descend in the lateral part of the reticular formation of the pons and medulla oblongata. One bundle of these fibers, the uncinate bundle of Russel, winds around the superior cerebellar peduncle before joining the others (Fig. 199). All of these bundles may be grouped under one name and designated as the *fastigiobulbar tract*. The fibers of this tract are intermingled with those of the vestibulocerebellar fasciculus (Fig. 163), descend close to the medial side of the inferior cerebellar peduncle and pass through the lateral and descending vestibular nuclei. The fibers end in these nuclei and in the reticular formation (Allen, 1924; Gray, 1926).

HISTOLOGY OF THE CEREBELLAR CORTEX

The cerebellar cortex differs from that of the cerebral hemispheres in possessing essentially the same structure in all the lobules. This would indicate that it functions in essentially the same way throughout, though as a result of different fiber connections the various lobules may act on different muscle groups. Briefly it may be stated that the afferent fibers reach the cortex where by various

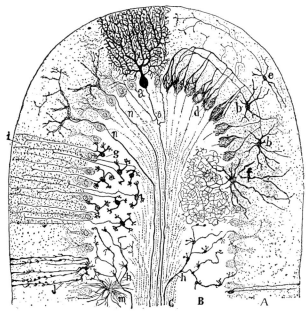

FIGURE 200. Semidiagrammatic transverse section through a folium of the cerebellum. (Golgi method): *A*, Molecular layer; *B*, granular layer; *C*, white matter; *a*, Purkinje cell; *b*, basket cells; *d*, pericellular baskets, surrounding the Purkinje cells and formed by the arborizations of the axons of the basket cells; *e*, superficial stellate cells; *f*, cell of Golgi Type II; *g*, granules, whose axons enter the molecular layer and bifurcate at *i*; *h*, mossy fibers; *j* and *m*, neuroglia; *n*, climbing fibers. (Cajal.)

means the impulses they carry are spread through intermediate neurons which connect with Purkinje cells, and these in turn send their axons to the central nuclei, from the cells of which extend the efferent cerebellar paths. There are patterns in these connections that allow diffusion and persistence of the effects of stimuli which have a bearing on the interpretation of cerebellar functioning. These patterns become evident as the microscopic structure is examined.

A section through the cerebellum, taken at right angles to the long axis of the folia, shows each folium to be composed of a central white lamina, covered by a layer of gray cortex. Within the white lamina the nerve fibers are arranged in parallel bundles extending from the medullary center of the cerebellum into the lobules and folia. A few at a time these bundles turn off obliquely into the gray matter, and there is no sharp demarcation between the cortex and the subjacent white lamina. The cortex presents for examination three well defined zones: a superficial molecular layer, a layer of Purkinje cells, and a subjacent granular layer.

The **cells of Purkinje** have large flask-shaped bodies and are arranged in an almost continuous sheet, consisting of a single layer of cells and separating the other two cortical zones (Fig. 200). In all there are upwards of 14 million Purkinje cells. They are more numerous at the summit than at the base of the folium. The part of the cell directed toward the surface of the cortex resembles the neck of a flask and from it spring one or two stout dendrites. These run into the molecular layer and extend throughout its entire thickness, branching repeatedly. This branching occurs in a plane at right angles to the long axis of the folium, and it is only in sections, taken in this plane, that the full extent of the branching can be observed. In a plane corresponding to the long axis of

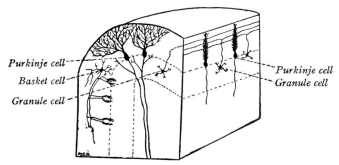

Purkinje cell
Basket cell
Granule cell

Purkinje cell
Granule cell

FIGURE 201. Diagrammatic representation of the structure of the cerebellar cortex as seen in a section along the axis of the folium (on the right), and in a section at right angles to the axis of the folium (on the left).

the folium the dendrites occupy a more restricted area (Fig. 201). In this respect the dendritic ramifications resemble the branches of a vine on a trellis. From the larger end of the cell, directed away from the surface of the cortex, there arises an axon which almost at once becomes myelinated and runs through the granular layer into the white substance of the cerebellum. These axons end in the central cerebellar nuclei. Near their origin they give off collaterals, which run backward through the molecular layer *to end in connection with neighboring Purkinje cells*—an arrangement designed to bring about simultaneous effects upon a whole group of such neurons, and to bring into action successively more and more Purkinje cells in the manner described by Cajal as "avalanche conduction."

Granules resembling the neurosecretory granules found in the diencephalon have been described in Purkinje cells but their function is unknown (Shanklin et al., 1957).

The **granular layer,** situated immediately subjacent to that which we have just described, is characterized by the presence of great numbers of small neurons, the *granule cells*. Each of these contains a relatively large nucleus, surrounded by a small amount of cytoplasm, and from each there are given off from three to five short *dendritic branches* with claw-like endings. These are synaptically related with the terminal branches of the mossy fibers, soon to be described, and form with them small glomeruli comparable to those of the olfactory bulb. Each granule cell gives origin to an unmyelinated *axon*, which extends toward the surface of folium and enters the molecular layer. Here it divides in the manner of a T into two branches. These run parallel to the long axis of the folium through layer after layer of the dendritic expansions of the Purkinje cells, with which they doubtless establish synaptic relations (Fig. 201). Besides the granules just described, this layer contains some large cells of Golgi's Type II (Fig. 200, *f*). Most of these are placed near the line of Purkinje cells and send their dendrites into the molecular layer, while their short axons resolve themselves into plexuses of fine branches in the granular zone.

The **molecular layer** contains few nerve cells and has in transverse sections a finely punctate appearance. It is composed in large part of the dendritic ramifications of the Purkinje cells and the branches of axons from the granule cells (Fig. 200). It contains a relatively small number of stellate neurons, the more superficial of which possess short axons and belong to Golgi's Type II. Those more deeply situated have a highly specialized form and are known as *basket cells*. From each of these there arises, in addition to several stout branching dendrites, a single characteristic axon, which runs through the molecular layer in a plane at right angles to the long axis of the folium (Fig. 201). These axons are at first very fine, but soon become coarse and irregular, giving off numerous collaterals which are directed away from the surface of the cortex. These collaterals and the terminal branches of the axons run toward the Purkinje cells, about which their terminal arborizations form basket-like networks (Fig. 85).

Nerve Fibers.   The axons of the Purkinje cells form a considerable volume of fibers directed away from the cortex. There are also two kinds of afferent fibers which enter the cortex from the white center, and are known as *climbing* and *mossy fibers* respectively. The latter are very coarse and give off numerous branches ending within the granular layer. The terminal branches are provided with characteristic moss-like appendages. These mossy tufts are intimately related to the claw-like dendritic ramifications of the granule cells. The *climbing fibers*, somewhat finer than those of the preceding group, pass through the molecular layer and become associated with the dendrites of the Purkinje cells in the manner of a climbing vine. Branching repeatedly, they follow closely the dendritic ramifications of these neurons and terminate in free varicose endings.

It would seem reasonable to suppose that the two kinds of *afferent fibers*, just described, have a separate origin and functional significance. It appears from experimental studies that mossy fibers are the terminations of fibers entering the cerebellum from without, as spinocerebellar, olivocerebellar, vestibulocerebellar and pontocerebellar fibers, while climbing fibers arise within the cerebellar nuclei and return to the cortex, or else are recurrent collaterals of efferent fibers (Carrea, Reissig, and Mettler, 1947). The *mossy fibers* transfer their impulses to the granule cells, and these, in turn, relay them, either directly or through the basket neurons, to the Purkinje cells. The *climbing fibers* transfer their impulses directly to the dendrites of the Purkinje cells.

The *efferent path* may be said to begin with the Purkinje cells, whose axons terminate in the central cerebellar nuclei. From these nuclei efferent fibers leave the cerebellum by each of the three peduncles. From the fastigial and the intermediate nuclei fibers pass into the brain stem reticular formation along the medial sides of the inferior and middle, and from the dentate nuclei flow the fibers forming the superior cerebellar peduncle.

By means of the axons of granule cells, basket cells, and neurons of Golgi Type II, as well as by the collaterals from the axons of Purkinje cells, an incoming impulse may be diffused through the cortex, and the effect of the stimulus maintained by the reverberating circuits involved. The recurrent axonic collaterals are interpreted by Retzlaff (1954) as being of two kinds, with probably separate functions: axo-axonic, which are inhibitory, and axo-dendritic, which are excitatory. The climbing fibers may supply a type of feedback by maintaining an enduring state of negativity in the dendrites (as suggested from the work of Bishop and Clare, 1953, with pyramidal cells of the cortex).

Many synaptic endings are to be found on the Purkinje cells, dendrites, and cell body; and with these conditions repetitive firing of the axon in the activity of such cells is explained; also by the arrangement of neurons in what Graham Brown called paired half-centers with the synapses on the axon hillock generating counter influences (Gesell et al., 1954). An impressive demonstration of the effectiveness of this mechanism for maintaining and diffusing a stimulus is produced when a point on the cerebellum is stimulated through a previously implanted electrode in an animal free from the effects of anesthesia. The motor effects which follow a brief stimulus may continue for five to fifteen minutes and show evidence of gradually involving more and more, perhaps all, of the cerebellar cortex. It is also of interest that such effects can be produced by mechanical means, as by a needle puncture of cerebellar cortex, emphasizing the responsibility of the cerebellar cortex itself in the reaction (Clark, 1938).

FUNCTION OF THE CEREBELLUM

The way the cerebellum functions has not been entirely clear. It is known that it deals with the synergy of skeletal muscle, and that it is not concerned with conscious sensation, nor can its functioning be said to be within the realm of consciousness. Other functions than control of synergy of skeletal muscle may become apparent as the various approaches to the study of cerebellar function are utilized. There is evidence of cerebellar effect in certain visceral mechanisms.

Cerebellar function has been studied from a variety of directions, among which are the following: (1) Study of the histologic picture, which shows the intimate connections of neurons. (2) Tracing paths into and from the cerebellum with study of their origin and distribution by methods involving degeneration of fibers and cells. (3) Tracing pathways to and from the cerebellum by electrical stimulation and recording of responses, the so-called physiologic neuronography. (4) Study of the development of the cerebellum on a comparative basis in different species of vertebrates, with attention to the muscle masses developed and utilized in the different animals with various styles of posture and progression. (5) Observation of the effects of experimental electrical stimulation of the cerebellum in the laboratory. (6) Study of symptoms or effects of removal or damage to parts of the cerebellum as seen in clinical cases and in laboratory experiments.

Some of the results attained with the first three methods listed have been discussed in the preceding pages in connection with the study of the internal structure of the cerebellum. It will be valuable to attempt to correlate these observations with other data from comparative studies, stimulation, and ablation of different parts of the cerebellum.

Comparative Morphology and Function.   The form of the cerebellum in a species of animal is apparently a reflection of the animal's style of posture and activities. In considering this relationship in any species it is important to take into account the position of the center of gravity of the animal in relation to its bulk and the points of its support; the type of progression employed; and the presence, development, and independent use of any limbs it may possess. It should be observed more than casually that the cerebrum varies also with the factors related to cerebellar variation.

Not only does the total mass of the cerebellum vary; portions of it show special development in different animals. In comparative studies it is seen that the middle portion of the cerebellum, corresponding to the vermis, is developed in those animals whose progressive movements and activity are largely dependent upon trunk musculature or symmetrical limb movements, as in birds and reptiles. The vermis which is acquired by the early bird is more highly developed in birds which fly than in the flightless ones like the ostrich. With the development of limbs and further with the degree of independence of limb movements in various animals, the hemispheres show development and variation.

Smaller subdivisions of the cerebellum vary in size with masses of muscle in different parts of the body of species of higher vertebrates and with the intricacy of muscle activity (Riley, 1929; Jansen, 1950). For example, the cerebellum of the giraffe with its highly developed neck and head mobility has a conspicuous lobulus simplex as in other species with mobility of the head. The lingula is relatively large in mammals that have proportionately large tails, as does the rat, but it is moderately well developed in the pig, which has a rather ineffectual tail (Larsell, 1952). The cat with excellent use of its extremities has a rather well developed ansoparamedian lobule; while in the narwhal with no external hind limbs and remarkably effective aquatic activity, Crus II of the ansoparamedian lobule is small. On the other hand the paraflocculus is very large (Larsell and Berthelsdorf, 1941). It has been argued from these and similar observations that the lobulus simplex is concerned with control of neck muscles, and that Crus I, and Crus II, of the ansoparamedian lobule are concerned respectively with the forelimb and hindlimb musculature. The paraflocculus is especially developed in aquatic forms having a high degree of coordination and synchrony in movements of axial and appendicular muscles.

In the primates with increasingly upright position, and especially in man with independent use of individual extremities, the hemispheres of the cerebellum are highly developed, and corticopontocerebellar connections are prominent. Much of the information from comparative studies such as these suggests localized responsibility of cerebellar parts but it has not been completely correlated with other observations.

Stimulation of the Cerebellum.   In considering evidence concerning cerebellar function as produced by stimulation of the cerebellum, it should be recalled that several synapses (neurons) are interposed between the cerebellar cortex and the final common path to skeletal muscle, or other effector neurons. Not only does such an arrangement allow other influences to be brought into play, but synaptic interruption in a pathway probably always provides means of multiplying the available routes from that point.

Effects follow stimulation of the cerebellum by either electrical or mechanical means, but the response is so affected by anesthesia and other conditions of stimulation that investigators have not always agreed upon the results.

The effects of stimulation have been described in several categories the most significant of which are:

1. Contraction of skeletal muscle in specific regions.
2. Inhibition of the excessive tone in decerebrate rigidity.
3. Disturbance of balance and posture.
4. Facilitation and inhibition of neuronal activity.
5. Effects upon activity of smooth muscle of visceral structures.

Some of the earliest investigators of stimulation of the cerebellum saw movement of skeletal muscle with evidence of specificity in different regions, and recent investigations support and elaborate this with modifications, but with less evidence of specificity than at first appeared. Sherrington's observation that stimulation of the cerebellum in the decerebrate animal inhibited the excessive tone of decerebrate rigidity so fixed the attention on this state that stimulation of the cerebellum in as nearly normal an animal as possible was neglected.

When the cerebellum is stimulated through an implanted electrode in an otherwise normal animal the visible motor results obtained, though they vary with the point stimulated, may occur in three phases (Clark, 1939). That is, there may be a response during the stimulus, a second response opposite in pattern immediately following cessation of the stimulus, and a third long effect in the nature of a very slow motor seizure lasting several minutes and involving successively all the animal's parts. The first two phases of this response occur commonly as movements that are "mirror images" of each other; the head, for example, moves during the stimulus toward the side stimulated, then toward the opposite side immediately following the stimulus. The second movement is apparently in the nature of a rebound to the first. This stimulus and rebound pattern is commonly produced by stimulation of the vermis or the region near it, or, to put it another way, in those cortical zones connected with the nuclei fastigii. Sprague and Chambers (1954) have elicited such reciprocal responses from stimulation of the reticular formation of the brain stem, and though the pattern is still present after acute removal of the cerebellum, it is lost if time is allowed for fibers connecting cerebellum and brain stem to degenerate. This would seem to prove the necessity of cerebellar connections for its occurrence.

The long after-effect (third phase of response) which lasts several minutes has been elicited from widespread areas of the cerebellum although not yet from the flocculonodular lobe. During the long after-effect movements occur in a series of patterns which suggest stimulus and rebound, as the movements in sequence are reversed in direction or alternate between sides. The body, for example, slowly becomes concave on one side, then the other; the hocks will be abducted and then gradually adducted until they scrape each other in walking; the tail will be arched to one side then the other, or over the back. Also during this phase of the response, as individual limbs are affected, there is dysmetria in walking with marked "over-stepping" comparable to that produced by cerebellar lesions. The effect sweeps through the animal's musculature in a definite sequence and suggests a diffusion by reverberating circuits through the cerebellar cortex. These movements appear to have no useful purpose, but are not like those of the common epileptic seizure.

Sherrington and others since have observed that stimulation of the anterior lobe of the cerebellum diminished the exaggerated extensor tonus of decerebrate rigidity, but other responses than mere inhibition of extensor tonus follow cerebellar stimulation in the decerebrate animal. Some very definite movements of extremities can occur which commonly show reversals of pattern with cessation of the stimulus as rebounds, with evidence of local representation of body parts.

Stimulation of the cerebellum in animals with intact brains can inhibit or facilitate movements produced reflexly or by cerebral cortical stimulation. The areas of the cerebellum which give this effect coincide generally with the areas receiving tactile impulses which also have connection with cerebral motor areas. The pathway for the facilitatory and inhibitory impulses is from cerebellar cortex to nucleus fastigii, thence to the bulbar reticular formation, and by reticulospinal paths to the cord (Snider and Magoun, 1949).

Since both facilitating and inhibiting influences spread from the cerebellum by closely associated pathways to skeletal muscle, and stimulus to the cerebellum of intact animals commonly displays quick reversals of movement as in stimulus-rebound, it may be assumed that the normal control of synergy of muscle action constantly involves such mechanisms nicely adjusted to momentary needs. The terms "reciprocal co-contraction," and "bridling action" have probably been well used in the description of the way the cerebellum controls muscle action.

An interesting commentary on methods of simultaneous excitation and inhibition may be apparent in the connections of Mauthner's cell, the large motor unit in the medulla of fishes. Retzlaff (1957) described single branched fibers of the eighth cranial nerve of fish as ending on the lateral dendrite and cell body of the homolateral Mauthner's cell and on the axon hillock of the contralateral Mauthner's cell. He supposes the impulses ending on the eighth nerve fibers from vestibular apparatus excited the homolateral cell while inhibiting the contralateral one. Here again the phenomenon of a state of enduring negativity on dendrites as described by Clare and Bishop may be involved.

It is not surprising that in this widespread control of the activity of voluntary muscle not only proprioceptive but various exteroceptive impulses should be provided to the centers concerned. The readjustment of the body in space demanded by each movement, large or small, requires a mechanism for complete orientation with its environment.

Except for pupillary dilatation, visceral responses have only recently been observed following cerebellar stimulation. Pupillary dilatation can be obtained from widespread areas and may not be specifically cerebellar, but pupillary constriction and contraction of the bladder with urination follow stimulation of small definite regions of the cerebellum (Chambers, 1943; McDonald, 1951). It has also been stated that the cerebellum has a relationship to vasomotor control, which keeps a balance between vasoconstriction and vasodilatation. Further investigation in this direction is needed. On hypothalamic stimulation there is a widespread electrical response from the anterior lobe and areas adjacent, which might imply autonomic relationship (Ban and Inoue, 1957).

Cerebellar Lesions.   The most conspicuous symptom following damage to the cerebellum or its connections is disturbance of coordination of movement in skeletal muscle. A number of clinical tests are employed to bring out one or another phase of this, and each demonstrates in its way the asynergia. There are differences in the pattern of deficit dependent upon the portion of the cerebellum affected by the lesion, but the effects of lesions can usually be analyzed in terms of disturbance of equilibrium, of posture, or of voluntary movement. Not only do lesions of the cerebellum itself show such deficits, but lesions of structures closely connected with it, as the inferior olivary nucleus, the cerebellar peduncles, and even the frontal cortex, may be accompanied by similar signs and symptoms.

There has been little opportunity in man to observe separately the function of the *anterior lobe* of the cerebellum, although animal experimentation has thrown light upon it. The anterior lobe has vestibular, spinal, and cerebral connections. Recent work with animals shows its relation to posture and limb movements with localization of functional responsibility in successive zones from the region of the primary fissure forward corresponding to face and head, forelimb, hindlimb, and tail.

Adjustment can be made to losses of the cerebellum or parts of it. A slowly growing destructive lesion may reach large size in the cerebellum without evident symptoms.

Operative removal of the whole cerebellum, if injury to the vestibular nuclei is avoided, produces less disturbance of movement than partial removal, apparently because of the amount of imbalance produced. Following partial removals not only does the part removed fail to function, the part remaining acts alone unopposed, as if were, instead of having its effect integrated with the function of the total cerebellum. In time the animal may adjust to this imbalance. Removal of one lateral half of the cerebellum results in constant falling or rolling of the animal toward the side of the removal. After several days, the hemidecerebellate animal learns to walk on a wide base although it will continue to fall more easily toward the side of operation for some time.

Removals of anterior or posterior "halves" of the cerebellum disturb the for-ward-backward equilibrium of an animal. Removal of small portions of the cerebellum result in temporary loss of synergy in the action of local muscle groups as in an extremity or one side, or the neck and head. Further controlled experiments are needed in this direction.

Lesions of the dentate nuclei are associated with ataxia of the extremities, while lesions of the fastigial nuclei are accompanied commonly by ataxia of axial musculature (Carpenter and Stevens, 1957).

The *flocculonodular lobe* is often involved by cerebellar tumors in children. As might be expected because of the vestibular connections of this lobe, a child with such a tumor shows a disturbance of equilibrium and is unsteady on his feet. When in bed the patient may show no incoordination in movements of the arms or legs and little if any tremor.

The *neocerebellar part of the posterior lobe* receives impulses from the cerebral cortex by way of the corticopontocerebellar path. The neocerebellum plays an important part in the coordination of muscular activity, especially that of the arms and legs. It is not concerned with the initiation of movement, but while movement is in progress its execution is regulated by the cerebellum and synergy maintained. *Synergy* means cooperation in action, as when several muscles function together in the production of a complex act, each muscle con-tracting at the right time and to the proper extent. Lack of synergy results in incoordination. In a patient with a neocerebellar lesion, movements are jerky and intermittent (ataxia) and overshoot the mark (dysmetria). If the patient tries to hold the elbow flexed while traction is being made at the wrist, the release of the wrist may result in sudden uncontrolled flexion at the elbow so that the hand may strike the face (rebound phenomenon). Movements may not take place in quite the right direction (spontaneous deviation or past-pointing). There may be difficulty in performing rapidly alternating move-ments such as repeated pronation and supination of both outstretched hands in unison (adiadochokinesis). An act which normally involves simultaneous movements at several joints may be dissected so that movement occurs first at one joint and then at another (decomposition of movement).

The symptoms resulting from damage to the neocerebellum in man include hypotonia and tremor. *Hypotonia* is evidenced by a diminished resistance to passive movement and by a wider than normal excursion of the distal segments of a hypotonic limb when the proximal segment is shaken. The *tremor* resulting from cerebellar lesions increases toward the end of a given movement and is associated with difficulty in stopping the movement at the proper point. The oscillations are coarser than those in multiple sclerosis. Fulton (1938) believes that an enduring pronounced tremor does not result from pure lesions of the cerebellar cortex but indicates an involvement of the nuclei. Carey (1957) has produced an action tremor which resembled cerebellar tremor during stimulation and after destruction of the red nucleus and areas near it, or of the thalamic nucleus lateralis ventralis. He interprets this as evidence of an elicited imbalance in cerebrocerebellar control. But the tremor and cerebellar asynergia from lesions of the red nucleus do not persist permanently (Carpenter, 1956).

Nystagmus is a more prominent symptom of cerebellar lesions in man than in animals. It occurs in patients with lesions in any part of the cerebellum except the posterior midline structures.

It has been elicited in the unanesthetized monkey by stimulation of the cerebellar cortex (Clark and Clark, 1958).

It is a common symptom of vestibular disturbance and with the large vestibular representation in the cerebellum would be expected to appear with at least some cerebellar lesions. Nystagmus occurs naturally following rotation of the head and its direction varies according to the alignment of the specific semicircular canals with the direction of rotation. The direction of the nystagmus is indicated by that of the quick component although the slow component is the true compensatory movement. Nystagmus when present in relation to a cerebellar or vestibular lesion can be elicited by having the patient follow the examiner's finger with his gaze, with head still, until the limit of eye deviation is reached. In normal people a slight nystagmus not long sustained may occur, while that indicating a lesion is usually sustained for some time.

An interesting commentary on the learning capacities dependent on the cerebellum is indicated by the fact that pigeons can become habituated to postrotational nystagmus, showing a shortening of the duration after successive standard times of whirling. This capacity to learn is lessened or abolished by removal of part of the cerebellum (Halstead, 1936).

Similarly adaptation to successive sound stimuli after the first in a rapid series is shown by diminution of the electrical responses of the cerebellum in the unanesthetized cat. After a pause of a half minute or more between single similar sounds of a series, the electrical response will return to its original height. Furthermore a new sound introduced between those of a series will elicit an electrical response of the usual height and may mask the response of the next one in the series.

Electrical responses of the cerebellum to flashes of light in the eye have been examined by Koella (1958) and disclose a relationship to quantity of illumination, and an adaptation to a series of flashes similar to that of a succession of auditory stimuli. The potentials are recorded after a brief delay from rather large areas at a single flash, but with some asynchrony as if there is a spread of the influence through the cortical connections. From these same areas it is possible to elicit postural adjustments on local stimulation.

From the various observations it becomes evident that representation in the cerebellum of body parts is strongly homolateral, but also bilateral, and that in both anterior and posterior lobes there is representation of body parts in reverse pattern. It can be pictured as if the animal were "suspended" at a midline point about the primary fissure and that with this point as a center each quadrant of the cerebellum is especially concerned with postural change of the animal toward a corresponding zone of its environment. Many types of sensory impulses (proprioceptive, exteroceptive, visual and auditory, and perhaps enteroceptive) give the necessary information of the animal's relation to the environment; and in response to alterations the adjustment of posture, in static or mobile situations, is influenced by cerebellar activity. Each quadrant of the cerebellum would thereby be related to activity of muscles in all parts of the body.

CHAPTER XV

The Diencephalon

The diencephalon, connecting as it does the cerebral hemispheres and the mesencephalon, has within it elements concerned with most bodily functions. In the axial portion about the third ventricle the diencephalon resembles the tegmentum of the mesencephalon with which it is continuous, but in it larger nuclear masses and pathways have developed with the greater cerebral development of man and the tendency to telencephalization. The diencephalon includes the thalamus, epithalamus, subthalamus, and hypothalamus and from it develop the retinae and optic nerves.

Upon the **thalamus,** if the geniculate bodies be included, converge the secondary afferent paths bearing sensory impulses of all types from the various receptors, special and general. Lying as it does in the middle of the cerebrum, it acts as a way-station where the afferent paths after interruption are relayed to cortical levels. The interruption of the pathways is not merely that, but there is thus made possible the diffusion and spread of impulses to centers other than cortical, and perhaps even a kind of integration, and the sending of impulses to regions lower than cortical that are capable of responding to the impulses received by the thalamus. Also it is accepted that at the thalamic level painful stimuli may appear in consciousness, whatever that may mean.

The thalamus is composed of several masses of nerve cells termed nuclei, which have diverse connections. As the details of their arrangement are examined it is well to keep in mind certain generalizations concerning their connections. Some of the nuclei serve to relay special and general afferent impulses from lower levels to the cortex; other nuclei have connections with lower levels but not the cortex; still other nuclei have connections with the cortex but not directly with lower levels. There is also significant connection between various thalamic nuclei. Topographically there is evidence of orderly relationship between cortex and thalamus, the more anterior portions of the thalamus having connection with more anterior portions of cortex and the more posterior parts corresponding, but the representation is not always as simple as that implies (Jasper, 1949; Rose and Woolsey, 1949).

What appears to be an almost constant rule in the nervous system is evident in thalamic connections with the cortex: there are corticothalamic fibers as well as thalamocortical ones, and these are commonly between the same regions of each. Such an arrangement probably allows for the principle of "feedback" as emphasized in electronic circuits and cybernetics.

Structure of the Thalamus.   The thalamus consists chiefly of gray matter, within which there may be recognized a number of nuclear masses. Its dorsal surface is covered by a thin layer of white matter which has been called the *stratum zonale*. On the lateral surface next the internal capsule but separated from it by a narrow zone of cells (the reticular nucleus) there are many myelinated fibers, which constitute the *external medullary lamina* (Figs. 202, 387). The medial surface is covered by a layer of *central gray matter*, continuous

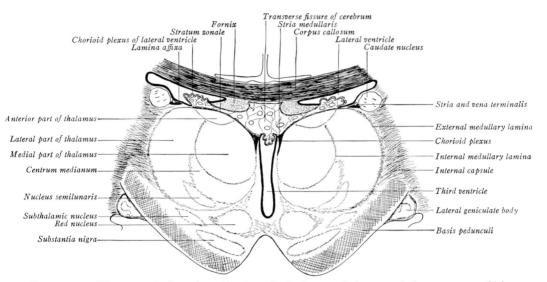

FIGURE 202.   Diagrammatic frontal section through the human thalamus and the structures which immediately surround it.

with that which lines the cerebral aqueduct, and forms part of the lateral wall of the third ventricle.

From the stratum zonale, which clothes its dorsal surface, there penetrates into the thalamus a vertical plate of white matter, the *internal medullary lamina*, which separates the thalamus into medial and lateral parts. At the rostral extremity of its dorsal border the internal medullary lamina bifurcates to surround partly the anterior part of the thalamus, which projects somewhat above the general level of the dorsal thalamic surface, forming the anterior tubercle. These laminae of fibers help to separate the nuclear groups whose connections they partly form.

The nuclei of the thalamus have been named by the comparative neurologists, the names being derived from their positions in the subdivisions of the thalamus. There has not been strict adherence to directions referable to the anatomical position of the human body in these names. The thalamus (and forebrain) is described as having a *dorsal* or superior surface which is toward the vertex of the head, and *ventral* or inferior surface opposite; *anterior* is toward the frontal poles of the cerebrum, *posterior* toward the occiput; medial and lateral areas as usual. Not all the named nuclei of the thalamus are referred to in this description. Further details may be found in the literature.

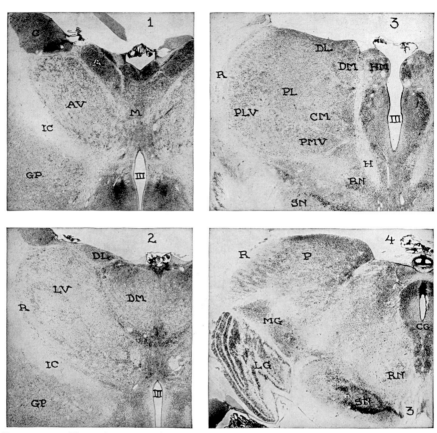

FIGURE 203. Photomicrographs from sections through the thalamus of the monkey: *A*, anterior thalamic nuclei; *AV*, anterior ventral nucleus; *C*, caudate nucleus; *CG*, central gray; *CM*, centrum medianum; *DL*, dorsal lateral nucleus; *DM*, dorsal medial nucleus; *GP*, globus pallidus; *H*, habenulo-peduncular tract; *HM*, medial habenular nucleus; *IC*, internal capsule; *LG*, lateral geniculate body; *LV*, lateral ventral nucleus; *M*, nuclei of the midline; *MG*, medial geniculate body; *P*, pulvinar; *PL*, posterior lateral nucleus; *PLV*, posterolateral ventral nucleus; *PMV*, posteromedial ventral nucleus; *R*, reticular nucleus; *RN*, red nucleus; *SN*, substantia nigra; *3*, third nerve; *III*, third ventricle.

The **nuclei of the thalamus** have been classified morphologically into five groups as follows:

(1) The *anterior thalamic nuclei* occupy the anterior part of the thalamus (Figs. 203, 226, 390, 396) and are separated from the remainder of it by the diverging limbs of the internal medullary lamina. The anterior group of nuclei receives fibers from the mammillothalamic tract and sends fibers to the cerebral cortex

connections with the corpus striatum and the amygdala. From experimental evidence it is stated that these nuclei, together with the reticular nucleus, form part of a reticular complex which has a widespread influence on the cortex. The reticular complex appears to constitute the upward extension of reticular relays ascending through the medulla, pons and mesencephalon, which on stimulation can cause generalized variations in the pattern of the electroencephalogram. The changes produced are in the direction of desynchronization of the electrical pattern and activation of the cortex. It has been suggested that this diffuse thalamic projection system is related to the state of wakefulness and sleep and so perhaps to consciousness. There is some disagreement as to which thalamic structures are chiefly responsible for the diffuse projection, but the concept of such a system is significant in the light of its possible regulatory effects on the cortex.

Collaterals from auditory and other somatic afferents in the brain stem enter the ascending reticular activating system and so contribute to an arousal system.

Increasing interest in the function of the thalamus has accompanied the development of the operation which severs the thalamofrontal radiation (leukotomy) in cases of severe depression. Selected cases have been used to trace thalamic connections, and have confirmed some of the results of investigation upon lower animals. Such studies have demonstrated the connection between the medial thalamic nucleus and Areas 9, 10, 11, and 12 of the frontal region; between the anterior thalamic nucleus and the medial surface of the cerebral hemisphere; and between the lateral group of nuclei and Areas 4, 6, and 8 on the cortex (Freeman and Watts, 1947).

Temporary disturbance of time sense, lasting a few days or weeks, in which the patients estimated poorly the memory of the length of times spent, and were confused as to time of day, dates, season, and even their own ages, has followed operative lesions on the dorsomedial nucleus of the thalamus (Spiegel et al., 1955). It was thought such lesions chiefly involved the connections within the frontal lobes, but there is some evidence that the anterior nucleus and its connections with the mammillary body are important to this, as well as perhaps other connections of thalamic nuclei with parietal lobes. Since the effect was transitory, it was thought that multiple structures are involved in this time sense, even memory of recent and past events.

Lesions in the lateral nucleus of the thalamus often cause, in addition to a loss or impairment of sensation on the opposite side of the body, intractable pain in the anesthetic regions. Any sensation evoked on the affected side may be extremely unpleasant or painful out of proportion to the stimulus and bring about an excessive emotional response. These peculiar sensory disturbances involved in the *thalamic syndrome* have not yet been adequately explained.

It is of interest that connections extend from cortex to thalamus as well as from thalamus to cortex, thus allowing for reverberating circuits between the two. Stimuli to the cortex, even though brief, may be maintained and amplified for proper response. It may also be that the cortex normally inhibits activity in the thalamus after the reception of stimuli, shutting down the activity of reverberating circuits. With connections with the cortex damaged or removed, unbridled activity in the thalamus may be the basis of the thalamic syndrome (Niemer and Jiminez-Castellanos, 1950).

THE SUBTHALAMUS

The subthalamus is situated between the (dorsal) thalamus and the tegmentum of the mesencephalon, and forms a zone of transition between these two structures. Lateral to it the internal capsule joins the basis pedunculi, and medial and rostral to it lies the hypothalamus. It includes white matter

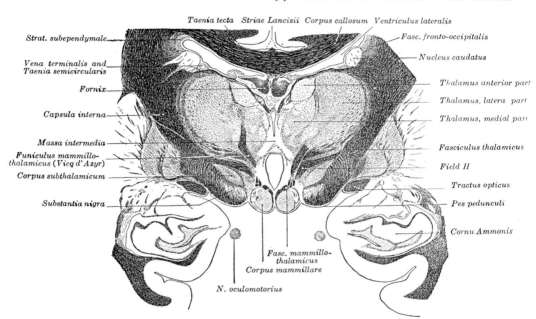

FIGURE 206.   Frontal section through the human diencephalon at the level of the mammillothalamic tract. Weigert method. (Villiger-Pierson.)

in subdivisions termed the fields H, H₁, and H₂ of Forel and the subthalamic nucleus. The red nucleus and substantia nigra project upward into it from the mesencephalon (Figs. 206, 207).

Partial responsibility for the regulation of motor activity resides in certain structures in this area, sharing this with the closely related basal ganglia (p. 424).

The *subthalamic nucleus* (corpus Luysii) is a biconvex mass of gray matter which lies upon the medial side of the transition zone between the internal capsule and basis pedunculi (Figs. 206, 216). This nucleus receives fibers from the external division of the globus pallidus and forms an important part of the descending pathway from the corpus striatum (see p. 317).

From the *internal* division of the globus pallidus a more dorsally placed bundle called *fasciculus lenticularis* (seen in Forel's field H₂) runs medially and is joined by other fibers from the globus pallidus which run in a ventrally placed bundle called the *ansa lenticularis*. (The ansa lenticularis runs nearly parallel to the optic tract which lies just below it.) These bundles plus some other fibers bend sharply in Forel's field H and continue as the thalamic fasciculus through field H_1 to the anterior ventral nucleus of the thalamus (Figs. 206, 214, 215, 225).

The ansa lenticularis is one of the bundles constituting the larger collection of fibers bundles known as *ansa peduncularis* (Figs. 209, 211), which bends about the posterior limb of the internal capsule where the latter is entering the basis pedunculi.

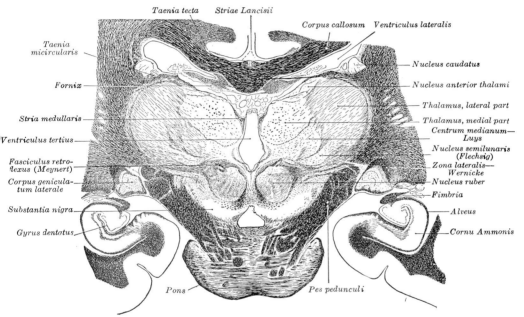

FIGURE 207.   Frontal section through the human diencephalon at the level of the centrum medianum. Weigert method. (Villiger-Piersol.)

The zona incerta is a continuation of the reticular formation of the mesencephalon. It has connections with nearby nuclei and receives fibers from the motor and premotor area of the cerebral cortex and from the temporal pole (Whitlock and Nauta, 1956). It lies just above the fasciculus lenticularis as a thin plate of gray matter. It is considered to be a correlation center for optic and vestibular impulses relayed to the outer part of the globus pallidus (Papez, 1951) (Figs. 215, *ZI*, 378, 396).

THE EPITHALAMUS

The epithalamus includes the pineal body, stria medullaris, and *habenular trigone*. The latter is a small triangular area located on the dorsomedial aspect of the thalamus rostral to the pineal body (Figs. 40, 41, 42). It marks the position of the *habenular nucleus,* an olfactosomatic correlation center, which receives fibers from the *stria medullaris,* a fascicle which runs along the border between the dorsal and medial surfaces of the thalamus subjacent to the taenia thalami (Figs. 41, 42). The stria medullaris takes origin from the olfactory centers on the basal surface of the cerebral hemisphere and, partially encircling the thalamus, reaches the habenular ganglion, in which it ends. Not all of the fibers terminate on the same side; some cross to the ganglion of the opposite side, forming a transverse bundle of myelinated fibers which joins the caudal end of the two ganglia together and is known as the *habenular commissure.* From the cells in this ganglion arises a bundle of fibers, known as the *fasciculus retroflexus* of Meynert or the tractus habenulopeduncularis. This bundle of fibers is directed ventralward toward the base of the brain and ends in the interpeduncular ganglion (Figs. 249, 357, 374, 375, 409). The stria medullaris, habenular ganglion and fasciculus retroflexus are all parts of an arc for olfactory reflexes. According to Edinger (1911) the cells, from which the stria medullaris arises, are intimately related to a bundle of ascending fibers from the sensory nuclei of the trigeminal nerve. If this be true, this olfactory mechanism may receive afferent impulses from the nose, mouth, and tongue and be concerned with feeding reflexes.

The **pineal body** is a small mass, shaped like a fir cone, which rests upon the mesencephalon in the interval between the two thalami. Its base is attached by a short stalk to the habenular and posterior commissures, and into the stalk there extends the small pineal recess of the third ventricle. The pineal body is a rudimentary structure and is not composed of nervous elements. In some vertebrates, certain lizards, for example, it is more highly developed, resembles in structure an invertebrate eye, and lies close to the dorsal surface of the head.

The **posterior commissure** is a large bundle of fibers which crosses the median plane dorsal to the point where the cerebral aqueduct opens into the third ventricle (Fig. 41). Some of its fibers serve to connect together the two superior colliculi, but the source and termination of most of its fibers remain obscure.

THE HYPOTHALAMUS

The hypothalamus lies ventral to the thalamus and forms the floor and part of the lateral wall of the third ventricle (**Fig. 40**). As seen on the ventral surface of the brain (Fig. 31) it includes the optic chiasma, corpora mammillaria, tuber cinereum, infundibulum, and neurohypophysis. The *mammillary bodies* are a pair of small spheric masses of gray matter, situated close together in the interpeduncular space rostral to the posterior perforated substance. The *tuber cinereum* is an elevated gray area rostral to the mammillary bodies. To it the hypophysis is attached by the funnel-shaped *infundibulum* (Fig. 40).

The Neurohypophysis. The enlarged upper end of the infundibulum, known as the median eminence, is attached to the tuber cinereum and forms a small part of the floor of the third ventricle (Fig. 208). At its lower end the infundibular stalk joins the neural lobe of the hypophysis, which with the pars intermedia forms what has been called the posterior lobe. The median eminence, infundibular stem and neural lobe (or infundibular process) constitute the neurohypophysis (Rioch, Wislocki, and O'Leary, 1940). All three parts have the same structure and contain modified neuroglial cells known as pituicytes.

The neurohypophysis develops as a downward evagination of the embryonic diencephalon. To it there becomes attached a glandular mass, the adenohypophysis, derived from the stomodeum. Both the neural and the glandular parts of the hypophysis function as endocrine glands.

Structure of the Hypothalamus. For convenience of description each lateral half of the hypothalamus may be divided into a medial part with many

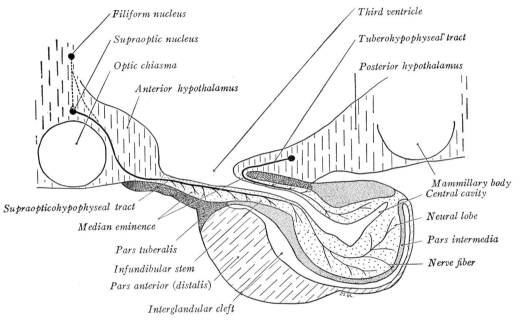

FIGURE 208. Diagram of a midsagittal section through the hypothalamus and hypophysis of the cat.

nuclei and few myelinated fibers and a lateral part, the lateral hypothalamic area, containing scattered nerve cells and many longitudinally coursing myelinated fibers. It may also be divided transversely into three parts: supraoptic, tuberal, and mammillary. Immediately in front of and not sharply marked off from the hypothalamus is the preoptic region, i. e., the region between the anterior commissure and optic chiasma (*AX* and *OX*, Fig. 209).

Nuclei. The nerve cells of the hypothalamus are not uniformly distributed but are arranged in more or less definite nuclear groups. Most of the cells are small and their grouping into nuclei is not always sharply defined. The *supraoptic nucleus* is an important exception. It is composed of large closely packed cells and forms a conspicuous mass overlying the beginning of the optic tract (Figs. 209–211, 217, *SO*). In the supraoptic portion of the hypothalamus there

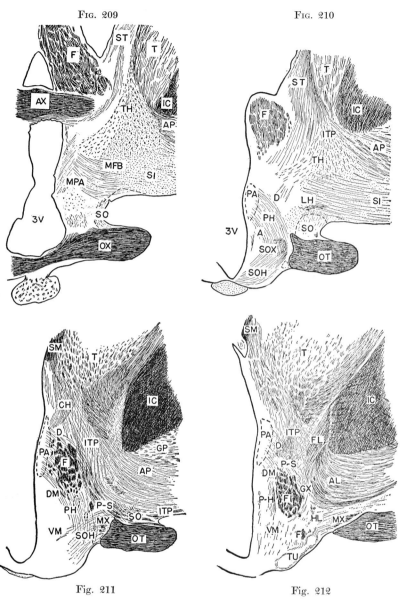

Fig. 209 Fig. 210

Fig. 211 Fig. 212

FIGURES 209–216. Semischematic drawings illustrating the fiber pattern and the location of nuclei in the human hypothalamus. The first seven figures represent transverse sections through successive rostrocaudal levels and Fig. 216, a parasagittal section. (Ingram, The Vegetative Nervous System, Vol. IX, Assn. for Research in Nervous and Mental Disease.) *A*, Anterior hypothalamic area; *AL*, ansa lenticularis; *AP*, ansa peduncularis; *AX*, anterior commissure; *CH*, corticohabenular fibers; *D*, dorsal hypothalamic area; *DESC*, fibers of the diffuse descending system; *DM*, dorsomedial hypothalamic nucleus; *F*, fornix; *FL*, fasciculus lenticularis; *FLD*, dorsal longitudinal fasciculus; *GP*, globus pallidus; *GX*, dorsal supraoptic commissure, pars dorsalis; *H*, *H₁*, fields of Forel; *HL* or *LH*, lateral hypothalamic area; *HP*, posterior hypothalamic area; *IC*, internal capsule; *Ic*, nucleus intercalatus; *IT*, fibers of nucleus tuberis; *ITP*, inferior thalamic peduncle; *MFB*, medial

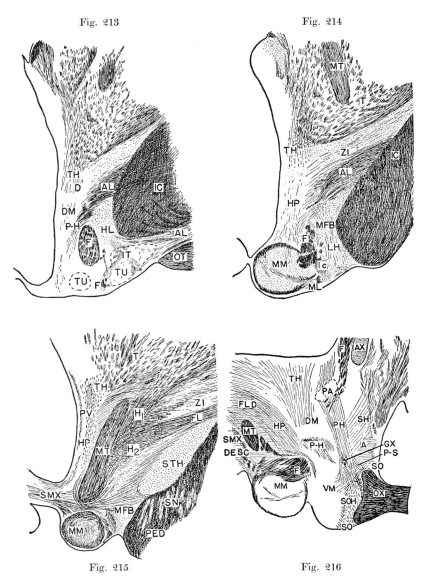

Fig. 213

Fig. 214

Fig. 215

Fig. 216

forebrain bundle; *ML*, lateral mammillary nucleus; *MM*, medial mammillary nucleus; *MPA*, medial preoptic area; *MT*, mammillothalamic tract; *MX*, dorsal supraoptic commissure, pars ventralis; *OT*, optic tract; *OX*, optic chiasma; *PA*, paraventricular nucleus; *PED*, cerebral peduncle; *PH*, paraventriculohypophyseal fibers; *P-H*, pallidohypothalamic fibers; *P-S*, paraventriculo-supraoptic fibers; *PV*, periventricular system; *SH*, septohypothalamic fibers; *SI*, substantia innominata; *SM*, stria medullaris; *SMX*, supramammillary commissure; *SN*, substantia nigra; *SO*, supraoptic nucleus; *SOH*, supraopticohypophyseal tract; *SOX*, supraoptic commissures; *ST*, stria terminalis; *STH*, subthalamic nucleus; *T*, thalamus; *TH*, thalamohypothalamic fibers; *TU*, nucleus tuberis laterale; *VM*, ventromedial hypothalamic nucleus; *ZI*, zona incerta; *3V*, third ventricle.

are in addition to the nucleus just described also the cells of the anterior hypothalamic area (Fig. 210, *A*), and the paraventricular nucleus (Figs. 210–212,
PA). In the tuberal region there are to be found the ventromedial hypothalamic
nucleus (Figs. 211, 212, *VM*), the dorsomedial hypothalamic nucleus (Figs. 211–
213, *DM*), and the cells of the dorsal hypothalamic area (Figs. 212, 213, *D*). In
the mammillary region are found the cells of the posterior hypothalamic area
(Figs. 214, 215, *HP*), and the nuclei of the mammillary body: the medial mammillary nucleus (Figs. 214, 215, *MM*), the lateral mammillary nucleus (Fig. 214,
ML), and the nucleus intercalatus (Fig. 214, *Ic*). The medial is much the largest
of these three nuclei in the mammillary body. The other two are small and
situated close to its lateral surface.

Lateral to the fornix throughout the length of the hypothalamus is the
lateral hypothalamic area (Figs. 210–212, *LH* or *HL*). The nerve cells which
it contains are small in the anterior part of the hypothalamus but they increase

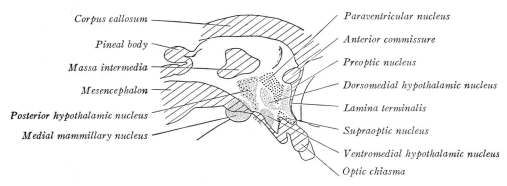

FIGURE 217.   The hypothalamic nuclei of man illustrated as if projected upon the lateral wall of the
third ventricle. (After Le Gros Clark.)

in size posteriorly, forming what Malone called the tuberomammillary nucleus.
A detailed account of the hypothalamic nuclei and fiber tracts has been published by Ingram (1940).

Afferent Nerve Fibers.   The *medial forebrain bundle* contains fine myelinated and unmyelinated fibers running from before backwards through the
lateral hypothalamic area. It forms a connection between the ventromedial areas
of olfactory cortex and the preoptic and hypothalamic areas. The lateral hypothalamic area also contains descending fibers which run from the hypothalamic
nuclei into the brain stem. The *fornix* is a large, heavily myelinated fascicle
which runs obliquely through the hypothalamus from above downward and
backward (Figs. 209–214, *F;* 232). It takes origin from the hippocampus and
ends in the medial and lateral mammillary nuclei, and some fibers are traceable
into the mesencephalic tegmentum. A small but well defined fascicle of myelinated fibers, the *pallidohypothalamic tract* (Fig. 214, *P-H*), takes origin from
the globus pallidus. After separating from the ansa lenticularis it runs medially
and ventrally through the hypothalamus to end in the ventromedial hypothalami nucleus (Ranson *et al.*, 1941). Corticohypothalamic and thalamohypo-

thalamic connections, either direct or indirect, exist but information on this subject is meager. Connections to hypothalamus have been traced from the frontal and limbic areas, the orbital, sensorimotor and auditory areas (Niemer and Jiminez-Castellanos, 1950). The *mammillary peduncle* contains fibers which ascend from the brain stem to end in the lateral mammillary nucleus. Fibers, which belong to the *stria terminalis,* run from the amygdaloid nucleus to the preoptic and hypothalamic regions.

The *supraoptic commissures* consist of fibers which cross the midline dorsal to the caudal border of the optic chiasma. Although in this part of their course they lie in the hypothalamus, these fibers make no connections with the hypothalamic nuclei (Magoun and Ranson, 1942).

Efferent Nerve Fibers. The *supraopticohypophyseal tract* arises from the cells of the supraoptic nucleus and runs through the median eminence and infundibular stem into the neural lobe of the hypophysis (Fig. 208). It distributes fibers to all parts of the neurohypophysis, including the median eminence and infundibular stem as well as the neural lobe (Fisher, Ingram, and Ranson, 1938; Magoun and Ranson, 1939). Fibers from the paraventricular nucleus and from the tuber also reach the neurohypophysis (paraventriculohypophyseal and tuberohypophyseal tracts).

Descending fibers from the hypothalamic nuclei enter the mesencephalon in medial and lateral bundles. The lateral fibers descend through the lateral hypothalamic area and reach the midbrain by passing dorsolaterally to the mammillary body (Magoun, 1940). The medial fibers descend in the periventricular system close to the wall of the third ventricle and form the *dorsal longitudinal fasciculus* ventral to the cerebral aqueduct (Fig. 166). This bundle has fibers which interconnect thalamic and hypothalamic nuclei; others which reach all the preganglionic cells of the cranial autonomic neurons; others passing to the motor nuclei of the cranial nerves other than those to the eye muscles; other fibers related to the periventricular gray matter of pons and medulla, as the dorsal nucleus of the raphe, the laterodorsal and dorsal tegmental nuclei. Some fibers are contributed to the dorsal longitudinal fasciculus by the latter gray masses and by the nucleus of fasciculus solitarius. By its connections its significance to visceral mechanism is emphasized. The *mammillothalamic tract* is a large well myelinated bundle which arises from the mammillary nuclei and ends in the anterior thalamic nuclei (Figs. 206, 242). The *mammillotegmental tract* is a descending bundle which branches off from the mammillothalamic tract and runs into the mesencephalon. Like the latter tract it arises from the mammillary nuclei.

FUNCTIONS OF THE HYPOTHALAMUS

The hypothalamus, representing but 4 grams of a total brain weight of around 1200 grams, is concerned with more fundamental functions than might be imagined. It is related to the hypophysis and to many endocrine interrelationships, to various autonomic functions, to emotional expression, and has a subtle influence on the cerebral cortex since it contains a sleep-regulating mechanism

It is of interest that stimuli applied directly to the hypothalamus have been employed to produce conditioned responses (Ban and Shinoda, 1956).

The **activity of the hypothalamus,** when released from cortical inhibition, furnishes information concerning the normal function of this part of the brain. Animals from which the cerebral cortex has been removed show on slight provocation signs of rage including struggling, piloerection, pupillodilatation, and increase in arterial blood pressure. This sham rage does not appear if the hypothalamus has been removed along with the cerebral hemisphere. The hypothalamus contains a center for the excitation and integration of the visceral and somatic responses which regularly form a part of the reaction pattern of fear and rage (Bard, 1934).

Electrical stimulation of the hypothalamus in anesthetized cats causes an increase in rate and depth of respiration, a rise in arterial blood pressure, pupillodilatation, and under some conditions also erection of hair. The sympathetic responses are accompanied by struggling and other activity of skeletal muscles suggestive of emotional excitement. It would thus appear that by electrical stimulation of the hypothalamus there is activated that mechanism for emotional expression which, when freed from cortical inhibition by decortication, gives rise to "sham" rage.

Functions related to parasympathetic activity are also represented in the hypothalamus. Stimulation of the hypothalamus affects the heart rate and the effect is different from stimulation of different regions; for example, stimuli applied to the lateral hypothalamic region gave effects similar to excessive vagus stimulation and this response was abolished by cutting the vagus nerves (Yuasa, Ban and Kurtosu, 1957).

Stimulation of the preoptic region causes contraction of the bladder and sometimes also other evidence of parasympathetic activity. It is believed that a pathway leads backward from this center through the hypothalamus (Ranson and Magoun, 1939).

Lesions of the hypothalamus cause impairment or abolition of certain normal activities. The functions, which are thus affected, may be ascribed to the hypothalamus although quite obviously the function may be one with which other parts of the brain and other organs may be involved. Bilateral lesions situated in the caudal part of the lateral hypothalamic area regularly cause *somnolence.* The explanation for this seems to be that these lesions interrupt the important pathway from the hypothalamus, which descends through the lateral hypothalamic area and enters the mesencephalon after passing dorsolateral to the mammillary body. It is assumed that the impulses, which descend along this pathway and which under certain conditions are able to cause the intense and widespread activation of the body seen in rage, are under ordinary conditions an important factor in maintaining that degree of activity of the brain stem and spinal cord which is essential for the waking state. At any rate it is certain on the basis of clinical as well as experimental evidence that lesions so placed as to interrupt bilaterally this descending pathway from the hypothalamus do cause somnolence (Ranson and Magoun, 1939; Collins, 1954).

That the hypothalamus may not be the highest level at which sleep mechanisms operate is implied in the common knowledge that in sleep consciousness is temporarily in abeyance, and by some observations indicating that disturbances in sleep may accompany pure cortical lesions.

It may well be that sleep occurs when impulses ascending from the hypothalamus and other lower levels toward the cerebral cortex are eliminated by the lesions described. Electroencephalographic evidence is strong that the hypothalamus and other parts of the diencephalon have marked effect on cortical rhythms. Lesions in the hypothalamus and some adjacent areas interfere with the animal's reaction to disturbing stimuli which would normally produce activation of the cortex (Koella and Gellhorn, 1954).

Disturbances in temperature regulation often result from hypothalamic lesions. Bilateral lesions in the posterior part of the lateral hypothalamus impair or abolish the capacity for regulation of body temperature. If the room temperature is in the usual comfortable range, the body temperature falls to a low level, but by the application of external heat the body can be easily overheated without bringing into play sweating or other means for dissipating heat. Bilateral lesions in the preoptic region do not impair the capacity to react to a cold environment by vasoconstriction and shivering, but they do eliminate the ability to reduce body temperature by sweating or panting. An animal with such anteriorly placed lesions can be easily overheated but chills no more readily than a normal animal. In man and animals acute bilateral lesions in the preoptic region often cause a rapid rise in body temperature, which may reach a fatally high level or may subside again within a day or two. Hyperthermia resulting from operations in the region of the optic chiasma is very troublesome for the neurosurgeon.

On the basis of all the available evidence it now seems clear that a center controlling heat-loss functions such as sweating and panting is situated in the preoptic region and that a pathway from this center runs backward through the lateral hypothalamus (Fig. 218). The center for preventing heat loss by vasoconstriction and for increasing heat production by shivering is situated in the hypothalamus proper, and its descending pathway also runs backward through the lateral hypothalamus. Both descending pathways run close together dorsolateral to the mammillary body and enter the mesencephalic tegmentum. Bilateral lesions in the caudal part of the lateral hypothalamus interrupt both pathways and interfere with both the heat-loss and the heat-conservation mechanisms. Bilateral lesions in the preoptic region destroy the heat-loss center leaving the heat-conservation mechanism intact; as a result, the body temperature either remains normal or may be temporarily elevated (Ranson, 1940; Beaton et al., 1943). Local heating of the anterior hypothalamus produces synchronous slow changes in potential from this region and not from other areas, and there is a correlation between these slow potentials and panting (von Euler, 1950).

Diabetes insipidus, a disease characterized by the passage of an excessive amount of sugar-free urine of low specific gravity, is caused by the interruption of the supraopticohypophyseal tract, the destruction of the supraoptic nuclei, or by the removal or destruction of the neurohypophysis. All three parts of the neurohypophysis, i. e., the median eminence, infundibular stem, and neural lobe (Fig. 208), have the same structure and constitute an endocrine gland which secretes an antidiuretic hormone. This hormone acts on the kidney to reduce the amount of urine. The supraoptic nuclei give rise to the supraoptico-hypophyseal tract, and this is distributed to the neurohypophysis. These three structures, nucleus, tract, and endocrine gland, are mutually interdependent. When one is destroyed the other two degenerate and diabetes insipidus results because of a deficiency of the antidiuretic hormone normally formed by the neurohypophysis. Clinically, the most common cause of diabetes insipidus is the

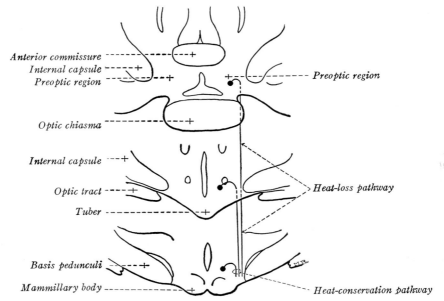

FIGURE 218. Diagrammatic representation of the mechanism for temperature regulation, superimposed upon schematic drawings of three transverse sections through the preoptic region and hypothalamus.

interruption of the supraopticohypophyseal tract in the floor of the third ventricle or in the infundibular stem. The disease has been produced in animals by interrupting the tract at one or the other of these two levels. It can also be produced in animals by removing all of the neurohypophysis, but, if the median eminence and infundibular stem are left, these may constitute a sufficient remnant of the gland to prevent the disease from developing (Fisher, Ingram, and Ranson, 1938; Magoun and Ranson, 1939). A small subcommissural organ beneath the posterior commissure shows relationship to water intake. Gilbert (1956) found that destruction of it was followed by diminished water consumption.

There is evidence (Bargman and Scharrer, 1951) that the pars nervosa of the hypophysis stores secretion which is produced by neurosecretory cells of the hypothalamus, rather than performing the actual secretion. The neurosecretory granules demonstrated in the supraoptic and paraventricular nuclei and along the nerve fibers leading to the hypophysis increase when an animal has excessive water intake and diminish when an animal is in a dehydrated state, implying the use of the antidiuretic principle. There is evidence that the neurosecretory granules also are responsible for the oxytocic and vasopressor substances related to the neurohypophysis. There is some indication that neurosecretory granules may be of more than one variety (D'Angelo et al., 1956; Ford and Kantounis, 1957).

An influence of hypothalamic areas on pregnancy in the rabbit implying an interaction with hypophysis and ovary has been demonstrated (Tsutsui et al., 1957). Destruction of an area including the ventromedial nucleus ("sympathetic zone") during pregnancy caused no disturbance, though the pregnancy might be prolonged a day or so; but destruction of the lateral hypothalamic area ("parasympathetic zone") was followed by abortion, which could, however, be prevented with adequate doses of progesterone.

Neurosecretory granules have been seen in the pars intermedia of the frog's hypophysis arranged in lines as if still in nerve fibers (Dawson, 1953). Because of the close association of the neurosecretory granules to capillaries of the hypophyseal portal system, it has been suggested that they may be the hormonal link between the nervous system and the adenohypophysis (Palay, 1953), but this may be merely a close relation to pituicytes that lie near the vessels (Rennels and Drager, 1955). The experiments of de Groot (1957) caused him to conclude that the neurosecretory material did not have a direct relationship to function of the adenohypophysis.

Disturbances in fat metabolism may result from hypothalamic lesions. In the rat and probably in some other animals and in man, lesions in the hypothalamus which do not in any way involve the hypophysis may result in adiposity (Hetherington and Ranson, 1942).

Lesions involving the hypothalamus or the paths to or from it may predispose to ulceration or hemorrhage in the alimentary tract. This has been demonstrated in both man and animals (French et al., 1952).

The Internal Structure
of the Cerebral Hemispheres

The surface anatomy and general topography of the interior of the cerebral hemispheres have been described in an earlier chapter, and now detailed relationships and connections must be considered before discussing the functions of the telencephalon and its parts. Since lesions of the great motor and sensory pathways form such important means of interpreting neurologic connections, the relations of these pathways are of paramount importance in each region of the central nervous system. In the telencephalon such pathways assume proportions which in some instances can be dissected and observed grossly. The gross relationships of these to masses of gray matter as well as the neuronal connections they form are worthy of study.

THE BASAL GANGLIA OF THE TELENCEPHALON

There are four deeply placed masses of gray matter within the hemisphere, known as the *caudate, lentiform,* and *amygdaloid nuclei,* and the *claustrum.* The two former, together with the white fascicles of the internal capsule which separate them, constitute the *corpus striatum* (Fig. 219).

The **caudate nucleus** (nucleus caudatus) is an elongated mass of gray matter bent on itself like a horseshoe, and is throughout its entire extent closely related to the lateral ventricle (Figs. 56, 220–226). Its swollen rostral extremity or *head* is pear-shaped and bulges into the anterior horn of the lateral ventricle. The remainder of the nucleus is drawn out into a long, slender, highly arched *tail.* In the floor of the central part of the ventricle the head gradually tapers off into the tail, which finally curves around into the roof of the inferior horn and extends rostrally as far as the amygdaloid nucleus. Because of its arched form it will be cut twice in any horizontal section which passes through the main mass of the corpus striatum, and in any frontal section through that body behind the amygdaloid nucleus (Figs. 219, 223, 226). The head of the caudate nucleus is directly continuous with the anterior perforated substance, and ventral to the anterior limb of the internal capsule it is fused with the lentiform nucleus (Fig. 220).

The **lentiform** or **lenticular nucleus** (nucleus lentiformis) is deeply placed in the white center of the hemisphere and intervenes between the insula, on the one hand, and the caudate nucleus and thalamus on the other (Figs. 219, 226, 228). In shape it bears some resemblance to a biconvex lens. Its lateral, moderately convex surface is nearly coextensive with the insula from which it is separated by the claustrum. Its ventral surface rests upon the anterior perforated substance and the white matter forming the roof of the inferior horn of the lateral ventricle (Figs. 221–223). Its sloping medial surface is closely applied to the internal capsule. The lentiform nucleus is not a homogeneous

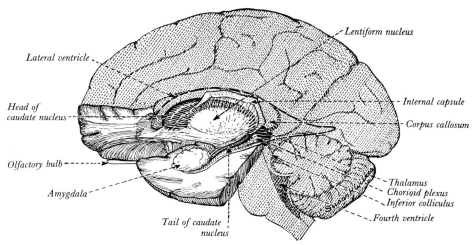

FIGURE 219. Drawing of a brain with left hemisphere dissected to expose the amygdaloid, lentiform and caudate nuclei. The internal capsule is shown as if transparent, extending between the lentiform nucleus laterally and the caudate nucleus and thalamus medially. The left lateral ventricle is shown with solid line where the wall is intact and with broken line where it has been dissected away. The only part of the left cerebral cortex remaining is shown in the temporal lobe and the inferior part of the frontal lobe.

mass, but is divided into two parts by the *external medullary lamina*. The more lateral zone is the larger and is known as the *putamen*. It is separated by this lamina from the smaller more medial zone, which, because its numerous myelinated fibers give it a lighter color, is known as the *globus pallidus*. The latter is subdivided by the *internal medullary lamina* into the internal and external divisions (Figs. 222, 225).

Especially in the anterior part of the internal capsule, bands of gray substance stretch across from the lentiform to the caudate nucleus, producing a striated appearance (Figs. 392, 393). This appearance, which is accentuated by the medullary laminae and the fine fiber bundles in the lentiform nucleus, makes the term *corpus striatum* an appropriate name to apply to the mass formed by the two nuclei and the internal capsule, which separates them.

The caudate nucleus and putamen have the same *histologic structure*. They are composed of small nerve cells among which are interspersed a few of medium

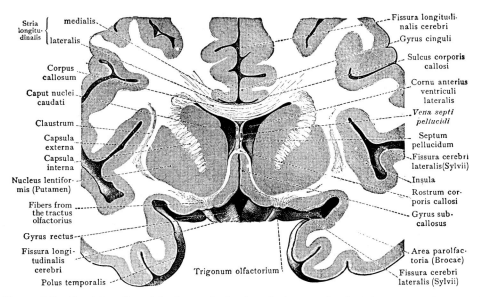

Stria longitudinalis { medialis
lateralis

Corpus callosum

Caput nuclei caudati

Claustrum

Capsula externa

Capsula interna

Nucleus lentiformis (Putamen)

Fibers from the tractus olfactorius

Gyrus rectus

Fissura longitudinalis cerebri

Polus temporalis

Fissura longitudinalis cerebri

Gyrus cinguli

Sulcus corporis callosi

Cornu anterius ventriculi lateralis

Vena septi pellucidi

Septum pellucidum

Fissura cerebri lateralis(Sylvii)

Insula

Rostrum corporis callosi

Gyrus subcallosus

Area parolfactoria (Brocae)

Fissura cerebri lateralis (Sylvii)

Trigonum olfactorium

FIGURE 220. Frontal section of the human brain through the rostral end of the corpus striatum and the rostrum of the corpus callosum. (Toldt.)

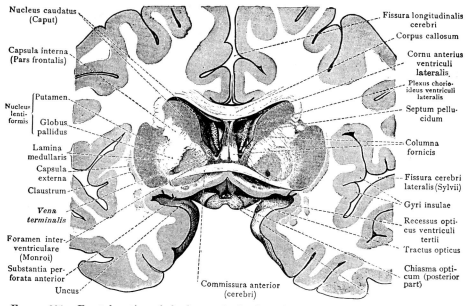

Nucleus caudatus (Caput)

Capsula interna (Pars frontalis)

Nucleus lentiformis { Putamen
Globus pallidus

Lamina medullaris

Capsula externa

Claustrum

Vena terminalis

Foramen interventriculare (Monroi)

Substantia perforata anterior

Uncus

Fissura longitudinalis cerebri

Corpus callosum

Cornu anterius ventriculi **lateralis**

Plexus chorioideus ventriculi lateralis

Septum pellucidum

Columna fornicis

Fissura cerebri lateralis (Sylvii)

Gyri insulae

Recessus opticus ventriculi tertii

Tractus opticus

Chiasma opticum (posterior part)

Commissura anterior (cerebri)

FIGURE 221. Frontal section of the human brain through the anterior commissure. (Toldt.)

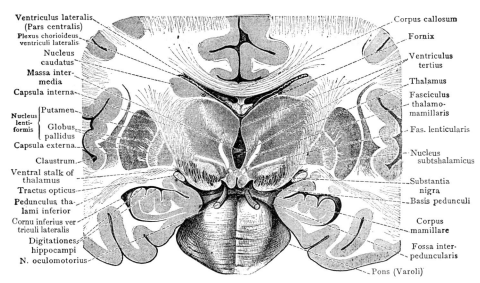

Ventriculus lateralis
(Pars centralis)
Plexus chorioideus
ventriculi lateralis
Nucleus
caudatus
Massa inter-
media
Capsula interna

Nucleus
lenti-
formis
Putamen
Globus
pallidus
Capsula externa

Claustrum

Ventral stalk of
thalamus
Tractus opticus
Pedunculus tha-
lami inferior
Cornu inferius ver
triculi lateralis
Digitationes
hippocampi
N. oculomotorius

Corpus callosum
Fornix
Ventriculus
tertius
Thalamus
Fasciculus
thalamo-
mamillaris
Fas. lenticularis
Nucleus
subtshalamicus
Substantia
nigra
Basis pedunculi
Corpus
mamillare
Fossa inter-
peduncularis
Pons (Varoli)

FIGURE 222. Frontal section of the human brain through the mammillary bodies. (Toldt.)

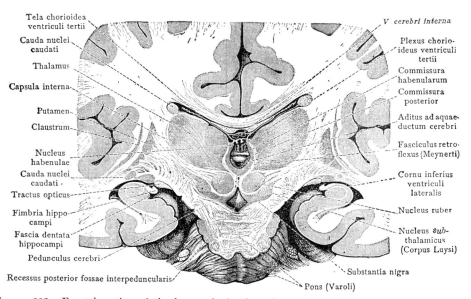

Tela chorioidea
ventriculi tertii
Cauda nuclei
caudati
Thalamus

Capsula interna

Putamen
Claustrum

Nucleus
habenulae
Cauda nuclei
caudati
Tractus opticus

Fimbria hippo-
campi
Fascia dentata
hippocampi
Pedunculus cerebri

Recessus posterior fossae interpeduncularis

V cerebri interna
Plexus chorio-
ideus ventriculi
tertii
Commissura
habenularum
Commissura
posterior
Aditus ad aquae-
ductum cerebri
Fasciculus retro-
flexus (Meynerti)
Cornu inferius
ventriculi
lateralis
Nucleus ruber
Nucleus sub-
thalamicus
(Corpus Luysi)
Substantia nigra
Pons (Varoli)

FIGURE 223. Frontal section of the human brain through the rostral part of the pons. (Toldt.)

size. The globus pallidus has a very different structure. Its cell are large, and it contains many more myelinated fibers than do the caudate nucleus and putamen. Because of this difference in structure between the putamen and globus pallidus, the lentiform nucleus is clearly a composite structure rather than a single nucleus. It is now customary to group the caudate nucleus and putamen together as the *striatum* (not to be confused with the corpus striatum which includes the globus pallidus) and to call the globus pallidum the *pallidum*. In man the pallidum is relatively larger than it is in lower animals.

Nerve Fibers. The two divisions of the striatum send fibers to the pallidum, which, in turn, gives rise to fibers which go to other parts of the nervous

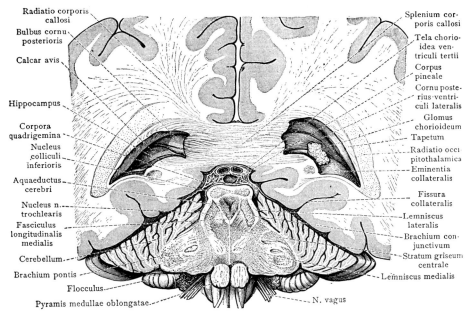

FIGURE 224. Frontal section of the human brain through the splenium of the corpus callosum. View into the posterior horn of the lateral ventricle. (Toldt.)

system (Fig. 225). The fibers which arise in the putamen converge like the spokes of a wheel before they end in the internal and external divisions of the globus pallidus. Other fibers are said to arise in the external and end in the internal division of the pallidum.

As illustrated in Fig. 225, fibers from the internal division of the globus pallidus run by way of the ansa and fasciculus lenticularis (H_2), and after passing through field H curve dorsally and then laterally through the thalamic fasciculus (H_1), to the anterior part of the ventral thalamic nucleus. A few fibers run ventromedially into the hypothalamus forming the pallidohypothalamic tract (Fig. 212). Fibers from the external division of the globus pallidus run to the subthalamic nucleus. These pallidosubthalamic fibers do not pass through field H, but reach the subthalamic nucleus after crossing the lower end of the internal capsule (Fig. 225). (Ranson et al., 1941, a, b.)

The corpus striatum receives fibers from the thalamus, and, according to Cajal, also fibers from the cerebral cortex. Physiologic evidence has been presented to show that fibers from the cortex go to the caudate nucleus and putamen (Dusser de Barenne, Garol, and McCulloch, 1942).

The corpus striatum and the substantia nigra are connected by fibers which have been thought to run a descending course and have been called strionigral fibers, but a study of Marchi preparations following injury to the substantia nigra in monkeys has shown that many of these fibers degenerate

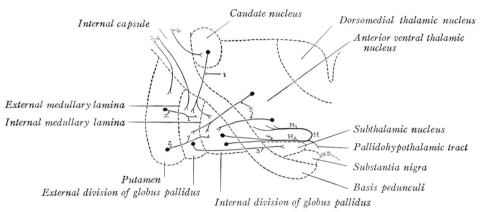

FIGURE 225. Diagrammatic representation of the fiber connections of the corpus striatum. H, H_1 and H_2, Fields of Forel; 1 and 2, fibers joining parts of the corpus striatum; 3, pallidosubthalamic tract; 4, fasciculus lenticularis; 5, thalamostriatal connection; 6 and 7, fibers from the cerebral cortex. The ansa lenticularis, which joins the field H without passing through H_2, is not shown in the diagram.

upward from the substantia nigra to the globus pallidus (Ranson et al., 1941). There are, however, fibers from the region of the corpus striatum which descend to the red nucleus (Laursen, 1955).

Function. Very little is known concerning the function of the corpus striatum except what may be inferred from the symptoms exhibited by patients in whom the basal ganglia are diseased. Some exhibit the Parkinsonian syndrome, characterized by tremor, which persists during rest, and by a plastic rigidity of all the skeletal muscles with resultant slowness of movement and a masklike face. In other patients disease of the basal ganglia results in bizarre involuntary movements (athetosis and chorea). Since the pathology in the diseases which produce these syndromes is widespread and since the symptoms have not been reproduced by damage to the corpus striatum in monkeys or other animals, it is not possible to draw from these clinical observations a clear picture of the function of the various parts of the corpus striatum. It has been said that stimulation of the caudate nucleus or putamen may inhibit phasic movements, induced by cortical stimulation, as well as spontaneous movements (Mettler, 1942). In the unanesthetized cat Ward (1952) has observed trunk

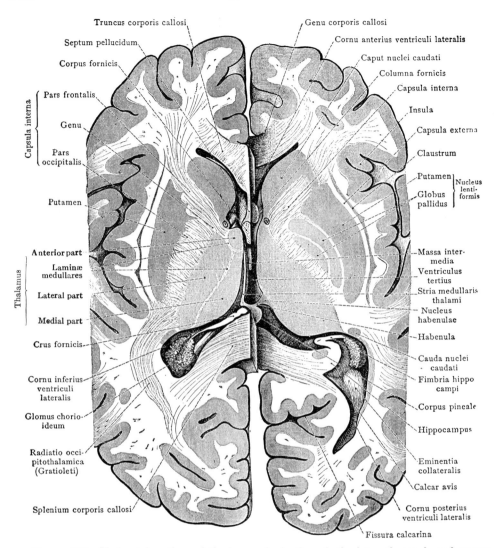

FIGURE 226. Horizontal sections of the human brain through the internal capsule and corpus striatum. The section on the right side was made 1.5 cm. farther ventralward than that on the left. (Toldt.)

movements, including head turning to the opposite side, accompanying stimulation of the head of the caudate nucleus, which occurred even in the absence of the primary cortical motor area.

The corpus striatum is generally regarded as an important link in an extrapyramidal motor path. The function of the corpus striatum and the course of descending pathways by which it can influence the activity of the spinal cord still remain largely unknown.

The **claustrum** is a thin plate of gray substance, which, along with the white matter in which it is embedded, separates the putamen from the cortex of the insula. Its lateral surface is somewhat irregular, being adapted to the convolutions of the insula, with which it is coextensive (Figs. 222, 226). Its concave medial surface is separated from the putamen by a thin lamina of white matter, known as the external capsule.

The claustrum in the usual horizontal slices of the cerebrum is only a thin gray lamina, but, in frontal sections through the cerebrum from the level of the optic chiasma back to the mammillary bodies, the claustrum appears as a large gray mass just lateral to the putamen and dorsolateral to the amygdaloid body, which also in this region shows its greatest dimensions (Figs. 392–396).

The Amygdaloid Body. In the roof of the terminal part of the inferior ventricular horn, at the point where the tail of the caudate nucleus ends, there is located a mass of gray matter, known as the amygdaloid body (Figs. 219, 393, 394). It is continuous with the cerebral cortex of the temporal lobe lateral to the anterior perforated substances (Fig. 235). Primitively, the amygdaloid body is developed within the caudal end of the lateral olfactory nucleus but is added to in reptiles from an area related to the pyriform cortex. In size it rivals the globus pallidus.

The **external capsule** is a thin lamina of white matter separating the claustrum from the putamen. Along with the internal capsule it encloses the lentiform nucleus with a coating of white substance.

THE INTERNAL CAPSULE

The internal capsule is a broad band of white substance separating the lentiform nucleus on the lateral side from the caudate nucleus and thalamus on the medial side (Fig. 226). In a horizontal section through the middle of the corpus striatum it has the shape of a wide open V with the apex of the V pointing medially. The angle, situated in the interval between the caudate nucleus and the thalamus, is known as the *genu.* From this bend the *frontal part* or *anterior limb of the internal capsule* extends laterally and rostrally between the lentiform and the caudate nuclei, while the *occipital part* or *posterior limb of the internal capsule* extends laterally and toward the occiput between the lentiform nucleus and the thalamus.

The **anterior limb of the internal capsule,** intervening between the caudate and lentiform nuclei, is broken up by bands of gray matter connecting these two nuclei. It consists of corticipetal and corticifugal fibers. The former belong to the *frontal stalk of the thalamus* or anterior thalamic radiation from the lateral nucleus of the thalamus to the cortex of the frontal lobe. The corticifugal fibers form the *frontopontile tract* from the cortex of the frontal lobe to the nuclei pontis (Fig. 227).

The **posterior limb of the internal capsule** intervenes between the thalamus and the lentiform nucleus, and is molded around the posterior end of the latter (Figs. 226, 228). It accordingly consists of three parts, designated as lenticulothalamic, retrolenticular, and sublenticular (Fig. 32). The *lenticulothalamic part* consists of fibers belonging to the *thalamic radiation* intermingled with others representing the great efferent tracts which descend from the cerebral cortex (Fig. 227). Of these, the *corticobulbar tract* to the motor nuclei of the cranial

nerves occupies the genu, and the *corticospinal tract* the adjacent portion of
the posterior limb. The fibers of the corticospinal tract are so arranged that
those for the innervation of the arm are nearer the genu than those for the leg.
Accompanying the corticospinal tract are descending fibers from the cortex of
the frontal lobe to the red nucleus, the *corticorubral tract*. Those fibers of the
thalamic radiation which run to the posterior central gyrus and convey general

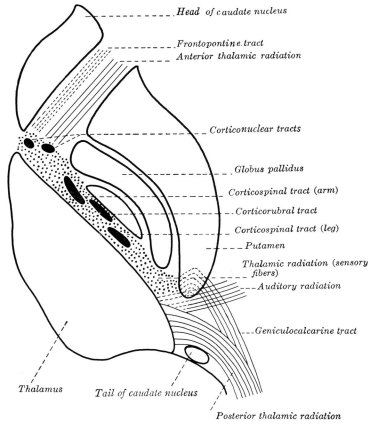

Head *of caudate nucleus*

Frontopontine tract
Anterior thalamic radiation

Corticonuclear tracts

Globus pallidus
Corticospinal tract (arm)
Corticorubral tract
Corticospinal tract (leg)
Putamen
*Thalamic radiation (sensory
fibers)*
Auditory radiation

Geniculocalcarine tract

Thalamus   *Tail of caudate nucleus*

Posterior thalamic radiation

Figure 227. Diagram of the internal capsule as shown in horizontal section (Fig. 226).

sensory impulses from the thalamus are situated behind the corticospinal tract.
The *retrolenticular part* of the internal capsule rests upon the lateral surface
of the thalamus behind the lentiform nucleus and contains the posterior thalamic
radiation. The *sublenticular part* of the internal capsule lies ventral to the
posterior extremity of the lenticular nucleus and contains the temporopontile
tract from the cortex of the temporal lobe to the nuclei pontis, the geniculocalcarine tract from the lateral geniculate body to the calcarine cortex, and the
auditory radiation from the medial geniculate body to the transverse temporal
gyrus (Fig. 369).

The fibers of the anterior limb run nearly horizontally forward; those of the several parts of the posterior limb run in different directions. The fibers of the lenticulothalamic part run nearly vertically upward, those of the retrolenticular part nearly horizontally backward, and those of the sublenticular part nearly horizontally lateralward. Where one part of the internal capsule becomes continuous with another there is a gradual transition in the direction of the fibers (Figs. 32, 227, 229).

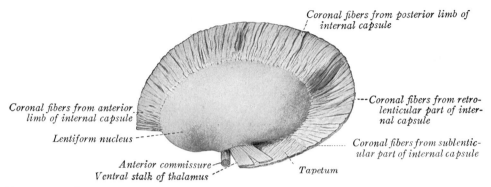

FIGURE 228. The lentiform nucleus and the corona radiata dissected free from the left human cerebral hemisphere. Lateral view.

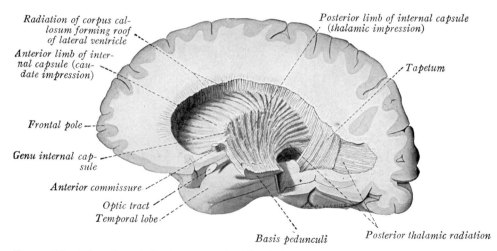

FIGURE 229. Dissection of the human cerebral hemisphere, showing the internal capsule exposed from the medial side. The caudate nucleus and thalamus have been removed.

Dissections of the Internal Capsule (Figs. 32, 228, 229).   A large part of the fibers of the internal capsule, including the corticopontile, corticobulbar, and corticospinal tracts, are continued as a broad thick strand on the ventral surface of the cerebral peduncle, with which we are already familiar under the name *basis pedunculi*. By removing the optic tract, temporal lobe, insula, and lentiform nucleus, this strand can easily be traced into the internal capsule where it is joined by many fibers radiating from the thalamus and spreads out in a fan-shaped manner (Fig. 32), forming a curved plate which partially encloses the lentiform nucleus. As seen from the lateral side, the line along which the fibers of the internal capsule emerge from behind the lentiform nucleus forms two-thirds of an ellipse (Fig. 228). Beyond the lentiform nucleus the diverging strands from the internal capsule, known as the *corona radiata*, join the central white substance of the hemisphere and intersect with those from the corpus callosum (Figs. 52, 272).

An instructive view of the internal capsule may also be obtained by removing the thalamus and caudate nucleus from its medial surface. It is then seen to bear the imprint of both of these nuclei, and especially of the thalamus, and between the two impressions it presents a prominent curved ridge (Fig. 229). This ridge is responsible for the sharp bend known as the genu, which is evident in horizontal sections at appropriate levels through the capsule. Many broken bundles of fibers, representing the thalamic radiation, are seen entering the capsule upon its medial surface.

THE MEDULLARY CENTER OF THE CEREBRAL HEMISPHERE

The medullary center of the cerebral hemisphere underlies the cortex and separates it from the lateral ventricle and corpus striatum. It varies greatly in thickness, from that of the thin lamina separating the insula and the claustrum (Fig. 226) to that of the massive centrum semiovale (Fig. 52). The myelinated nerve fibers of which it is composed are of three kinds: namely, association fibers, projection fibers, and commissural fibers. It is becoming increasingly apparent that the principle of feedback is common in the nervous system. Frequently it can be shown that two regions of gray matter are mutually interconnected, although the fibers carrying impulses in one of the directions may be more conspicuous. At times this feedback is by direct connection, and at other times, it is circuitous over interrupted neuronal paths. There are conspicuous cortico-ponto-cerebellar paths, and in return cerebello-thalamo-cortical ones, for example. Such connections, while not always clear in their implications, can often be shown to be useful in integrating the functions of the connected parts.

Commissural Fibers. There are three commissures joining together the cerebral hemispheres. Of these, the *corpus callosum* is by far the largest and its radiation contributes largely to the bulk of the centrum semiovale (Fig. 52). The fibers which compose it arise in the various parts of the neopallium of each hemisphere; they are assembled into a broad compact plate as they cross the median plane, and then spread out again to terminate in the neopallium of the opposite side. As they spread through the centrum semiovale they form the radiation of the corpus callosum. The majority of the fibers connect symmetrical areas in the two hemispheres (Curtis, 1940). Some cortical areas are better supplied with these fibers than others, few, if any, being associated with the visual cortex about the calcarine fissure (Van Valkenburg, 1913). The *anterior* and *hippocampal commissures* connect portions of the rhinencephalon in one hemisphere, with similar parts on the opposite side. The anterior commissure traced by degeneration in the monkey shows a division into two limbs, an anterior and a posterior. The anterior limb is very small and is distributed to the olfactory tubercle, anterior olfactory nucleus, and olfactory bulb. The posterior limb contains most of the fibers and is distributed for the most part to the middle temporal gyrus (Fox, Fisher, and Desalva, 1948), (Figs. 221, 233, 234). The hippocampal commissure is composed of fibers which join together the two hippocampi by way of the fimbriae and the psalterium (Fig. 240).

Projection Fibers.   Many of the fibers of the medullary white center connect the cerebral cortex with the thalamus and lower lying portions of the nervous system. These are known as projection fibers, and may be divided into two groups according as they convey impulses to or from the cerebral cortex. The corticipetal or *afferent projection fibers* include the following: (1) the *geniculocalcarine tract*, which arises in the lateral geniculate body and ends in the visual cortex about the calcarine fissure; (2) the *auditory radiation*, which arises in the medial geniculate body and terminates in the auditory cortex of the anterior transverse temporal gyrus; (3) the *thalamic radiation*, which unites the thalamic nuclei with various parts of the cerebral cortex. The lateral olfactory stria, which conveys impulses from the olfactory bulb to the pyriform area, is not a projection system in the strict sense of the word, since it begins and ends within the telencephalon.

Efferent projection fibers convey impulses from the cerebral cortex to the thalamus, basal ganglia, brain stem, and spinal cord. They represent the axons of pyramidal cells. The most important groups are those of the *corticospinal* and *corticonuclear (corticobulbar) tract*, which together form the great motor or pyramidal system. These fibers begin in the motor cortex of the anterior central gyrus, in part as axons of the giant cells of Betz. Entering the white medullary center of the hemisphere, they are assembled in the corona radiata and enter the internal capsule (Fig. 32). A few such fibers have been seen to run from the cortex, cross in the corpus callosum and extend through the pyramid of the opposite side (Walberg and Brodal, 1953). Their course beyond this point has been traced in the preceding chapters. They convey impulses to the primary motor neurons of the opposite side of the brain stem and spinal cord. Another important group of corticifugal fibers is contained in the *corticopontile tracts*. Of these there are two main strands. The *frontopontile tract* consists of fibers which begin as axons of cells in the cortex of the frontal lobe, traverse the centrum semiovale, corona radiata, frontal part of the internal capsule and medial one-fifth of the basis pedunculi, and finally terminate in the nuclei pontis. The *temporopontile tract* has a similar origin from the cortical cells of the temporal lobe and possibly of the occipital lobe also, passes through the sublenticular part of the internal capsule and lateral one-fifth of the basis pedunculi, and finally terminates in the nuclei pontis (Figs. 32, 161). Fibers from the temporal lobe reach the putamen, pulvinar, and dorsomedial nucleus of the thalamus, pretectal area, medial geniculate body, superior colliculus, tegmentum of the mesencephalon, tail of the caudate nucleus and anterior commissure (Whitlock and Nauta, 1956). The ascending thalamic radiation is paralleled by descending *corticothalamic fibers,* which should be included among the efferent projection systems, although their physiologic significance is not fully understood. A *corti-*

corubral tract descends from the frontal lobe through the posterior limb of the internal capsule to end in the red nucleus of the mesencephalon. According to Cajal (1911), collaterals from the corticospinal fibers are given off to the corpus striatum. The efferent projection tracts which we have considered all have their origin in the neopallium.

There are several *projection tracts from the rhinencephalon*, and of these the most important is the fornix. The fibers of this fascicle take origin in the hippocampus, follow an arched course already described and, entering the diencephalon, terminate in part in the mammillary body and in part in the tegmentum of the brain stem (Figs. 242, 248).

The *medial forebrain bundle* arises in the basal olfactory centers and runs caudally through the lateral part of the hypothalamus.

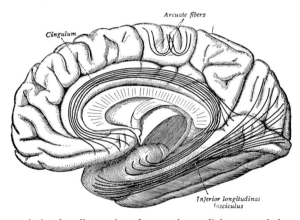

Figure 230.   Some association bundles projected upon the medial aspect of the cerebral hemisphere. (Sobotta-McMurrich.)

Association Fibers.   The various parts of the cortex within each hemisphere are bound together by association fibers of varying length. The *short association fibers* are of two kinds: (1) those which run in the deeper part of the cortex and are designated as *intracortical*, and (2) those just beneath the cortex, which are known as the *subcortical fibers*. The greater number of these subcortical association fibers unite adjacent gyri, curving in U-shaped loops beneath the intervening sulci, and are accordingly often designated as arcuate fibers (Fig. 230). Others unite somewhat more widely separated gyri. The *long association fibers* form bundles of considerable size, deeply situated in the medullary center of the hemisphere, and unite widely separated cortical areas. There are four of these which may be readily displayed by dissection of the human cerebral hemisphere, namely, the uncinate, inferior occipitofrontal, and superior longitudinal fasciculi, and the cingulum. Another, known as the fasciculus occipitofrontalis superior, is less easily displayed.

The *cingulum* is an arched bundle which partly encircles the corpus callosum not far from the median plane (Figs. 52, 230). It begins ventral to the rostrum of the corpus callosum, curves around the genu and over the dorsal surface of that commissure to the splenium, and then bends ventrally to terminate near the temporal pole. It is closely related to the gyrus cinguli and the hippocampal gyrus and is composed for the most part of short fibers, which connect the various parts of these convolutions.

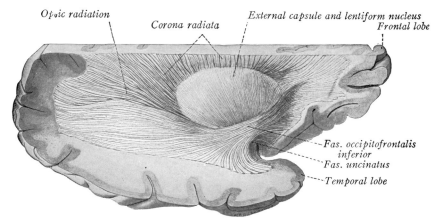

FIGURE 231. Lateral view of a dissection of a human cerebral hemisphere. The dorsal part of the hemisphere has been cut away. On the lateral side the insula, opercula, and adjacent parts have been removed.

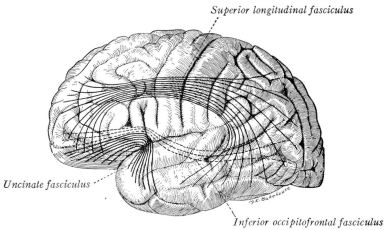

FIGURE 232. Some of the long association bundles projected upon the lateral aspect of the cerebral hemisphere.

The *uncinate fasciculus* connects the orbital gyri of the frontal lobe with the rostral part of the temporal lobe. It is sharply bent on itself as it passes over the stem of the lateral fissure of the cerebrum (Figs. 231, 232).

The *superior occipitofrontal fasciculus* runs in an arched course close to the dorsal border of the caudate nucleus and just beneath the corpus callosum. It is separated from the superior longitudinal fasciculus by the corona radiata (Fig. 233).

The *inferior occipitofrontal fasciculus* runs from the occipital to the frontal lobes along the ventrolateral border of the lentiform nucleus (Figs. 231, 232). It can be displayed by dissection, but this method cannot be regarded as giving a satisfactory demonstration that it is composed of long fibers joining the frontal and occipital lobes. It is included in the external sagittal stratum (Figs. 399, 401).

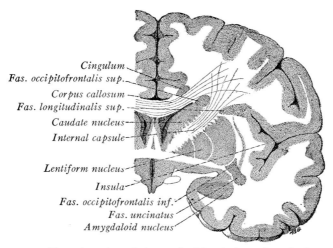

FIGURE 233. Frontal section of the cerebral hemisphere through the anterior commissure showing the location of the long association bundles.

The *superior longitudinal fasciculus* (fasciculus arcuatus) is a bundle of association fibers which serves to connect many parts of the cortex on the lateral surface of the hemisphere (Fig. 232). It sweeps over the insula, occupying the base of the frontal and parietal opercula, and then bends downward into the temporal lobe (Fig. 52). It is composed for the most part of bundles of rather short fibers which radiate from it to the frontal, parietal, occipital, and temporal cortex.

An *inferior longitudinal fasciculus* has been described as a large bundle which runs through the entire length of the temporal and occipital lobes (Fig. 230). It forms part of the external sagittal stratum (Figs. 399, 402) and it consists chiefly of geniculocalcarine projection fibers.

into the hemisphere the olfactory tract forms a triangular enlargement, the *olfactory trigone.*

From the point of insertion of the olfactory bulb or tract a band of gray matter, the *medial olfactory gyrus,* can be seen extending toward the medial surface of the hemisphere (Figs. 234, 235). A similar gray band, the *lateral olfactory gyrus,* runs caudalward on the basal surface of the sheep's brain.

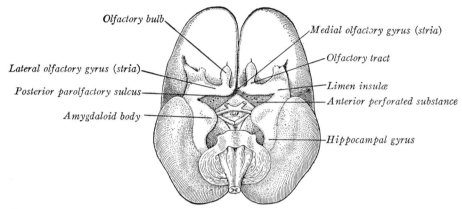

FIGURE 235. Brain of a human fetus of 22.5 cm. Ventral view. (Retzius, Jackson-Morris.)

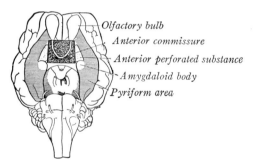

FIGURE 236. Ventral view of a sheep's brain, pyriform area shaded and anterior commissure exposed.

Along its lateral border it is separated from the neopallium by the rhinal fissure, while its medial border contains a band of fibers, the *stria olfactoria lateralis* (Fig. 234). The same gyrus is seen in the brain of the human fetus, but here it is directed outward toward the insula (Fig. 235). In the adult human brain these olfactory convolutions are very inconspicuous, and with the fibers from the olfactory tract which accompany them are usually designated as the *medial* and *lateral olfactory striae* (Fig. 31).

Between the olfactory trigone and the medial olfactory gyrus, on the one hand, and the optic tract on the other, is a depressed area of gray matter known as the *anterior perforated substance,* through the openings of which numerous small arteries reach the basal ganglia (Figs. 31, 234). The part immediately rostral to the optic tract forms a band of lighter color, known as the diagonal gyrus of the rhinencephalon or the *diagonal band* of Broca (Fig. 234). This can be followed on to the medial surface of the hemisphere, where it is continued as the *paraterminal body* or subcallosal gyrus (Fig. 237). Rostral to this gyrus the *hippocampal rudiment,* which corresponds in part to the subcallosal area, extends as a narrow band from the rostrum of the corpus callosum toward the medial olfactory gyrus. In those mammals which possess an especially rich innervation of the nose and mouth, the region of the anterior perforated space is marked by a swelling, sometimes of considerable size, called the *tuberculum*

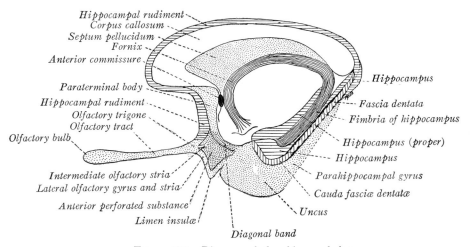

FIGURE 237. Diagram of the rhinencephalon.

olfactorium. According to Retzius, a small oval mass is present in the anterior perforated substance of man immediately adjacent to the olfactory trigone, which represents this tubercle.

The Pyriform Area. The lateral olfactory gyrus is continuous at its caudal extremity with the hippocampal gyrus (Figs. 234, 235), and the two together form the pyriform area or lobe (Fig. 236). In the adult human brain it is more difficult to demonstrate the continuity of these parts. As the temporal lobe is thrust rostrally and the insula becomes depressed, the pyriform area is bent on itself like a **V** (Fig. 235). The knee-like bend forms the *limen insulae,* and with the rest of the insula becomes buried at the bottom of the lateral fissure. The continuity of the pyriform area is not interrupted in the adult, though part of it is hidden from view. It includes the *lateral olfactory stria* and the *cortex subjacent* to it (or lateral olfactory gyrus), the *limen insulae,* the *uncus,* and at least a part of the *parahippocampal gyrus* (Fig. 237). It is not easy to determine just how much of the human parahippocampal gyrus should be included. Cajal (1911) apparently includes the entire gyrus, while Elliot Smith (1915) limits it to the part of the gyrus dorsal to the rhinal fissure. In Fig. 237 we have followed the outlines of the hippocampal region as given by Brodmann (1909).

The Amygdaloid Body. This nuclear group, which is sometimes referred to as the archistriatum, is blended with the gray matter near the tip of the inferior horn of the lateral ventricle (Fig. 219). In lower mammals it lies on the floor of this horn but in higher mammals occupies the rostral wall. Belonging to the olfactory secondary centers, it has non-olfactory connections of considerable quantity. Like other basal nuclei the amygdaloid complex has a primitive component and a more recently acquired portion which developed in higher mammals having more cerebral cortex. The amygdaloid complex includes subdivisions or nuclei termed: lateral, basal (and accessory basal), central, medial, cortical, and a nucleus of the lateral olfactory tract. The lateral and basal nuclear divisions of the amygdaloid complex are the most recent in origin.

The comparative history of the amygdala implies greater functional significance than would be expected from its apparent lack of prominence in the human brain. In lowly vertebrates a primordial striatum occurs which is heavily connected to the thalamus and to olfactory nuclei. Out of this primitive striatum appears an olfactostriatum, in relation to the amygdaloid complex and pyriform cortex, and a somatostriatum (the future lentiform nucleus) with strong thalamic connections. In later vertebrates the hypopallium develops related to the neopallium anteriorly and the pyriform cortex posteriorly. In mammals the anterior part of the hypopallium is added to the olfactostriatum to make the caudate nucleus, and the posterior part becomes part of the amygdala. The amygdaloid body is a roughly ovoid mass (measuring around 2 cm. in length) lying at the anterior end of the inferior horn of the lateral ventricle (Figs. 393–396). It lies in part beneath the uncus and reaches the surface of the brain in a limited area adjacent to the anterior perforate substance. In Fig. 395 the close relationship of the dorsal aspect of the amygdala and the ventral surface of the lentiform nucleus is shown where the anterior commissure passes between them. Its anterior pole is closely related to the ventral edge of the claustrum. The main efferent pathway of the amygdala is the stria terminalis, and the chief source of those fibers is the large celled basal nucleus (Fox, 1943). The function of the amygdala is obscure, but for that matter so is that of the caudate nucleus (Crosby and Humphrey, 1944; Brodal, 1947; Jiminez-Castellanos, 1949). However, in animal experiments destruction of the amygdala can result in a gentling effect, diminishing the animal's tendency to rage and development later of a hypersexual behavior (Schreiner and Kling, 1956). In man, damage in the periamygdaloid area (uncus of hippocampus, amygdaloid nucleus, claustrum, insula) may result in a type of epilepsy showing automatisms during which the patient loses memory for what he is doing. From this it has been suggested that the periamygdaloid area has a diffuse regulatory effect on other parts of the brain since it is apparently involved in the process of memory recording and maintenance of the conscious state (Feindel and Penfield, 1954). This region, along with other portions of the limbic lobe, appears to have a definite relationship to emotional responses and alerting reactions.

Connections of the amygdala have been studied with electrical stimulation and recording and compared with previous anatomical descriptions by Gloor (1955). This author points out that, while the stria terminalis (Fig. 243) repre-

sents a clearly defined efferent pathway from the cortico-medial part of the
amygdala, the basolateral part is connected by shorter paths to subcortical
projection areas; but there are internal connections between amygdaloid parts.
The amygdala through these routes or by multisynaptic chains can project
to neocortical parts (anterior temporal and insular regions of man), paleocortex
(pyriform area), and archicortex (hippocampus). The functions attributed to
this system are reminiscent of the control of fundamental integrative mechanisms of both somatic and visceral activities of lower forms before the large
cortical and thalamic development of higher forms occurred in relation to their
sensory and motor systems and capacity for a greater variety of responses to
changes in environment.

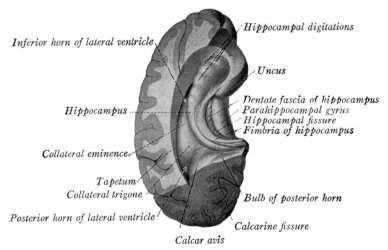

FIGURE 238. Part of temporal lobe of human brain showing inferior horn of lateral ventricle and
the hippocampus. Dorsal view. (Sobotta-McMurrich.)

The Hippocampus. An olfactory center of still higher order is represented
by the hippocampus, which was seen in connection with the study of the lateral
ventricle. If we turn again to the floor of the inferior horn of the lateral
ventricle, we shall see a long curved elevation projecting into the cavity (Figs.
57, 238). This is the hippocampus and is formed by highly specialized cortex
which has been rolled into the ventricle along the line of the hippocampal
fissure (Fig. 246). It is covered on its ventricular surface by a thin coating of
white matter, called the *alveus,* which is continuous along its medial edge with
a band of fibers known as the *fimbria of the hippocampus.* This, in turn, is continuous with the fornix (Figs. 238, 239). In Fig. 238 there may be seen, along
the border of the fimbria, a narrow serrated band of gray matter, the *fascia
dentata,* which lies upon the medial side of the hippocampus. It is separated
from the parahippocampal gyrus by a shallow groove, called the *hippocampal
fissure,* that marks the line along which the hippocampus has been rolled into
the ventricle.

The hippocampus and fascia dentata belong to the archipallium. In the marsupials and monotremes this extends dorsally on the medial surface of the hemisphere in a curve, which suggests that of the corpus callosum (Fig. 239). In the higher mammals the presence of a massive corpus callosum seems to inhibit the development of the adjacent part of the hippocampal formation, which remains as the vestigial indusium griseum, or supracallosal gyrus. This *hippocampal rudiment* is a thin layer of gray matter on the dorsal surface of the corpus callosum, within which are found delicate strands of longitudinal fibers. Two of these strands, placed close together on either side of the median plane, are more conspicuous than the others, and are known as the *medial longitudinal striae* (Fig. 52). On either side, where the supracallosal gyrus bounds the sulcus of the corpus callosum, there is a less distinct strand, the lateral

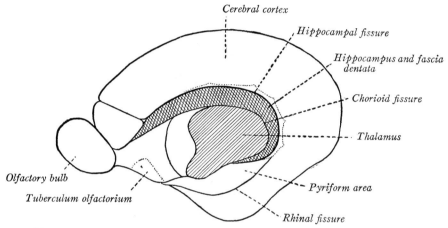

FIGURE 239. Median view of the cerebral hemisphere of a monotreme Ornithorhynchus. (Elliot Smith.)

longitudinal stria. The hippocampal rudiment can be traced upon the medial surface of the hemisphere from the region of the medial olfactory gyrus (or stria) toward the rostrum of the corpus callosum, then around the dorsal surface of that great commissure to the splenium, behind which it becomes continuous with the hippocampus proper, where this comes to the surface in the angle between the fascia dentata and the parahippocampal gyrus (Fig. 237; Elliot Smith, 1915). Research increasingly reveals functions other than olfactory with which the hippocampus is associated (Brodal, 1947). In addition to the points mentioned in connection with the periamygdaloid area, selective destruction of the hippocampus in animals has been found to eliminate certain previously established conditioned emotional responses and reconditioning in such animals is difficult (Brady, 1956).

The Fornix. Within the hippocampus fibers arise which run through the white coat on its ventricular surface, known as the *alveus*, into the *fimbria*. This is a thin band of fibers, running along the medial surface of the hippocampus and joining with the alveus to form the floor of the inferior horn of the lateral ventricle (Figs. 238, 246). The fimbria increases in volume as it is traced toward the splenium of the corpus callosum, to the under surface of which it becomes applied, where, together with its fellow of the opposite side, it forms the fornix. There is some evidence that the fornix also carries fibers arising in the septal region and passing to the anterior temporal cortex (Maclardy, 1955). Nauta (1956) has traced direct hippocampal pathways to the septal region, the preoptic region, the midline and anterior nuclei of the thalamus, mammillary and other hypothalamic areas.

The *fornix*, which is represented diagrammatically in Fig. 240, is an arched fiber tract, consisting of two symmetric lateral halves, which are separate at either extremity, but joined together beneath the corpus callosum. This medially placed portion is known as the *body of the fornix*. From its caudal extremity the fimbriae diverge, and one of them runs along the medial aspect of each hippocampus. In man the hippocampus does not reach the under surface of the corpus callosum, and the part of the fimbria which joins the body of the

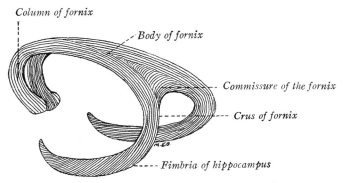

FIGURE 240.   Diagram of the fornix.

fornix, being unaccompanied by hippocampus, is known as the *crus fornicis*. Rostrally the fornix is continued as two arched pillars, the *columnae fornicis*, to the mammillary bodies.

The *body of the fornix* is triangular, with its apex directed rostrally. It consists in large part of two longitudinal bundles of fibers, representing the continuation of the fimbriae, widely separated at the base of the triangle, but closely approximated at the apex, whence they are continued as the columnae fornicis. At the point where these longitudinal bundles diverge toward the base of the triangle they are united by transverse fibers which join together the two hippocampi by way of the fimbriae. These fibers constitute the commissure of the fornix (Fig. 58). This part of the fornix, because of its resemblance to a harp, was formerly known as the psalterium.

The *columnae fornicis* are round fascicles which can be traced ventrally in an arched course to the mammillary bodies (Figs. 240, 242). They are placed on either side of the median plane. Each consists of an initial free portion, which forms the rostral boundary of the interventricular foramen, and a covered part, which runs through the gray matter in the lateral wall of the third ventricle to reach the mammillary body.

The *relations of the fornix* are well shown in Figs. 202, 237, and 242. The body of the fornix intervenes between the corpus callosum, septum pellucidum, and cavity of the lateral ventricle on the one hand, and the transverse fissure of the cerebrum and the thalamus on the other. The fimbria and body of the fornix form one boundary of the chorioid fissure. This fissure, which is shown but not labeled in Fig. 242, represents the line along which the chorioid plexus is invaginated into the lateral ventricle. When this plexus has been torn out, the fissure communicates with the interventricular foramen.

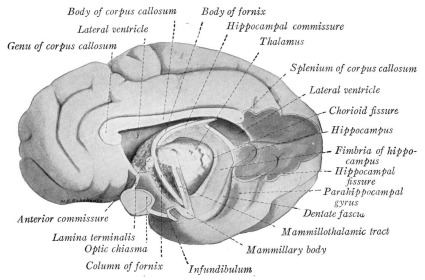

Body of corpus callosum   Body of fornix
Lateral ventricle   Hippocampal commissure
Genu of corpus callosum   Thalamus
                             Splenium of corpus callosum
                             Lateral ventricle
                             Chorioid fissure
                             Hippocampus
                             Fimbria of hippo-
                                 campus
                             Hippocampal
                                 fissure
                             Parahippocampal
                                 gyrus
                             Dentate fascia
Anterior commissure   Mammillothalamic tract
Lamina terminalis   Mammillary body
Optic chiasma
Column of fornix   Infundibulum

FIGURE 241.   Dissection of the cerebral hemisphere of the sheep to show the fornix and hippocampus.
Median view.

The **septum pellucidum** is the thin wall which separates the two lateral ventricles and fills in the triangular interval between the fornix and the corpus callosum (Fig. 242). It consists of two thin vertical laminae separated by a cleft-like interval, the cavity of the septum pellucidum (Fig. 56). Each lamina forms part of the medial wall of the corresponding hemisphere and the cavity, although sometimes called the fifth ventricle, develops as a cleft within the lamina terminalis and, therefore, bears no relation to the true brain ventricles, which are expansions of the original lumen of the neural tube.

Posteriorly is found at times another space called the sixth ventricle (of Verga) limited laterally by the crus of the fornix, dorsally by the corpus callosum, posteriorly by the splenium, and ventrally by the hippocampal commissure. Like the cavum septi pellucidi it is not a part of the ventricular system.

The **anterior commissure,** like the hippocampal commissure, belongs to the rhinencephalon. It is a rounded fascicle which crosses the median plane in the dorsal part of the lamina terminalis just rostral to the columnae fornicis (Fig. 242). In a frontal section of the brain, like that represented in Fig. 221, it can be traced lateralward through the most ventral part of the lentiform nucleus. It consists of two parts (Fig. 243). Of these, the more rostral is shaped like a horseshoe and joins together the two olfactory bulbs with fibers also passing to the anterior olfactory nucleus and the olfactory tubercle. This part can be readily dissected out in the sheep's brain (Fig. 236), but is poorly developed in man. The remaining portion, and in man the chief component, joins the pyriform areas of the two hemispheres together (Cajal, 1911). Fox et al. (1948) have traced in the monkey brain with the Marchi method the larger posterior

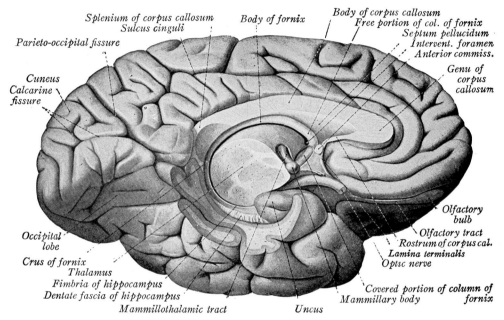

FIGURE 242. Dissection of the human cerebral hemisphere to show the fornix. Median view. (Sobotta-McMurrich.)

part of the anterior commissure to the external capsule and observed its distribution for the most part to the cortex of the middle temporal gyrus. In the rat it has been shown that other fibers reach parts of the amygdaloid nuclei and the pyriform area (Brodal, 1948).

Cajal has carried out extensive investigations concerning the structure and connections of the olfactory parts of the brain both in man and the smaller macrosmatic mammals, especially the mouse. His results, which differ in many respects from the ideas previously current, have been brought together in his "Histologie du Système Nerveux," Vol. II, pp. 646-823. The account which follows is largely based on his work.

Structure and Connections of the Rhinencephalon. In the olfactory portion of the nasal mucous membrane there are located *bipolar sensory cells,* each with a thick peripheral process, the ciliated extremity of which reaches the surface of the epithelium. These are the olfactory neurons of the first order, and their slender central processes are the unmyelinated axons which constitute the olfactory nerves. These fibers are gathered into numerous small bundles, the filaments of the *olfactory nerve,* which pass through the cribriform plate of the ethmoid bone and immediately enter the olfactory bulb (Fig. 244). Here they form a feltwork of interlacing fibers over that surface of the bulb which is in contact with the cribriform plate.

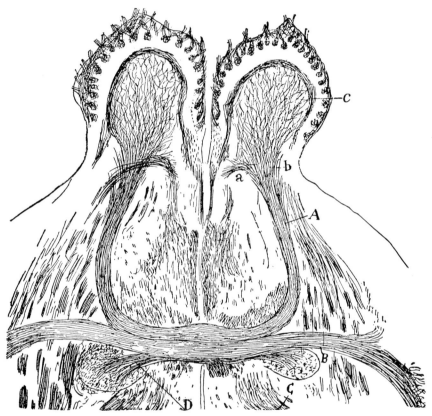

FIGURE 243.   Horizontal section of the rostral portion of the cerebral hemispheres of a mouse to show the anterior commissure. Golgi method. *A*, Anterior and *B*, posterior portions of anterior commissure; *D*, fibers from the stria terminalis; *C*, anterior column of the fornix. (Cajal.)

It has been reported that in the frog the olfactory epithelium and its contained neurons will regenerate after removal, and fibers of the olfactory nerve grow from the newly regenerated epithelium back to the olfactory bulb. This is remarkable since it implies the development of nerve cells from epithelial cells in the adult amphibian. Such an occurrence in mammals is probably not to be expected (Smith, 1951).

The **olfactory bulb** of man is solid, and the original cavity is represented by a central gray mass of neuroglia. This is surrounded by a *deep layer of myelinated nerve fibers* passing to and from the olfactory tract. Superficial to this are *several layers of gray matter* of very characteristic structure, and this, in turn, is covered with the *superficial layer of unmyelinated fibers* from the olfactory nerve filaments. Within the gray matter of the bulb are found three types of *neurons*, the mitral, tufted, and granule cells. The large *mitral cells* are the most characteristic element, and their perikarya are closely grouped together, forming a well defined layer (Fig. 245, *C*). The *tufted cells* are smaller and more super-

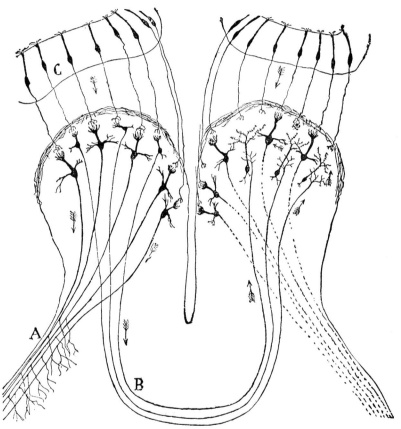

FIGURE 244.   Diagram showing the direction of conduction in the olfactory nerve, bulb and tract: *A*, lateral olfactory stria; *B*, anterior portion of the anterior commissure; *C*, bipolar cells of the olfactory mucous membrane. (Cajal.)

fically placed (Fig. 245, *B*). The larger dendrites from both these types of neurons are directed toward the superficial fiber layer. Each of these dendrites breaks up into many branches, which form a compact, rounded, bushy terminal. The terminal ramifications of olfactory nerve fibers interlace with these dendritic branches, and the two together form a circumscribed, more or less spheric *olfactory glomerulus* (Fig. 245, *A*). These relations were demonstrated by Cajal, in 1890, and possess considerable theoretic and historic interest. Since in these glomeruli the olfactory nerve fibers come into contact with only the dendritic ramifications of the mitral and tufted cells, it is evident that these dendrites must take up and transmit the olfactory impulses. That is to say, these glomeruli furnished positive proof that the dendrites are not, as had been thought by many investigators, merely root-like branches which serve for the nutrition of the cell. The mitral cells are larger than the tufted cells

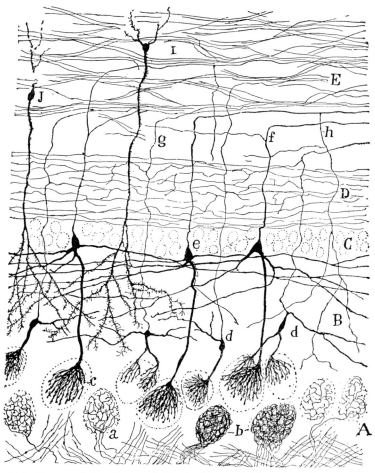

FIGURE 245. Section of the olfactory bulb of a kitten. Golgi method. *A*, Layer of glomeruli; *B*, external plexiform layer; *C*, layer of mitral cells; *D*, internal plexiform layer; *E*, layer of granules and white substance; *I*, *J*, granule cells; *a*, *b*, glomeruli, showing the terminations of the olfactory nerve fibers; *c*, glomerulus, showing the terminal arborization of a dendrite of a mitral cell; *d*, tufted cells; *e*, mitral cell; *h*, recurrent collateral from an axon of a mitral cell. (Cajal.)

and their axons are thicker. These coarse *axons* are directed for the most part into the lateral olfactory stria, while the finer axons of the tufted cells pass through the anterior commissure to the opposite olfactory bulb (Fig. 244, Allison, 1953). The axons of the deeply placed granule cells are relatively short and are directed toward the surface of the bulb.

The **olfactory tract** consists of fibers passing to and from the olfactory bulb. Through it each bulb receives fibers from the other by way of the anterior commissure as well as from the hippocampal cortex. The fibers leaving the olfactory bulb are the axons of the mitral and tufted cells. By far the greater number of the axons of the mitral cells are continued into the lateral olfactory stria. A much smaller number terminates in the olfactory trigone and in the tuberculum olfactorium within the anterior perforated substance. Other fibers pass by way of the medial olfactory stria to the parolfactory area of Broca, to the subcallosal gyrus, and to the septal area. The fibers of the *lateral olfactory stria* run upon the surface of the *lateral olfactory gyrus,* also known as the frontal olfactory cortex, to which they give off collaterals (Fig. 244). Fibers are distributed to the central and medial amygdaloid nuclei. The terminal fibers reach the *uncus* and part of the hippocampal gyrus. The chief olfactory centers of the second order are, therefore, found in the *pyriform area.* Prominent among the secondary centers in most mammals is the anterior olfactory nucleus, which occupies an area where the olfactory tract reaches the hemisphere, lying just anterior to the olfactory tubercle, and in lower forms extending along the tract and even into the olfactory bulb.

According to Cajal (1911), the *parahippocampal gyrus* may be subdivided in man, as in the mammals, into five areas: (1) the external region near the rhinal fissure; (2) the principal olfactory region, the most salient part of the convolution; (3) the presubiculum, a transitional area between 2 and 4; (4) the subiculum, near the hippocampal fissure, and (5) the caudal olfactory region, including the caudal part of the parahippocampal gyrus. Of these five regions, Cajal finds fibers from the lateral olfactory stria going to the second or principal olfactory region only. The presubiculum and subiculum and the caudal olfactory region represent olfactory association centers. The subiculum is characterized by the presence of a thick layer of myelinated fibers upon its surface.

The **hippocampus,** which constitutes an olfactory center of a still higher order, is directly continuous with the portion of the parahippocampal gyrus known as the subiculum (Fig. 246), and is formed by a primitive portion of the cortex that has been rolled into the ventricle along the line of the hippocampal fissure. Upon its ventricular surface it is covered by a thin layer of white matter, known as the alveus, through which the fibers arising in the hippocampus reach the fimbria and the fornix. Beginning at the line of separation from the fascia dentata, we may enumerate the constituent layers of the hippocampus as follows: the molecular layer, the layer of pyramidal cells, and the layer of polymorphic cells (Figs. 246, 247).

The *molecular layer* contains a superficial stratum of *tangential fibers* derived from the corresponding layer of the subiculum and from bundles of fibers that perforate the cortex of the subiculum (Fig. 247). More deeply placed is another fiber layer, containing collaterals from the pyramidal cells as well as collateral and terminal fibers from the alveus, and known as the *stratum lacunosum.* The molecular stratum in the hippocampus resembles that in other parts of the cortex in containing the terminal branches of the apical dendrites from the pyramidal cells, and a few nerve cells which for the most part belong to Golgi's Type II.

The Layer of Pyramidal Cells. The pyramidal cells are all of medium size and their fusiform bodies are rather closely packed together, forming a well

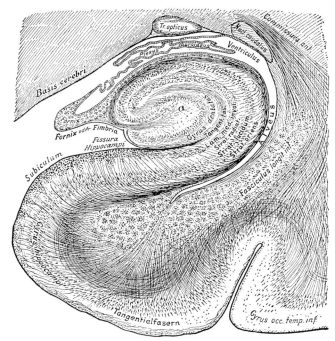

FIGURE 246. Cross-section of the hippocampus and parahippocampal gyrus of man. (Edinger.)

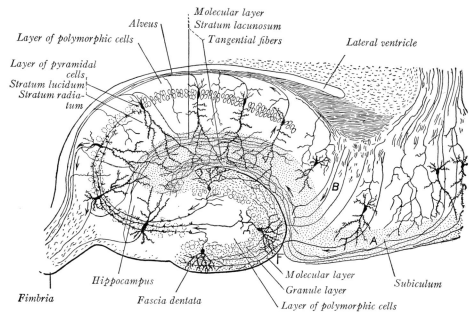

FIGURE 247. Diagram of the structure and connections of the hippocampus. The arrows show the direction of conduction; *A*, molecular layer, and *B*, pyramidal cell layer of the subiculum; *F*, hippocampal fissure. (Cajal.)

defined zone, the *stratum lucidum*. Their apical dendrites are directed toward the molecular layer and form the chief constituent of the *stratum radiatum*. The axons of these cells, after giving off collaterals, enter the alveus.

The *layer of polymorphic cells,* also known as the *stratum oriens*, contain cells of Martinotti, which send their axons into the molecular layer, and still other cells the axons of which enter the alveus.

The *alveus* is a thin white stratum which separates the preceding layer from the ventricle. It is continuous, on the one hand, with the white center of the hippocampal gyrus, and on the other with the fimbria. Through it the efferent fibers of the hippocampus enter the fimbria and fornix. The fibers of the commissure of the fornix are also carried in the fimbria and enter the hippocampus through the alveus.

The **fascia dentata** also belongs to the archipallium and is closely related to the hippocampus, which it resembles somewhat in the structure of its three strata: the *molecular layer, granule layer,* and *layer of polymorphic cells* (Fig. 247). The *granules* may be regarded as modified pyramidal cells of small size, ovoid or fusiform in shape. Each possesses instead of a single apical dendrite two or three branching processes which extend into the molecular layer. The axons are directed into the layer of pyramidal cells of the hippocampus. Originally this layer of pyramidal cells was continuous with the granule layer of the fascia dentata, but in all the higher mammals a break in this cellular stratum has occurred at the point of transition between the two divisions of the archipallium.

THE OLFACTORY PATHWAYS

The general pattern of connection of the olfactory tracts has been briefly described earlier in this chapter. Some additional points relating to cortical connections and efferent paths are of interest.

Impulses reach the glomeruli of the olfactory bulb along the fibers of the olfactory nerve and are here transferred to the dendrites of the mitral cells. Axons arising from these cells and running in the lateral olfactory stria transmit the impulses to the pyriform area (Fig. 244), whence they are conveyed to the hippocampus and fascia dentata by fibers entering the molecular layer in both of these parts of the hippocampal formation (Fig. 247).

According to Cajal, the fibers of the lateral olfactory stria terminate in the principal olfactory region of the parahippocampal gyrus, and there are present within the cortex of the pyriform area sagittal association fibers which unite the principal olfactory region with the caudal olfactory region of the hippocampal gyrus. From this latter region fibers reach the hippocampus and fascia dentata. These are relatively thick fibers which are found at first in the angle of the subiculum and can be traced through all the layers of that center into the molecular layer of the hippocampus and fascia dentata (Fig. 247, *B*). Within the molecular layer the impulses are transferred from these fibers to the dendrites of the pyramidal and granule cells.

The **efferent fibers from the hippocampus** represent the axons of the pyramidal cells. These penetrate the stratum oriens and enter the alveus (Fig. 247). Thence they are continued into the fimbria and fornix. They include both commissural and projection fibers. The *commissural fibers* serve to unite the two hippocampi and run through the commissure of the fornix as the transverse fibers of the psalterium. The *projection fibers* are continued rostrally, and in their course through the body of the fornix they form on either side of the median plane a longitudinal bundle, which is continued into the columna fornicis (Fig. 240). The latter bends caudally into the hypothalamic region, giving off fibers to the *mammillary body* where most of them end. The remaining fibers undergo a decussation just behind the mammillary body and are continued in the reticular formation of the brain stem (Fig. 248). It will be obvious that the fornix is the efferent projection tract of the archipallium and serves to convey

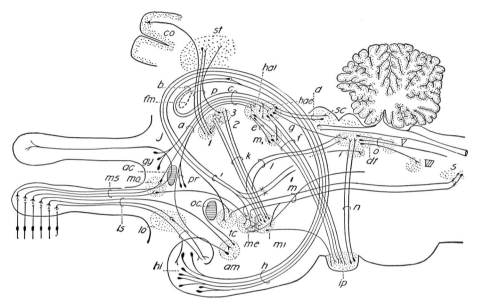

FIGURE 248. Olfactory connections of the diencephalon: *a*, Olfactohabenular fibers; *ac*, anterior commissure; *am*, amygdaloid nucleus; *b*, septohabenular and corticohabenular tract; *c*, stria medullaris; *co*, cortex; *d*, tectohabenular and habenulotectal fibers; *dt*, dorsal tegmental nucleus; *e*, habenulodiencephalic and thalamohabenular fibers; *f*, habenulopeduncular fibers; *fm*, interventricular foramen; *g*, habenulotegmental fibers; *gy*, gyrus subcallosus; *h*, fimbria; *hae*, external habenular nucleus; *hai*, internal habenular nucleus; *hi*, hippocampus; *i*, fornix; *ip*, interpeduncular nucleus; *j*, corticohypothalamic (and septohypothalamic) fibers; *k*, mammillothalamic fibers; *l*, mammillotegmental fibers; *lo*, lateral olfactory area; *ls*, lateral olfactory stria; *m*, mammillary peduncle; *m₁*, nucleus of Meynert's habenulopeduncular tract; *me*, external mammillary nucleus; *mi*, internal mammillary nucleus; *mo*, medial olfactory area; *ms*, medial olfactory stria; *n*, pedunculotegmental fibers; *o*, dorsal longitudinal fasciculus of Schultze; *oc*, optic chiasm; *pr*, preoptic area; *s*, bulbar centers; *sc*, superior colliculus; *st*, striatum; *tc*, tuber cinereum; *V*, motor nucleus of the fifth nerve; *VII*, motor nucleus of the seventh nerve; *1*, anterior dorsal nucleus; *2*, anterior medial nucleus; *3*, anterior ventral nucleus. (Huber and Crosby.)

impulses from the hippocampus to the hypothalamus and reticular formation of the brain stem. Through the mammillary bodies olfactory impulses are relayed along the mammillothalamic tract to the anterior nucleus of the thalamus, and along the mammillotegmental bundle to the tegmentum of the pons and medulla oblongata (Fig. 248, *k, l*).

The **medial forebrain bundle** (Fig. 209, 214, *MFB*) connects the ventromedial olfactory centers with the hypothalamus and with the preoptic area rostral and dorsal to the optic chiasma. It runs caudalward through the lateral part of the hypothalamus into the mesencephalic tegmentum (Fig. 213, *HL*).

Physiologic evidence indicates that the medial forebrain bundle is joined by descending fibers arising in the hypothalamus. The bundle carries both ascending and descending fibers and is apparently concerned with the correlation of olfactory impulses with visceral afferent impulses and so with appropriate activities involving these. It contains an ancient descending pathway from the olfactostriatum, which is the precursor of the head of the caudate nucleus, and another from the amygdala and pyriform lobe, the olfactory projection tract of Cajal.

The **stria medullaris thalami** consists of fibers which arise in the medial olfactory area, subcallosal gyrus, preoptic area, and amygdaloid nuclei. The fibers converge to form a bundle that runs backward to the habenular nucleus (Fig. 248, *a*). For some distance in front of the habenular trigone the stria medullaris lies along the dorsomedial border of the thalamus (Figs. 41, 42).

The **stria terminalis** is a delicate fascicle of nerve fibers which lies in the sulcus between the thalamus and caudate nucleus (Fig. 56), and accompanies the tail of the latter in the roof of the inferior horn of the lateral ventricle. It contains commissural fibers, joining the amygdaloid nuclei of the two sides, and projection fibers, the majority of which take origin from the amygdaloid nucleus, particularly the basal nucleus. After following the curved course of the caudate nucleus, it bends ventrad toward the anterior commissure to which it contributes fibers. The majority of the fibers, however, enter the preoptic region and hypothalamus.

The **anterior perforated substance,** or at least its more rostral part, which corresponds to the tuberculum olfactorium of macrosmatic mammals, receives besides fibers from the olfactory tract other afferent fibers which, according to Edinger (1911), come from the pons, perhaps from the sensory nucleus of the trigeminal nerve. It is probably "especially concerned with the feeding reflexes of the snout or muzzle, including smell, touch, taste, and muscular sensibility, a physiologic complex which Edinger has called collectively the 'oral sense'" (Herrick, 1918).

The reception of olfactory and gustatory impulses and of visceral afferent impulses can not be set apart as isolated functions of portions of the brain. The hippocampus is not exclusively olfactory nor is the rest of the somatic cortex unrelated to olfactory associations. Many of the subconscious activities of visceral structures are influenced by the olfactory mechanism, and somatic activities in feeding mechanisms must be intimately related to it.

The rhinencephalon is not as conspicuous clinically as the fundamental importance of its connections might imply. The testing of olfactory sensibility is commonly neglected, and a patient may even be unaware of his own anosmia. But there is a clinical entity associated with lesions within or in the neighborhood of the anterior end of the hippocampus (the uncus or gyrus uncinatus). Such lesions may be associated with attacks called *uncinate fits,* characterized by olfactory hallucinations, usually disagreeable, and a sense of unreality, plus at times actual convulsions and transient loss of the sense of smell and taste. In Penfield's experience olfactory sensations resulting from cortical stimulation in conscious patients are commonly disagreeable.

CHAPTER XVIII

The Cerebral Cortex

The study of the cerebral cortex is of interest to the psychologist who examines it through the normal behavior of the individual; the psychiatrist, who has an added interest in abnormal behavior; the physiologist, who is concerned with the function of specific parts, and the anatomist, whose interest allows a description of many, but not all as yet, of the details of its structure. Even this segregation of interests is artificial since here as much as in any bodily part function and structure are inseparable companions. However, the study of the gross and microscopic structure of the cortex can be a useful beginning to a consideration of its functions.

But as this study is undertaken we should remain aware of two significant points of view: First, this is the region of the brain with which we eventually come to deal when considering the higher thought processes, memory, speech and consciousness. It is therefore the portion of the brain which must study itself. Its accomplishments, if listed, would include all the artifacts of civilization, including the libraries and the contents of the printed pages they contain. Second, as anatomists and physiologists we assume that the entire gamut of functions of the brain depends wholly upon the transmission of nerve impulses over neurons. It might appear that the functions thus contemplated would be too numerous for the neurons contained, but it is worth noting that even in the shrew with a brain weight of about one quarter of a gram the neurons number 11×10^6 (Ryzen et al., 1955). Man's cortex has 7,000 million neurons (Shariff, 1953).

It is of further interest in contemplating the changes, mental and physical, that occur in man with age that the number of cells in the cerebral cortex decreases with increasing age, the change being chiefly in the granular cell layers (Brody, 1955).

The cerebral cortex forms a convoluted gray lamina, covering the cerebral hemisphere, and varies in thickness from 4 mm. in the anterior central gyrus to 1.25 mm. near the occipital pole. About half of the cortex forms the walls of sulci and so is unexposed on the surface. The organization of the cortex in the higher mammals is similar to that in man, and the increase in fissures and gyri in man is accompanied by an increase in cortical surface area rather than cortical thickness (Harman, 1947; Krieg, 1949). When sections through a fresh brain are examined macroscopically, the cortex is seen to be composed of alternating lighter and darker bands, the light stripes being produced by aggregations of myelinated nerve fibers (Fig. 249).

Nerve Fibers. In addition to a very thin superficial white layer of *tangential fibers,* there are in most parts of the cerebral cortex two well defined white bands, the *inner and outer lines of Baillarger* (Figs. 249, 252). These two bands contain large numbers of myelinated nerve fibers running in planes parallel to the surface of the cortex. In the region of the calcarine fissure only the outer line is visible; but this is very conspicuous and is here known as the *line of Gennari.* Myelinated fibers enter the cortex from the white center in bundles that in general have a direction perpendicular to the surface of the cortex. These bundles radiate into each convolution from its central white core and separate the nerve cells into columnar groups, thus giving the cortex a radial striation (Fig. 252).

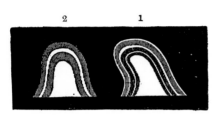

2   1

FIGURE 249. Schematic sections of cerebral gyri showing the alternate lighter and darker bands which compose the cerebral cortex: 1 shows the layers as seen in most parts of the cerebral cortex: 2, the layers as seen in the region of the calcarine fissure. (Baillarger, Quain's Anatomy.)

Many of the fibers in these radial bundles are *corticifugal,* representing the axons of the pyramidal and fusiform cells of the cortex. Within the medullary center they run (1) as association fibers to other parts of the cortex of the same hemisphere, (2) as commissural fibers through the corpus callosum to the opposite hemisphere, or (3) as projection fibers to the thalamus and lower lying centers. The others are *corticipetal* and are derived in part from the thalamic radiation, but an even greater number of them are the terminal portions of association and commissural fibers from other parts of the cortex. Many of these fibers end in the most superficial stratum of the cortex, the molecular layer, where the terminal branches of the apical dendrites of the pyramidal cells are widely expanded (Fig. 251). Others terminate as indicated in Fig. 250, where they are seen forming a close network of unmyelinated fibers. Enmeshed in the dense fiber plexus indicated at *B*, Fig. 250, are the pyramidal cells illustrated in Layer III of Fig. 252.

The **nerve cells** of the cortex are disposed in fairly definite layers as indicated in Fig. 252. We may enumerate five well recognized varieties: (1) pyramidal, (2) granule, (3) fusiform cells, (4) the horizontal cells of Cajal, and (5) the cells of Martinotti.

The **pyramidal cells** are the most numerous and are classified as small, medium, large, and giant pyramidal cells (Fig. 252). From the base of a pyramidal cell body an axon extends toward the subjacent white matter, giving off collaterals which ramify in the adjacent cortex (Fig. 80). The dendrites are of two kinds: a large apical dendrite and numerous smaller ones attached to the base and sides of the pyramid. The apical dendrite appears as an extension of the cell body and is directed toward the surface of the cortex, near which it ends in spreading branches. Its length varies with the depth of the cell body from the surface. To an even greater extent than other dendrites it is provided with short thorny processes called "spines" or "gemmules."

The **granule cells,** also known as stellate cells, are for the most part of small size, and their short axons branch repeatedly and terminate in the neighborhood

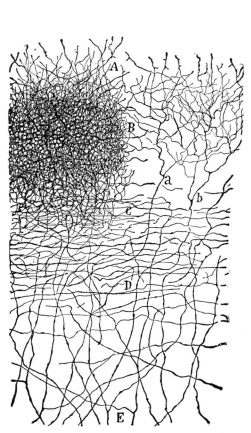

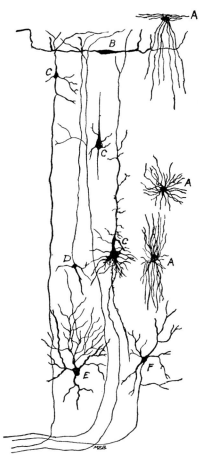

FIGURE 250. From the anterior central gyrus of the human cerebral cortex, showing the terminations of corticipetal fibers; *a, b,* Afferent fibers; *B,* dense network produced by the terminal branches of such fibers. Golgi method. (Cajal.)

FIGURE 251. Nerve cells and neuroglia from the cerebral cortex: *A,* Neuroglia; *B,* horizontal cell of Cajal; *C,* pyramidal cells; *D,* cell of Martinotti; *E,* stellate cell; *F,* fusiform cell.

of the cell of origin. That is to say, they are cells of Golgi's Type II. Although they occur in most layers of the cortex, they are especially numerous in the second and fourth strata which are accordingly designated as external and internal granular layers (Fig. 251,*E*; 252).

The **cells of Martinotti,** which are also found in most of the cortical strata, have this as their distinguishing characteristic, that their axons are directed toward the surface of the cortex and ramify in the superficial layer (Fig. 251, *D*).

The **horizontal cells of Cajal,** which are present only in the superficial layer, are fusiform, with long branching dendrites directed horizontally. Their axons form tangential fibers in the superficial layer (Fig. 251,*B*).

Fusiform or polymorphous cells are found in the deepest stratum of the cortex (Figs. 251, 252). Their axons enter the subjacent white matter.

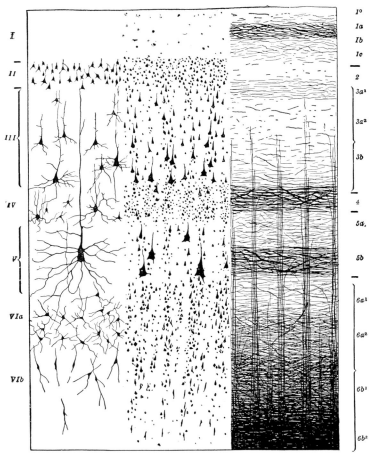

FIGURE 252.   Diagram of the structure of the cerebral cortex: *I*, Molecular layer; *II*, external granular layer; *III*, layer of pyramidal cells; *IV*, internal granular layer; *V*, ganglionic layer; *VI*, layer of fusiform or polymorphic cells; *3a¹*, band of Bechterew; *4*, outer band of Baillarger; *5b*, inner band of Baillarger. (Brodmann.)

Lamination.   The size and type of cells found in the cortex vary at different depths from the surface, that is to say, the cells are disposed in fairly definite layers. As already indicated, many of the myelinated fibers are arranged in bands parallel to the surface. By means of this cell and fiber lamination Brodmann (1909) recognized six layers in the cerebral cortex (Fig. 252). Other authors, notably Campbell (1905) and Cajal (1906), numbered these layers somewhat differently. Moreover, the arrangement varies in different parts of the cortex. In certain regions one or more of the strata may be reduced, enlarged, or subdivided. The six layers are as follows:

1. The **molecular layer** (plexiform layer) is the most superficial. It contains the superficial band of tangential myelinated fibers and many neuroglia cells. The nerve cells, which are not numerous, are of two kinds: horizontal cells of Cajal, and granule cells. Within this layer ramify the terminal branches of the apical dendrites from the pyramidal cells of the deeper layers.

2. The **external granular layer,** also known as the layer of small pyramidal cells, contains a large number of small nerve cells. Some of these are small pyramids with axons running to the white center of the hemisphere. Others belong to the short-axoned group (Golgi's Type II or granule cells).

3. The **layer of pyramidal cells** may be subdivided into two substrata, the more superficial stratum containing chiefly medium-sized pyramids and the deeper one chiefly large pyramids. There are also present granule cells and cells of Martinotti. According to Cajal (1900–1906) and Campbell (1905), it is within this layer that the outer stripe of Baillarger is located, but Brodmann places this line in the next layer.

4. The **internal granular layer** or layer of small stellate cells is characterized by the presence of a large number of small multipolar cells with short axons (granule cells of Golgi's Type II). Scattered among these are small pyramids. Brodmann places the outer line of Baillarger in this stratum, as does von Bonin.

It is within the outer stripe of Baillarger that the axons forming the stripe synapse with the basal dendrites of the deeper pyramidal cells of layer three (axo-dendritic synapses).

The fourth layer is at times subdivided, and in its outer layer it is considered that synapses occur between axons in the outer stripe of Baillarger and the body of the deeper pyramidal cells (axo-somatic synapses).

5. The **ganglionic layer** or deep layer of large pyramidal cells contains pyramidal cells, which in most parts of the hemisphere are smaller than those in the deeper strata of the third layer. Axons of some pyramidal cells in this layer give off collaterals which ramify in the cortex and then course to subcortical regions as projection fibers. In the motor region it contains the giant pyramidal cells of Betz, which give origin to some of the fibers of the corticospinal tract. The apical dendrites of these cells are very long and, like those of the more superficial pyramidal cells, reach and ramify within the molecular layer. Axons of some of the inner cells of this layer appear to run through the corpus callosum to the opposite cortex. The horizontal fibers of Baillarger's internal line are found in this layer in most of the cortical areas, though it is sometimes considered to belong to layer 6.

6. The **layer of fusiform or polymorphic cells** contains irregular fusiform and angular cells, the axons of which enter the subjacent white matter.

The internal granular layer (4) and the two supragranular layers (2 and 3) are probably receptive and associative in function and most of the afferent fibers of the cortex terminate in them (Fig. 250). The infragranular layers (5 and 6) are mainly corticifugal and commissural (Kappers, 1909).

The cells and connections in the cortex cerebri have an arrangement which, however complicated in appearance, can be shown to possess certain principles that are common to other regions of the nervous system. The early observations of Cajal and the recent ones of Lorente de Nò have emphasized them.

Reverberating Circuits.   There is in the branching of fibers that enter the cortical layers from other sources a mechanism of spreading the entering impulses to a number of cells whose cell bodies and dendrites are in the area. Further extension and continuation of such an influence is made possible through the intrinsic cells with short axons that branch about in the various layers. From a region thus activated efferent impulses may be started on their way toward adjacent cortical areas or along corticifugal fibers, the axons of pyramidal cells. However, this does not end the matter for when an impulse passes from the cortex by way of a pyramidal cell axon, it can also return to the cortex nearby along collateral branches of the original axon, and activate neighboring cells, which can in a similar manner perpetuate the activity. The smaller intrinsic neurons of the cortex are likewise organized so that reverberating circuits may maintain cortical activity. With commissural and the shorter and longer association neurons impulses may after entering the cortex be sent about for a considerable time and involve a large number of nerve cells. A brief sensory experience sending impulses into the cortex may be followed by prolonged activity there in addition to the external response. Perhaps even memory may be explainable in this "storage" of impulses in reverberating circuits.

Electrical evidence of the activity of the cerebral cortex is available in the study of the electroencephalographic recording. Alterations in the electrical variations recorded from the cerebral cortex are produced by attention, mental work, sleep; chemical alterations in the blood, as for example, the level of blood sugar; cortical damage; physiologic alteration of other parts of the nervous system which may impress their rhythm on the cortex. Eccles (1951) suggests that the common 10-per-second rhythm in the resting electroencephalogram can be explained by circulation of impulses in closed self-reexciting chains. He points out that after the discharge of an impulse a neuron develops a positive after-potential, associated with depressed excitability which is deepest about 0.015 second after the impulse passes. The recovery of the neuron is gradual, being about complete one-tenth of a second after the impulse. It is then ready for activation by the impulses circulating in the closed circuits with which it is connected. Entrance of other influences from outside the region could alter both the frequency and amplitude of the rhythm by increasing or decreasing the synchrony. Such a theory would still allow for the occurrence of spontaneous rhythmic activity in neurons which may be basic to the electroencephalogram.

Cortical Areas.   The cerebral cortex does not have a uniform histologic structure throughout all parts of the hemisphere. Due to the work of Campbell (1905), Brodmann (1909), and von Economo (1929), and others, many different cortical areas have been described as having individual characteristics. These areas differ from one another in the thickness and composition of the cellular layers, in the thickness of the cortex as a whole, in the number of afferent and efferent fibers and in the number, distinctness, and position of the white striae. The existence and general boundaries of some of these regions are now well established, and as a result of experimental and pathologic research it is known that specific differences in function are correlated with these differences in structure. The differences in thickness of the cortex and in the arrangement of the white striae can in some instances be detected with the unaided eye.

From the cyto-architecture three general types of cortical areas can be identified, the *homotypical, heterotypical* and *koniocortex* (von Bonin, 1950). The homotypical cortex is the commonest pattern with the usual six layers and radial columns, the subdivisions of it showing only minor differences. It makes up the major part of the frontal, parietal and temporal lobes. The heterotypical cortex includes portions with structure that departs widely from the first type by having an indistinct laminar pattern due largely to the scarcity of cells of the fourth layer (agranular cortex). Fifth layer pyramidal cells may be quite large, as in the motor area. In the koniocortex the cells are generally small and so appear closer together. The postcentral sensory area is of this type as are the visual and auditory areas.

The maps of cortical areas based on the arrangement of cells made by different investigators do not all agree. Although definite differences are readily visible in the major projection areas, finer distinctions are disputed (Lashley and Clark, 1946). Descriptions have ranged from the elaborate subdivisions of von Economo to the somewhat radical implication that there is little to be gained from cyto-architectonic studies. The truth should be somewhat between. Newer painstaking analyses of the histology, correlated with the tracing of impulses to and from specific areas by electronic apparatus (physiologic neuron-ography) combined with observations of the results of direct stimulation, and the tracing of fibers by methods of degenerations have been of help and will continue to clarify the studies.

While more than a hundred structurally different areas have been distinguished, some of these resemble others very closely and all can be classified in one or the other of five fundamental types (Fig. 253, 1 to 5). Cortex of Type 1 lacks, more or less completely, the two layers of small granule cells and for this reason may be designated as agranular. It is also characterized by its great thickness and the large number of typical pyramidal cells. The regions in which it is found are shown in maps made by von Economo (Fig. 254). Types 2 and 3 occupy extensive areas in the frontal, parietal, and temporal lobes and they both have well developed granular layers. Cortex of Type 4 is relatively thin, and has well developed granular layers and large numbers of medium sized pyramidal cells. Since it is found near the frontal and occipital poles, it has been designated as polar cortex. Type 5 consists chiefly of closely packed small granule cells. Even the pyramidal cells and fusiform cells are small and do not form well defined layers. Cortex of this type is found in the areas which receive the sensory projection fibers. While the structural plans illustrated in Fig. 253, 1, 2, 3, 4, and 5, are in a general way characteristic of the corresponding areas shown in Fig. 254, each of these areas is composed of subdivisions with their

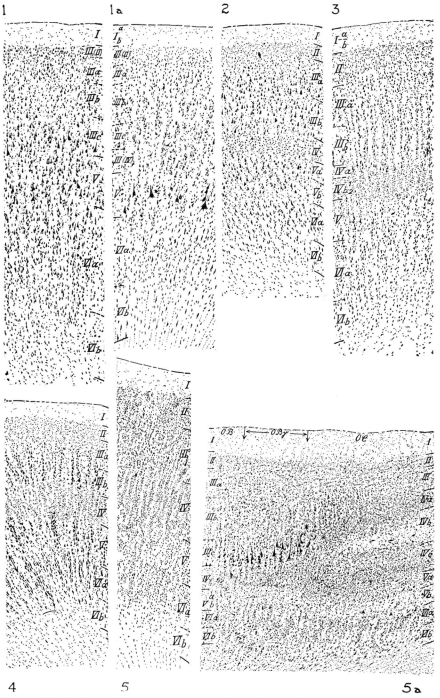

FIGURE 253. Sections of the cerebral cortex of man showing the arrangement of nerve cells in each of five cortical types the distribution of which on the surface of the hemisphere is shown in Fig. 254. Each section is enlarged to the same extent so that the thickness of the different types

own peculiarities. But all the subdivisions belonging to a given type show a
family resemblance. As illustrations of such variations within types, the auditory
cortex of the transverse temporal gyrus (Fig. 253, 5) may be compared with
the visual cortex of the area striata (Fig. 253, 5a, right half). It will be seen
that the family resemblance consists in the absence of large neurons and the

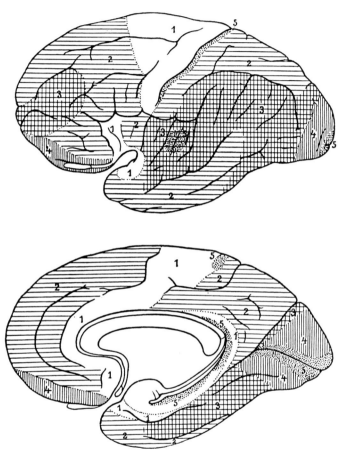

FIGURE 254. Maps showing the distribution of the five types of cortex illustrated in Fig. 248.
(von Economo.)

great number of closely packed granule cells. The visual cortex is the thinner
of the two and has a zone relatively free from cells (IVb) corresponding to the
position of the line of Gennari. Another illustration of the individual differences

of cortex can be directly compared. 1, From the posterior part of the superior frontal gyrus (Type
1); 1a, from the anterior central gyrus, motor cortex (a variety of Type 1); 2, from the middle
part of the middle frontal gyrus (Type 2); 3, from the supramarginal gyrus (Type 3); 4, from the
lateral surface of the occipital lobe (Type 4); 5, from the anterior temporal gyrus, auditory cortex
(Type 5); 5a, oc, the striate area, visual cortex (a variety of Type 5). Note the sharp transition
from striate to peristriate cortex. (von Economo.)

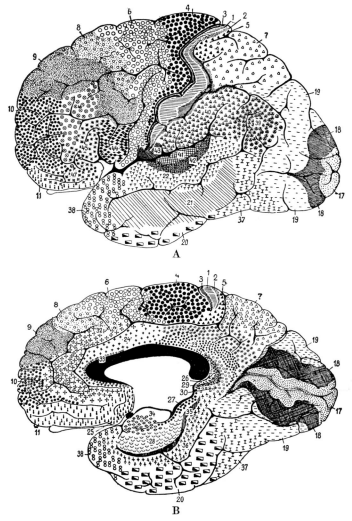

FIGURE 255. Areas of the human cerebral cortex each of which possesses a distinctive structure: A, lateral view; B, medial view. (Brodmann.)

within a given type is furnished by a comparison of the two sections represented by 1 and 1a. The former was taken from the posterior part of the superior frontal gyrus, the latter from the motor cortex of the anterior central gyrus. In both the cortex is thick and lacks the two granular layers, but the motor cortex is distinguished by the presence within the fifth layer of the giant pyramidal cells of Betz.

    At the borders separating certain of the cortical areas there occurs a very abrupt change in structure; at other points the change is quite gradual. In Fig. 253, 5a, there is seen a remarkable alteration in cellular layers at the border of the striate cortex.

CORTICAL LOCALIZATION OF FUNCTION

The Motor Cortex. The idea that specific areas of the brain had special functions is ancient, but it was given its strongest support with the demonstration by Fritsch and Hitzig in 1870 that electrical stimulation of what has come to be called the motor area resulted in movements of body parts. With the repetition and extension of these experiments by Ferrier (1886) and others since then it was easy for the belief in specific functional areas to become fixed. As the study of the cortex shows less and less evidence of complete dependence on small areas for specific functions, it becomes evident that the important demonstration of a motor cortex has perhaps delayed final analysis of the method of

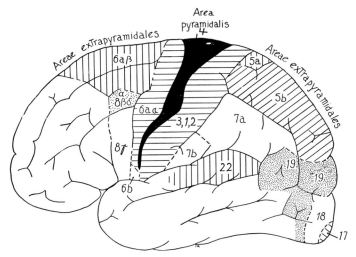

FIGURE 256. Lateral view of the human cerebral hemisphere showing the areas of electrically excitable cortex. (Redrawn after Foerster.) The motor cortex proper (Area 4) is represented in black; the other regions from which movements of the limbs and trunk can be elicited are lined; and the eye fields ($8\alpha\beta\delta$ and 19) are stippled. The numbering of the areas is somewhat different, from that in Brodmann's figures, and follows the pattern used by the Vogts.

cortical function by causing a strong belief in the attachment of specific functions to isolated cortical areas.

The region commonly referred to as the motor area is Area 4 of Brodmann's chart, the location of the giant pyramidal cells of Betz, which until recently were considered the only source of fibers in the corticospinal or pyramidal tract. As a result of the pioneer work on this area it is frequently referred to as if voluntary muscular action originated in it. Such a view is unjustifiable, for the nervous system normally works as a whole, and a voluntary muscular action may be influenced not only by thoughtful consideration of its desirability and its consequences, but by a host of influences which we are accustomed to think of as occurring on a reflex level involving many paths and centers in all parts of the nervous system, all aiding in the nicety of control of the muscles involved. It is not to be denied that Area 4 is important to voluntary action since destructive lesions in it result in paralysis of voluntary muscle.

The area of giant pyramidal cells is located in the anterior wall of the central sulcus, in the adjacent part of the anterior central gyrus, and in that part of the paracentral lobule which lies rostral to the continuation of the central sulcus on the medial surface of the hemisphere (Fig. 256). The part of Area 4 which is exposed to view is triangular in shape, tapering to a long drawn-out point where the central sulcus approaches the lateral fissure and widening to include almost the entire anterior central gyrus at the dorsal border of the hemisphere.

The *structure* of the cortex in Area 4 is characteristic. Here the gray matter is thick (3.5 to 4.5 mm.) and the lines of Baillarger are broad and diffused. The

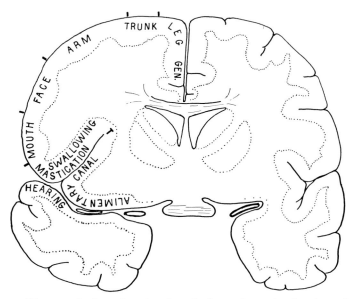

FIGURE 257.   Diagram of a frontal section through the cerebrum showing the major subdivisions of the pattern of representation of motor and sensory areas and the alimentary system as determined by cortical stimulation (modified from Penfield and Rasmussen, 1950). *T,* Tentative location of area representing taste. *Gen.,* Genital region.

two granular layers (II and IV) are lacking or are indistinguishably fused with the layer of pyramidal cells (III) which is unusually wide (Fig. 253, 1a). The ganglionic layer (V) contains the giant pyramidal cells of Betz, from which arise the larger fibers of the corticospinal and corticobulbar tracts.

The different regions of the body musculature are represented in Area 4 rather specifically. A rough approximation to this distribution could be shown by the picture of a man head down along the precentral gyrus. The sequence of representation has at least two breaks in it, the more conspicuous being that the face and head are represented "right side up." Hughlings Jackson pointed out that areal allotments in the cortex are not proportional to the amount of muscle in a region of the body but more to the elaborateness of movement the parts may show. The hand, mouth, and face have proportionately larger representations than the arm, leg or foot (Fig. 270).

In man with the brain exposed under local anesthesia stimulation of Area 4 produces specific movements involving contralateral muscle groups, small or large, the result depending on the type, strength, and duration of stimulus, the immediately preceding experience of the cortex, and the depth or absence of anesthesia. A threshold stimulus results in single movements not prolonged beyond the stimulus. Prolonging the stimulus or increasing its strength may bring into action additional muscles, and the effect may continue after cessation of the stimulus. If the stimulus is sufficient the after-effect may spread to muscle groups over the entire body producing a "march" as in Jacksonian epilepsy, with the sequence of involvement of body parts being related as in the pattern of representation of the body in the motor area.

Irritative lesions in the area can be the basis of epileptic attacks which start in a particular part of the body but involve finally all of its musculature. Observation, therefore, of the *beginning* of seizures a patient may exhibit is important in the planning of surgical intervention. If an epileptic seizure is generalized, that is, if the clonic movements appear throughout the body at once or even in bilaterally symmetrical portions simultaneously, the irritative focus may be at some distance from the motor area. Such seizures probably are commonly focal, and the spread of the epileptic pattern, as indicated by an original aura or by symptoms other than motor which precede the muscular outburst, may give a clue to the point of origin. Electrical activity as indicated by the brain waves (electroencephalogram) before and during a seizure may be useful in localizing the epileptogenic focus.

Removal or local destruction of Area 4 in man results in immediate paralysis of corresponding voluntary muscles. The paralysis is at first flaccid and there is loss or impairment of reflexes. Within a day or two changes begin which, after a few days or weeks, result in restoration of reflexes with a tendency to exaggeration of the response and the appearance of the type of reflex responses usually associated with upper motor neuron lesions, and the paralysis becomes "spastic" (though from animal experiments this implies involvement of the region 4S anterior to 4, not yet well recognized in man). Gradually the paralysis may diminish, and if the lesion is very small and is confined to Area 4 the deficit in motion may be impossible to discover with ordinary tests (Pilcher, Meacham, and Holbrook, 1947). With even larger portions of the body showing paralysis, compensation may proceed until only skilled movements show deficiency. In the monkey the degree of the initial paresis is less, the rate of recovery is greater, and the paralysis remains flaccid unless Area 4S is encroached upon by the lesion.

There is evidence from stimulation experiments of bilateral representation in the cortex, most in those muscles which act bilaterally as in the trunk, eyelids, and jaw; less in the muscles of the limbs; and least representation of the ipsilateral cortex in movements of fingers and toes. But even those movements involving simultaneous use of bilateral muscular groups may have a leading side, as in chewing movements with side to side grinding motions. In artificial stimulation of the brain of ruminants different cortical points are related to the original direction of deviation of the jaw in chewing. Ipsilateral movement has also been seen in response to cortical stimulation in the face (Lauer, 1952). Following bilateral removal of Area 4 compensatory recovery is not as great in a particular extremity as after unilateral removal.

Some clinical observers have maintained that the motor disturbances resulting from isolated destruction of Area 4 in man do not differ to a detectable degree from those caused by the combined destruction of both Areas 4 and 6aα (Foerster, 1936). After the initial period of shock has passed, in which the muscles may be flaccid and reflexes may be absent or weak, increased resistance to passive movement and increased tendon reflexes are characteristic of the paralysis resulting from lesions of the motor cortex and pyramidal tract in man but not in the monkey. The reason for this difference is not known.

It should be remembered that the lesions in man resulting from tumors, hemorrhages, and other "natural" causes are not as well controlled as those made in the laboratory on experimental animals, although the surgically produced lesions in man are often like well controlled laboratory experiments. Bucy (1957) states that cutting the central half of the cerebral peduncle which contains the corticospinal tract is not followed by spastic paralysis and hyperactive reflexes, and the patients (operated upon because of abnormal involuntary movements) may retain rather well coordinated movements of the digits. Nor does cutting the lateral or medial part of a peduncle appreciably affect normal or abnormal movements. Careful analysis of the symptoms in human cases will continue to be valuable in interpreting motor function. There is, of course, no regeneration of nerve cells and fibers of the central nervous system, but after a vascular accident to the brain absorption of hemorrhage and edema which had been interfering with transmission of nerve impulses by pressure allows restoration of function in intact nerve fibers.

Other Cortical Areas with Motor Functions. Area 6, immediately in front of Area 4, is the premotor region of Fulton (1935). In histologic structure it closely resembles Area 4 except for the absence of the large motor cells (Fig. 253, 1). Lesions restricted to this territory cause a temporary loss of acquired skills. Forced grasping is frequently seen after such lesions (Hines, 1937).

Areas 4 and 6aα (Fig. 256) both respond to electrical stimulation by isolated movements of individual parts of the opposite side of the body, but to obtain these effects from Area 6aα considerably stronger stimulation is needed. The isolated movements obtained from 6aα are called forth by impulses transmitted to Area 4 and thence conveyed downward in the pyramidal tract. When Area 4 is excised or the pyramidal tract interrupted. Area 6aα no longer gives rise to isolated movements but responds to strong faradic stimuli by mass movements of the whole contralateral half of the body similar to those described in the next paragraph.

Area 6aβ, when stimulated by strong faradic currents, gives rise to a complex movement of all parts of the contralateral half of the body. Head, eyes, and trunk turn to the contralateral side and the contralateral arm and leg are usually flexed. This response persists after removal of Area 4 and after interrupting the pyramidal tract. Centers for conjugate deviation of the eyes to the opposite side are located in Area 8αβδ and in Area 19. Separate portions of the frontal eye field respond to stimulation with specific direction of movement of eyes, which are duplicated in mirror image fashion in opposite hemispheres. But there is also a duplication of the pattern of movement in a single hemisphere in mirror image fashion concerned especially with the upward and downward components of the conjugate deviation (Crosby et al., 1952). Stimulation of Area 6b produces coordinated rhythmic movements of the lips, tongue, jaw, and larynx as in mastication and swallowing.

On the medial aspect of the hemisphere a **supplementary motor area** has been described from the observations of Penfield. It lies just anterior to the motor region in the intermediate frontal area. Stimulation of this supplementary motor zone results in bilaterally synergic movements; the opposite arm and hand are raised and the head and eyes turn as though following the hand. Change in the size of the pupil may occur and vocalization (not speech) has followed stimulation in this area. Inhibition of voluntary activity also is frequently the result of stimulation.

It is interesting that the movements produced from stimulus are bilateral alterations in postures and complex maneuvers, giving homolateral as well as contralateral effects. Removal of the motor area in the precentral gyrus did not prevent the occurrence of the usual effects of stimulating the supplementary motor area (Penfield and Welch, 1951; Bates, 1953).

Motor responses may also be elicited by electrical stimulation of areas posterior to the central sulcus, though the sensory receptor areas predominate here. Stimulation of Area 5 produces effects similar to those from Area $6a\beta$ with, however, a tendency for effects in homolateral limbs to follow more quickly the contractions elicited from the contralateral side. In the monkey, movements of body parts have followed stimulation of Areas 5 and 7 even in the absence of the pre- and postcentral areas (Fleming and Crosby, 1955).

Cortical Representation of Motion. With the differences in motor responses to stimulation from the various cortical zones it is appropriate to ask what in terms of motion is represented in the cortex. Hughlings Jackson asserted movements were represented and this is in general agreement, but "What movements?" might be asked. Hines (1944) points out that with proper control of conditions movements of individual muscles can be elicited by stimulation of the precentral gyrus but warns that this is not likely to be the usual way the cortex functions. However, action on the part of certain individual muscles may be the only requirement for some movements. Foerster observed movements of apparently individual muscles from man's motor area. The organization of the cortical elements and the arrangement of muscles about joints allows the production of larger movements involving several muscles by electrical stimulation of the cortex, and these are the type usually observed. Even rhythmically repeated movements of an extremity can be produced from specific points (Bucy, 1933; Clark and Ward, 1937), and rhythmic movements associated with chewing and swallowing are readily elicited from distinct cortical regions. The rhythmic motions require prolonged stimuli which is no doubt true in normal functioning also.

Ward (1938) from experiments on unanesthetized cats with electrodes implanted on the cortex was able to show that the character of the movement of a limb accompanying stimulation of a given fixed cortical point varied with the previous position of the limb and of the head. Stimulation of a given point of the motor zone controlling foreleg movements, for example, caused the contralateral foreleg to assume a "final position," making whatever preliminary adjustments that were necessary to attain it. Depending on the position previous to stimulation the limb might begin its approach to the final position with protraction or retraction, movements exactly opposite in direction. Such results go far toward explaining the phenomena of reversal and deviation in the response of a given cortical point described by Sherrington, and others since, as instability of a cortical point. Furthermore, when stimulation of a single cortical point in an experimental animal causes a limb to move to a definite position regardless of its previous pose, and then perform rhythmic action (as, for example, a series of stepping movements) which requires alternate contraction and relaxation of antagonistic groups of muscles, it appears unreasonable to try to assign to that particular point responsibility for the contraction of a single muscle. And since stimulation of a neighboring point on the cortex will produce comparable rhythmic action involving the same general groups of muscles but with slightly different pattern (as, for example, a batting movement of the paw), it becomes obvious that individual muscles may be under the control of more than one cortical point.

It appears likely that there is a mosaic of representation in the motor cortex, with the zones related to individual movements appropriately overlapping or being in close connection with each other, and all subject to influences from the receptive mechanisms and other neuronal connections that may instigate motion or contribute to the nicety of its control. Further evidence of overlap in cortical representation comes from the report that small lesions in the hand area (in monkeys) caused degeneration in the corticospinal tract as far caudalward as the lumbar region (Glees and Cole, 1950).

That the sensory side of the nervous system plays an important part in motor mechanisms is emphasized by the reported observation that bilateral removal of all the parietal cortex in monkeys results in complete immobilization of the animal. Kennard (1944), however, reported that flaccidity of muscles without impairment of their capacity for movement, and even increased tendon reflexes, have followed removal of the parietal areas alone. It is stated that in animals section of all the dorsal roots supplying the arm results in more voluntary motor deficit than unilateral removal of the opposite motor cortex; if, however, only one dorsal root to the brachial plexus is left intact the motor impairment is less and appears only as clumsiness or weakness. But section of the dorsal roots does not prevent the elicitation of rhythmic and other movements of the involved extremity by cortical stimulation.

It would appear then, that while motion of the most complicated type or of very simple pattern may be elicited by artificial or natural stimulation of the motor cortex, such motions can hardly be said to be completely dependent upon the activity of this area. The connections made with other cortical and subcortical structures in addition to the sensory mechanisms bring into play influences which affect the character of the resultant motion. The descending paths from higher levels concerned with the control of activity in voluntary muscle are generally referred to as the pyramidal and extrapyramidal pathways.

Pyramidal and Extrapyramidal Motor Pathways. For years the corticospinal tract has been called the pyramidal tract because it formed the bulk of the pyramids of the medulla; since it was believed to arise from Area 4, the region of large pyramidal cells, this area was associated with the term. With the knowledge that there were other influences on voluntary motion than those from Area 4, and with Sherrington's name for anterior horn cells, the *final common path*, emphasizing this, the term *extrapyramidal pathways* began to be used to refer to tracts other than the one called corticospinal. With subsequent recognition that cortical areas other than 4 were concerned with problems of motion the term "extrapyramidal areas" was used (Foerster, 1936).

There are according to Lassek's analysis (1940) about 34,000 Betz cells in Area 4 of one human hemisphere and approximately the same number of large fibers (9 to 22 micra in diameter) in one pyramid in the medulla. This constitutes only 2 to 3 per cent of the total number of fibers in the pyramid. When, however, Area 4 is destroyed, not only these large fibers but a total of 27 to 40 per cent of all the fibers in the pyramid degenerate, which implies that Area 4 contributes many smaller fibers which are probably the axons of smaller pyramidal cells in this area. But this is not all, as evidence from experiments on animals, not yet confirmed for man, indicates that a significant number of fibers in the pyramids arise from areas posterior to the central sulcus (Levin and Bradford, 1938; Peele, 1942). In the cat, fibers have been traced from the temporal and occipital cortex through both homolateral and contralateral pyramids and finally into the gray matter of the cord (Walberg and Brodal, 1953).

Tower (1944) in reviewing the work on the pyramidal tract points out that cortical Areas 4, 3, 1, 2, 5, and 7 in the monkey have been shown to contribute fibers to the pyramidal tract, and that in man there is proof of origin from Area 4 and possibly Area 6. However, there are some fibers in the pyramids whose origin is still unaccounted for. These fibers, according to Tower, are descending, but it is not known whether they arise from the cortex or from lower levels. Walshe (1942) strongly supports the latter possibility.

There is no general agreement as to what the term extrapyramidal includes, and, as Bucy (1957) points out, there is no single entity with which the "pyramidal tract" can be identified. This is more evident when it is seen that many of the fibers in the corticospinal path in the pyramids do not arise from Area 4 and that certainly only a small per cent of them arise from the Betz cells. Some may even arise from centers below the cerebral cortex. In any case the term "pyramidal" appears to be coming to include only those influences originating from Area 4, and logically all other influences playing on the primary motor neurons would be extrapyramidal. These should include paths from the cortex or any level below. For clear understanding paths should be named to indicate origin, destination, and direction of impulse, as corticospinal, and it would seem desirable, if possible, to avoid the use of such terms as pyramidal and extrapyramidal in situations in which ambiguity is introduced.

Descending paths arising from several cortical areas can be traced. Based on evidence of degeneration or electrical response (or both) (Levin, 1944), they may be summarized somewhat as follows: (1) *Corticostriate* fibers, from cortical Areas 4S, 6, and 8 (also 24, 2, and probably 19, i. e., all the "suppressor" areas) and 9 also to the caudate nucleus; from 4, 6 and 8 to the globus pallidus.

(2) *Corticothalamic* paths parallel to thalamocortical fibers; many to the ventral lateral nucleus to which come fibers of the brachium conjunctivum and from which go fibers to the motor cortex. Areas 10, 11, and 12 send fibers to the medial thalamic nucleus; 9 and 11 to septal nuclei; and 9 to medial and lateral thalamic nuclei; 8 to the medial thalamic nucleus; 6 to septal nuclei, medial and lateral thalamic nuclei; 4 to lateral thalamic nuclei.

(3) *Corticohypothalamic* fibers, thought to be largely from the hippocampus, and so related to olfactory connections. Fibers also reach the hypothalamus from frontal (Area 6), orbital, sensorimotor, and auditory cortex.

(4) A few fibers from Areas 4, 4S, and 6 to the *zona incerta* and the anterior small-celled portion of the *red nucleus*, and from 6 to the ipsilateral subthalamic nucleus.

(5) *Corticonigral* paths largely from Areas 4, 4S, 6, and 8. Fibers from substantia nigra go mainly to the corpus striatum. Ranson and Ranson traced them in the monkey to the globus pallidus.

(6) Areas 4 and 6 project to tegmental regions, the nuclei pontis and the inferior olivary nuclei; in addition to the well known projection of Area 4 to the spinal cord.

In the rat, the striate cortex has homolateral projections to lower levels, as the lateral geniculate body, thalamus, superior colliculus, zona incerta and pons, though these are not to be considered motor fibers in the usual sense (Nauta and Bucher, 1954).

Suppressor Zones. Recent inclusions in the specialized areas of the cortex, but with the significance not yet clear, are the suppressor areas described in the monkey and other animals. According to McCulloch (1944), who has contributed largely to a knowledge of them, on the architectonic map they are Areas 4S (the strip area of Hines), 8, 2, 19, and 24. When one of them is stimulated electrically, or mechanically, or is strychninized, there follows a suppression of the electrical evidence of cortical activity, first in areas near the point stimulated then gradually in more remote regions. The time relations are of great interest, since a half hour may be used in the spread to distant areas though by this time recovery has occurred near the original focus. In addition to the electrical evidence stimulation of Area 8, for example, can result in immediate relaxation of muscular contractions, the holding off of motor evidence of after discharge, and it will cause suppression of the motor response to a stimulus from other cortical areas. Smith (1945) observed in monkeys cessation of somatic movement on stimulation in part of Area 24 on the gyrus cinguli, but there were also some visceral responses and vocalization. Removal of Area 24 in monkeys is said to increase tameness temporarily. Fibers from the superior frontal convolution (Areas 4, 6, 9, and 10) have been found entering Area 24, and fibers from it pass to the septal region, the subcallosal gyrus, and the posterior part of gyrus rectus. From the posterior, part of 24 fibers pass to the anterior nucleus of the thalamus.

Some of these suppressor areas receive impulses from several other cortical areas and send efferent fibers to Areas 31 and 32 on the medial surface of the hemisphere. Difficulties have been encountered in tracing connections to the basal ganglia, but by strychninization experiments in animals it has been shown that Areas 4S, 8, 24, 2, and probably 19, send impulses to the caudate nucleus. By this means also it was shown that Area 6 sends impulses to the putamen and the lateral portion of the globus pallidus while fibers from Area 4 go to the putamen. McCulloch points out that large lesions of the caudate nucleus do not prevent suppression of the motor response from Area 4S, for example, although it is known that this motor suppression is dependent on descending paths, the exact course of which is unknown. Stimulation of the reticular formation in the medulla stops motor activity induced reflexly by brain stem mechanisms or from the motor cortex (Magoun, 1944). It has been found that suppression from cortical stimulation can still occur when any one of the following structures is destroyed: caudate nucleus; putamen; globus pallidus; substantia nigra and cerebellum.

According to some observers suppression of motor activity has followed stimulation of other areas than those identified as "suppressor," and the existence of true suppressor areas has been seriously questioned. No specific cytoarchitectonic pattern has been assigned to them. It should be pointed out also that the word "suppression" has been used at times to describe cessation or inhibition of muscular activity and at times to describe diminution of recorded electrical activity of the cortex. The reader should note the meaning implied in each case. The phenomenon may or may not differ from the so-called spreading depression, which is a spreading diminution of electrical activity in exposed cortex accompanied by visible vasodilatation. The explanation of this is obscure but is believed to be dependent on exposure of the brain surface (Marshall and Essig, 1951). Ochs (1958) has shown this to be blocked temporarily by shallow cuts in the cortex and believes it dependent upon contiguity of apical dendrites of pyramidal cells.

Clarification of the influence of the various cerebral centers on motion is gradually appearing from experimental stimulation in intact animals, with observation on both reflex action and cortically evoked movement. It appears that anatomic overlap in the course of pathways and the distribution of cell bodies may be responsible for conflicting results, emphasized in the difficulty of separating inhibitory and facilitating influences at various levels. It appears probable that in connection with voluntary acts corticospinal (and corticobulbar) projections not only act through primary motor neurons to induce contraction of muscles appropriate to a movement, but facilitate subcortical systems which would aid in the accomplishment of the movement.

From experimental evidence pathways for unilateral *inhibition* of motor activity (contralateral to cerebral centers) have been proposed which would originate in the suppressor cortex; pass by way of the caudate nucleus, putamen, and globus pallidus; then to the nucleus ventralis anterior of the thalamus; and then to the motor cortex. For bilateral inhibition influences can arise in the gyrus cinguli, pass to septal nuclei, and midline thalamic nuclei, then into the hypothalamus to reach the medial reticular formation, and from this to primary motor neurons (Hodes, Peacock, and Heath, 1951).

Pathways for *facilitation* of reflex muscular activity of both sides of the body can apparently originate in the diencephalon and be transmitted caudally. (Midline, intralaminar, and medial thalamic nuclei to hypothalamus, to lateral reticular formation, and then to primary motor neurons.) Facilitating influences in cortically induced movement may begin in the cortex, as the gyrus cinguli, then to diencephalic centers, as the head of the caudate nucleus, then to the globus pallidus, to the nucleus ventralis anterior of the thalamus, then to the motor cortex. Facilitating effects may also go from the gyrus cinguli to septal nuclei, through midline thalamic nuclei, and then to the reticular nucleus of the thalamus and then to the motor cortex.

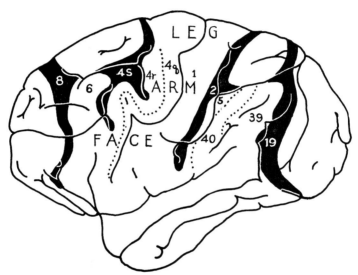

FIGURE 258.   Diagram of the brain of a chimpanzee showing the suppressor zones (in solid black) on the lateral surface. (After Bucy.)

Cortical Autonomic Representation.   Fibers extend from Area 24 in the gyrus cinguli to other cortical areas, which are perhaps suppressor in function, and some fibers have been traced from it through the medial part of the cerebral peduncles to the medial reticular formation in the tegmental part of the pons. On stimulation of points in this region, autonomic effects and effects on skeletal muscle, both of suppression and tonic movements, occur. It has been suggested that this region and related ones are concerned with the mechanism of emotions (Ward, 1948). While the hypothalamus is closely related to regulations of visceral functions it is becoming increasingly evident that the cerebral cortex is also directly involved. Kennard (1944) in a review of the question points out that in the frontal lobe, Area 6, and to a less extent Areas 8 and 4 have influence upon the pupil, bladder, vascular system, gastrointestinal tract, and pilomotor system. While less definite than the foci concerned with the control of skeletal muscle there is a tendency for localization in the cortex corresponding roughly to the somatic pattern. A vasodilator effect in skeletal muscles in the dog was observed after stimulation of the posterior part of the motor area (Eliasson et al, 1952).

Autonomic foci also appear on the orbital surface of the frontal pole. Bilateral removal of this area may affect gastric motility and blood pressure as well as respiration. It has been shown that stimulation of the frontal region of the cat brain under proper conditions produces transient elevation of blood pressure and renal cortical ischemia from vasoconstriction. The kidney may be damaged by repeated experiences.

Alterations in blood pressure follow cortical stimulation in the temporal poles, as well as the posterior part of the orbital region of the frontal pole, and from cortex continuous with these areas through the anterior part of the insula, the gyrus cinguli, the subcallosal region, the uncus and anterior perforated space. While not autonomic, since the muscles involved are voluntary, respiratory responses also follow stimulation of these cortical areas (Chapman et al., 1950; Poirier and Shulman, 1954).

From animal experiments it appears that the hypothalamus is not involved in the pathway of all descending routes from the cortex affecting blood pressure. Section of the pyramid abolishes the blood pressure changes resulting from stimulation of the sensory-motor cortex (Kaada, Pribram, and Epstein, 1949).

Stimulation of the gyrus cinguli anteriorly or of the orbital region affects the movement of the pyloric part of the stomach. Sensory as well as motor visceral representation occurs in the insula, particularly in relation to the alimentary canal, stimulation in man producing sensations of abdominal discomfort, as fullness, nausea, and the like (Pool and Ransohoff, 1949; Babkin and Kite, 1949; Penfield and Rasmussen, 1950) (Fig. 257).

In lower animals visceral afferent impulses from stimulation of the splanchnic nerves reach primarily cortical zones in sensory Areas I and II in the portions related to the trunk. Stimulation of the central end of the cut vagus nerve results in electrical activity in the region of orbital gyri showing afferent connections of viscera here.

Smith (1945) reported that stimulation of gyrus cinguli in monkeys (Area 24) was followed by cardiovascular changes, piloerection, dilatation of the pupils, respiratory arrest, cessation of somatic movements, and vocalization.

Clinical cases showing the effects of cortical lesions commonly include alterations in blood flow in the extremities and in sweating.

The Sensory Projection Centers. These are the areas within which terminate the sensory projection fibers bringing impulses of vision, hearing, smell, and the general sensations from the surface of the body and deeper tissues. In each of these centers the cortex is characterized by numbers of closely packed small granule cells and belongs to von Economo's Type 5.

The **somesthetic area** receives by way of the thalamus impulses subserving general body sensibility from the skin and deeper tissues, including the muscles, joints, and tendons, on the opposite side of the body (Fig. 205). It occupies the *posterior central gyrus*. The parts of the body are represented in this gyrus in the same inverted order as in the motor cortex. In general it may be said that the sensory representation of any part of the body lies directly across the central sulcus from its motor representation.

A *histologic description* of the cortex of the posterior central gyrus is complicated by the fact that this gyrus is composed of three distinct strips (Fig. 255, 1, 2, 3). The cortical strip forming the posterior wall of the central sulcus (Area 3) has the structure characteristic of sensory cortex (Type 5 of von Economo, Fig. 254). It is relatively thin, measuring about 2 mm. The pyramidal cells are very small so that layers II, III, IV, and V look like one broad granular layer. In layer V there is a thick network of myelinated fibers.

When points in the posterior central gyrus are electrically stimulated during an operation on an unanesthetized patient, there are evoked *sensations* of numbness and tingling or paresthesia at points in the opposite half of the body. Movements are elicited from electrical stimulation of these areas in man, as might be expected from their close connection with motor zones. It is also true, as mentioned above, that sensory impressions result from stimulation of Area 4. According to Penfield and Boldrey, sensory impressions follow stimulation of the precentral gyrus more than motor results follow stimulation of the postcentral gyrus.

Cortical stimulation practically never results in a painful sensation as reported by the patient, and it is possible that an occasional report of pain could be due to stimulation of nerve fibers in pia mater or along small blood vessels. Perhaps it is significant in this connection, however, that pain does not result from cutting the lateral spinothalamic tracts in conscious patients.

Normal highly specialized sensations are aroused only by afferent impulses which have passed through the thalamus, activating it and being modified by it before reaching the cortex. Tactile stimuli applied to the skin evoke electrical action potentials in the somesthetic area. Ablation of parts of the posterior central gyrus produces severe impairment of sensation on the opposite side of the body. All modalities of sensation may be lost at first in the affected areas. But with the lapse of time there is considerable recovery, pain being the first to return. Recovery is the least in the case of light touch. This recovery may be due in part to the existence of some ipsilateral representation, part of the function of the damaged cortex being assumed by the corresponding area of the opposite hemisphere. It is probable also that the thalamus may have, or may acquire after its cortical connections have been severed, the capacity for appreciation of simple sensory impressions.

Another possible explanation for this recovery, namely that the somatic sensory cortex may not be limited to the posterior central gyrus but may include all of the parietal lobe and all but the most anterior part of the frontal lobe, is based on the fact that the application of strychnine in the monkey to any point in this large area of cortex causes the monkey to behave as if an unpleasant stimulus were being applied to the opposite side of the body (Dusser de Barenne, 1924).

In addition to the primary sensory area in the posterior central gyrus a smaller secondary sensory region has been demonstrated in Penfield's cases about the lower end of the central sulcus, with foot and hand on the opposite side distinctly represented. There was also in the area the suggestion of motor representation from the results of stimulation, but removal of the area resulted in no motor or sensory loss. The secondary sensory area corresponds generally to a similar region previously demonstrated in animals by electrical methods.

The significance of such secondary areas is not clear, but comparable ones occur in relation to the visual and auditory receptive areas, and probably the olfactory. No doubt they represent a region of connection allowing correlation of incoming afferent impulses with cerebral mechanisms generally. Pinching of foot and of ear gave electrical responses from the limbic system similar in character to those produced by olfactory stimuli (McLean et al., 1952).

The distribution in the cerebral cortex of fibers from the thalamus throws additional light on the question of the location and limits of the somesthetic cortex. It has been mentioned in a preceding chapter that the fibers from the posteromedial ventral and posterolateral ventral nuclei of the thalamus, which relay to the cortex impulses from the spinothalamic tract, medial lemniscus, and secondary sensory tracts of the fifth nerve, terminate in the posterior central gyrus (Figs. 205, 261). It is this gyrus, therefore, that receives the direct projection of the somatic sensory paths.

There is reason to believe that pain and perhaps some other simple sensory modalities may enter consciousness at the thalamic level. The cerebral cortex is concerned especially with those aspects of sensation which require comparison and judgment: (1) recognition of differences in weight, (2) spatial discrimination as of two closely juxtaposed points, (3) tactile localization, (4) appreciation of size and shape, and (5) of similarities or differences in temperature. A patient whose left posterior central gyrus has been damaged may sense an object placed in his right hand but will not know whether it is smooth or rough, round or square, large or small, warm or cool. But if it were unpleasantly hot or in any way painful to hold he would be aware of the discomfort.

The **visual receptive center** or striate area (Area 17 of Fig. 255) is located in the cortex forming the walls of the *calcarine fissure* and in the adjacent portions of the *cuneus* and the *lingual gyrus*. Rostral to the point where the calcarine is joined by the parieto-occipital fissure the visual cortex is located only along the ventral side of the former. Sometimes the center may extend around the occipital pole onto the lateral surface of the brain. The structural peculiarities of the visual cortex are very evident. The outer line of Baillarger is greatly increased in thickness and known as the line of Gennari (Fig. 259). Because of the prominence of this line the region is known as the area striata. It is surrounded by cortex of quite different structure, and nowhere can the differences in adjacent cortical areas be better illustrated than at its border, where the prominent line of Gennari is seen to terminate abruptly. At this border there is also a sudden change in the character of the cellular lamination (point marked with an asterisk in Fig. 253, 5a).

The visual cortex is relatively thin, averaging 2 mm. in thickness. Like other sensory fields it conforms to von Economo's Type 5 in which the pyramidal and fusiform cells are small and inconspicuous as illustrated in the right half of Fig. 253, 5a. The fourth or internal granular layer is thick and is separated by a light zone into superficial and deep parts. The light zone is seen in appropriately stained sections to be occupied by myelinated fibers belonging to the line of Gennari.

The *fibers of the geniculocalcarine tract* from the lateral geniculate body terminate in the visual center. These fibers carry impulses from the temporal side of the corresponding retina and the nasal side of the opposite one. The visual cortex of one hemisphere, therefore receives impressions from the objects on the opposite side of the line of vision (Figs. 191, 193).

Evidence from the study of the visual fields of soldiers suffering from lesions of the occipital lobes indicates that:

1. The center for macular or central vision lies in the posterior extremities of the visual areas near the occipital poles (Fig. 193).

2. The center for vision subserved by the periphery of the retinae is situated in the anterior end of the visual area, and the serial concentric zones of the retinae from the macula to the periphery are represented in this order from behind forward in the visual area.

3. The upper half of the retina is represented in the upper part of the visual areas, and the lower half of the retina in the lower part of the visual areas. For example, the right upper quadrant of each retina is represented in the upper part of the visual area of the right hemisphere and the left lower quadrant of each retina is represented in the lower part of the visual area of the left hemisphere (Holmes and Lister, 1916; Fulton, 1938).

The lower half of Area 17 which receives visual impressions from objects in the upper visual field connects with adjacent parts of Area 18 and this with the upper part of Area 19; from here corticotectal paths extend to the rostral medial portion of the superior colliculus, which has connections with the rostral part of the nucleus of the oculomotor nerve. Similar connections can be traced from the upper half of Areas 17 to 18 and to lower 19 and so to the caudal part of the oculomotor nucleus and the trochlear nucleus. Middle portions of Area 19 are related to conjugate movements of the eyes to the opposite side in a horizontal plane. The para-abducens nucleus is concerned in these movements, along with the nucleus for the lateral and the medial rectus.

The eye movements just discussed in relation to the cortical visual areas are cortical automatisms. Stimulation in the occipital cortex in either the primary (Area 17) or secondary (18, 19) visual fields produces visual images unlike ordinary objects, but which include bright stars or flashes of lights which may be colored and may move. Removal of an occipital pole results in complete homonymous hemianopsia with sparing of the macula in the blind field. Removal of the secondary visual cortical fields alone is not followed by blindness. There is evidence of bilateral vision in the secondary areas from the results of electrical stimulation (Penfield and Rasmussen, 1950).

The **auditory receptive center** is located in the two *transverse temporal gyri* and chiefly in the more anterior of the pair (Fig. 52). For the most part this area lies buried in the floor of the lateral fissure, but it comes to the surface near the middle of the dorsal border of the superior temporal gyrus (Fig. 259). It receives the auditory radiation from the medial geniculate body. The cortex in this area, measuring about 3 mm. in depth, is slightly thicker than that in the other sensory fields. Like them it belongs to Type 5, contains no large pyramidal cells, and is characterized by a wealth of small cells in all layers (Fig. 253, 5).

Stimulation of this cortical area during an operation without anesthesia causes the patient to hear buzzing, chirping, and roaring sounds.

Stimulation further along on the first temporal convolution in what must be the secondary auditory area is similar in effect, but there is sometimes added to the simple sounds an interpretation of them by the patient. Stimulation in the auditory area also has an effect on hearing, sometimes resulting in increase or decrease or change of character of sounds coming to the patient's ear at the time.

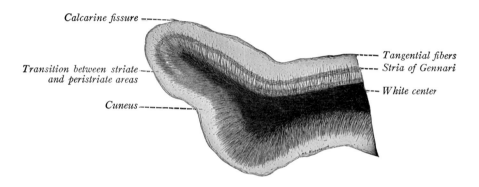

Calcarine fissure

Transition between striate
and peristriate areas

Cuneus

Tangential fibers
Stria of Gennari

White center

FIGURE 259. Section through the most rostral part of the Cuneus. Pal-Weigert method.

Each ear appears to be bilaterally represented in the cortex. A man with one temporal lobe removed shows very little or no impairment of hearing. Since removal of both temporal lobes in man does not entirely abolish hearing, it seems probable that there must be some appreciation of sound at or below the thalamic level. Decorticate cats and dogs respond readily to auditory stimuli and the decorticate cat is able to localize accurately the source of the sound (Bard and Rioch, 1937). Tunturi (1944) has shown that in the auditory reception area of the dog's cortex tones of high frequency are represented anteriorly and low tones posteriorly, with successive octaves in orderly arrangement. Numerical considerations become interesting here. There are, according to Chow (1951), in the monkey 88 thousand cells in the cochlear nuclei and ten million in the cortical acoustic area.

A **vestibular receptive center** probably also exists in the temporal lobe. When this region is stimulated in man either electrically or by disease, sensations of dizziness are aroused. In Penfield's cases sensations of disturbed equilibrium occurred when the first temporal convolution near the lateral fissure was stimulated, but the zone was not clearly defined from the auditory one. Following electrical stimulation of the vestibular division of the eighth nerve in the cat, projection of impulses to the cortex occurred in a region overlapping the somato-sensory area for the face and arms anteriorly and the auditory area posteriorly (Kempinsky, 1951). It would not be unreasonable to assume that the cortical centers for the two divisions of the eighth nerve would be situated close together (Spiegel, 1934).

The Olfactory and Gustatory Areas. Very little has been learned concerning the cortical centers for smell and taste from either clinical or experimental investigations. On anatomic grounds the archipallium may be assumed to contain the olfactory center because of its connections with the olfactory nerve (Fig. 260). The uncus and adjacent portion of the parahippocampal gyrus constitute the principal olfactory area of Cajal. Clark (1947) found the lateral olfactory tract ending in the cortex of the pyriform lobe and the periamygdaloid cortex. Even less is known about the gustatory area, but there is some

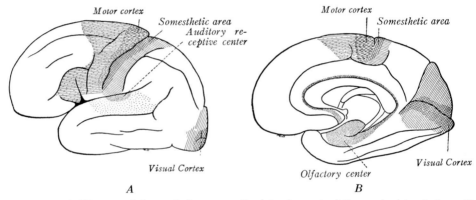

FIGURE 260. *A*, Diagram of the cortical areas on the lateral aspect of the cerebral hemisphere. *B*, Diagram of the cortical areas on the medial aspect of the cerebral hemisphere.

evidence that it may be located at the lower end of the posterior central gyrus (Börnstein, 1940) (Fig. 257).

Thalamocortical Connections. The somesthetic radiation joins the postero-medial and posterolateral ventral nuclei with the cortex of the posterior central gyrus. The geniculocalcarine tract joins the lateral geniculate body with the area striata, and the auditory radiation joins the medial geniculate body with the auditory cortex in the temporal lobe. The lateral ventral nucleus, within which the fibers of the brachium conjunctivum end, sends its fibers to the motor and premotor cortex (Brodmann's Areas 4 and 6 of the human brain, Fig 255). To the parietal lobe behind the posterior central gyrus go fibers from the dorsal and posterior lateral nuclei and pulvinar, the fibers from the latter being distributed behind those from the two former. The posterior part of the temporal lobe also receives fibers from the pulvinar. On the basis of the studies of the chimpanzee brain it is probable that in the human brain the fibers from the posterior lateral nucleus go to Brodmann's Areas 5, 7, and 40 and those from the pulvinar to Brodmann's Areas 37, 39, anterior part of 19, and posterior part of 7. The small-celled part of the dorsomedial nucleus sends its fibers to the granular cortex of the frontal lobe (Areas 9, 10, 11, 45, 46, and 47 of Brodmann's map, Fig. 255).

The gyrus cinguli receives fibers from the anterior nucleus of the thalamus which in turn receives the mammillothalamic tract. Not only do nerve fibers extend from thalamic nuclei and other subcortical areas to the cortex, but there are also connections from the cortex to these areas. For example, in the case of the temporal lobe, each of the three temporal gyri send fibers to the pulvinar of the thalamus and to the putamen; the superior and middle temporal gyri send fibers to the superior colliculus; the middle and inferior gyrus send fibers to the dorsomedial nucleus of the thalamus and to the tail of the caudate nucleus, and the superior temporal gyrus supplies fibers to medial geniculate body and the tegmentum (Whitlock and Nauta, 1956). This type of two-way connection is compatible with an interpretation of neurological mechanisms on the feedback principle of electronics.

Functional Significance of the Cerebral Cortex. To attempt to clarify entirely the functions of the cerebral cortex with the information available would be presumptuous. But some functions that have been attributed to the cortex on the basis of physiologic experiment, or as a result of analysis of morphologic details or study of the behavior of animals possessing more or less cortex, can be identified. One of the difficulties in the way of complete clarification must be that the very instrument to be used in the analysis is the same cortex which is being subjected to scrutiny. If we could only read between the lines of Baillarger with accuracy!

An obvious principle in the structure of the nervous system is the steady increase in the number of neurons successively involved in the stations on paths that ascend to the great suprasegmental areas, tectum, cerebellum and cerebrum. Many thousands of primary afferent neurons are concerned in bringing information into the central nervous system. (An optic nerve carries a million fibers.) But in the cerebellar cortex and cerebral cortex are many million of cells. (There are upwards of 14 million Purkinje cells in the cerebellar cortex in addition to the granule cells, basket cells, etc., and around 7,000 million cells in the cerebral cortex). Descending paths from these areas become funnelled again into smaller numbers of neurons as can readily be seen in the smaller size of the brain stem and cord. (Each pyramid has about two million fibers in it.) It appears obvious therefore that specific functions may not be ascribed to small collections of cortical neurons beyond those in the primary projection centers (auditory, visual, motor, etc.), where local specific responsibility is expected.

Another general principle of nervous connections that is significant functionally exists in the common pattern of feedback. A center or cell group that receives fibers from another source is quite likely to have fibers extending in the reverse direction. There are, for example, corticothalamic paths as well as thalamocortical projections, reticulocerebellar and the reverse. The larger paths from cerebellum to thalamus to cortex are more or less paralleled by corticopontocerebellar connections, and so on. Even on a microscopic level there are commonly collaterals of axons leaving an area that returns to the area. Such collaterals are found on the axons of anterior horn cells, Purkinje cells and cortical pyramidal cells. Reverberating circuits involving several neurons are also common.

Whatever impulses that arise from a system so well interconnected must be the resultant of the circulation of impulses from a variety of sources, and the electrical phenomena detectable as arising spontaneously from cellular collections must be involved in the total activity; though as yet the exact significance of these is not fully known.

Some of the fundamental physiology of the cortex has been revealed by study of the effects of brief stimuli applied to motor or sensory areas. Repetition of a subliminal stimulus to a specific point on the motor or sensory cortex within a few seconds of the original stimulus may bring forth a response by *facilitation*. The effect may be enhanced with continued quick repetition of the stimulus, even to the extent of producing an after-discharge. Furthermore, when such primary facilitation has been obtained, the same effect may be produced from nearby points if the interval between stimuli is kept brief. This is termed *secondary facilitation*, and can be elicited from points that do not respond with the same effect if they are stimulated in advance of the original point or after a longer interval. The second point stimulated may thus have its primary effect inhibited. It is also true that repeated stimuli can be applied to a given point in such a way as to produce fatigue or extinction, and the effect is progressively diminished. Originally described from experiments on animals, such effects have been well demonstrated by Penfield and Welch on the human sensorimotor cortex and reflect what has been called instability of a cortical point. Though the principles are conspicuously applicable to motor effects, these authors suggest that sensory inhibition and facilitation play a part in the normal analysis of sensory experiences, as in the sense of localization of stimuli to the body surface.

The cortical areas discussed in preceding paragraphs have been called sensory receptive centers because they receive the afferent impulses which evoke conscious sensations. Destruction of these areas abolishes or in the case of hearing greatly impairs sensation by preventing afferent impulses from acting on the cerebral cortex. Through association fibers the sensory receptive areas are linked with other parts of the cortex and it is probable that any conscious sensation involves widespread cortical activity. Some indication of this may be found in the electrical changes in the electroencephalogram with visual stimulus or other attention-getting mechanism. The pattern over large areas of cortex may be suddenly changed by merely opening the eyes, or concentration on a mental problem.

Association fibers and paths may not be as widespread or as numerous as has been thought. Bailey and associates (1943) found in the chimpanzee only a few long association tracts, capable of only one-way conduction and connecting a minority of the functional divisions of the cortex. Even the corpus callosum in man has been found not indispensable (Smith and Akelites, 1942). Lashley (1944) tested the efficacy of association paths in the retention of maze problems in rats by making longitudinal and transverse cuts through the cerebrum which isolated regions connected with known thalamic nuclei. He found that the operations affected the rats' maze learning only by the amount of cortical damage or by the interruption of thalamocortical paths. Lashley (1952) has also emphasized the necessity for considering the neurological activity of a psychological event as dependent upon many elements and in no way simpler than the psychological activity with which it is concerned. In a discussion of visual pathways Le Gros Clark (1944) stated that the association fibers from the cortical visual area were very short, extending only into Area 18, and this area was connected with 19 by additional short association fibers. Area 19 incidentally is one of the "inhibitory areas," stimulation of which suppresses the electrical activity of the entire cortex.

The interesting studies on man following removal of cortical areas at operation or cutting frontothalamic pathways have been of great value in interpretation of cortical function. Unilateral removal of a large part of the frontal lobe, including Areas 9, 10, 11 and 12 of Brodmann, causes no obvious disability in man but bilateral removal results in detectable changes in behavior and personality and in memory for recent events. Somewhat similar operations termed lobotomy, or leukotomy, are designed to disconnect part of the frontal cortex from the thalamic nuclei. Bilateral operations of this type are often effective in relieving severe depression and have been used to relieve intractable pain. The pain may not be abolished by such an operation, but the patient may no longer seem concerned about it.

Watts and Freeman, who have had a large experience with lobotomy, offer comments about the normal functioning of parts of the brain from their observations of patients experiencing the operation. They believe it likely that the effects of prefrontal lobotomy are due to degeneration of the thalamus which is related markedly to affective experience.

They suggest that the cortex at the base of the frontal lobe is responsible for general awareness of self, primitively largely visceral, but potentially on higher planes of the personal and the spiritual self. "Intelligence" does not appear to belong to the prefrontal regions alone and may not be affected by the operation. The frontal lobes add to man's mind foresight and insight, and patients after lobotomy may be too contented with things, and lack the drive to pursue a planned course with adequate adaptation to unexpected turns. The desirable effects of lobotomy, or its modification, topectomy, on man have also been produced by operations on the ventromedial quadrant of the frontal lobe by cutting or coagulation of the white matter (Grantham, 1951; McIntyre et al., 1954). This procedure leaves the lateral part of the frontal lobes without injury and attacks those areas ventromedially where increasingly it is thought emotional phenomena are involved (Fulton, 1953), and known connections with visceral activity occur (p. 366). The close association of visceral activity and emotional states is of significance here, and part of the anatomical background for the beneficial effects of the operation may lie in connections that are known to exist. The hypothalamus has marked visceral connections and it has two way connections with the dorsomedial nucleus of the thalamus, which projects to the cortex in the orbito-tempero-insular region. It will be recalled that the James-Lange theory of emotions implicated visceral activity, which Cannon showed was unnecessary since emotions appeared without a sympathetic outflow. But this does not exclude visceral connections from being involved and there is common knowledge of the influence of emotions on visceral function and vice versa.

With the use of tranquilizing drugs has come additional interest in humoral substances produced in the body such as serotonin that have effect on functions of the nervous tissue. For example, evidence has been presented that the administration of reserpine causes liberation of serotonin from tissues which usually retain it (Brodie et al., 1955) such as the brain tissues. The serotonin is then broken down; it has been suggested that the effects of administering reserpine are really due to serotonin.

In man and higher animals modification of behavior as a result of individual experience is due to cortical activity. If a bell is rung each time a dog is fed and this sequence is repeated many times the sound of the bell alone will ultimately cause the dog to salivate. This is a conditioned reflex (Pavlov, 1927), and is mediated through the cerebral cortex. Such responses can be impaired or abolished in the dog by removal of appropriate cortical areas: acoustic and visual conditioned reflexes by removal of posterior portions of the cerebral cortex, tactile conditioned reflexes by removal of the anterior half of the cerebral cortex, and auditory conditioned reflexes by removal of the temporal lobes. The cortex is not necessary for all conditioned responses, however. The possibilities in the use of conditioning experiments to study the importance of local areas to specific functions are numerous. Meyer and Woolsey (1952) have indicated how studies on frequency and intensity of sound can be so used.

Before it was known how widespread are the thalamic connections in the cerebral cortex and how numerous are the cortical areas which give rise to motor reactions (Fig. 256) or from which descending fibers can be traced to lower-lying parts of the nervous system (Mettler, 1935), it was customary to designate as **association centers** those parts of the cerebral cortex which were supposed to have only connections with other parts of the cortex. In late years the term has been used very little and carries no very precise connotation.

The granular cortex in the anterior part of the frontal lobe receives fibers from the dorsomedial nucleus of the thalamus, and the parts of the parietal lobe behind the posterior central gyrus receive fibers from the dorsal lateral and posterior lateral nuclei and the pulvinar. Since these thalamic nuclei receive no impulses from incoming sensory paths but serve as correlation centers for impulses coming from other thalamic nuclei, it is probable that these frontal and parietal association areas receive from the thalamus highly integrated impressions representing total situations rather than isolated sensations. From experiments on animals with lesions in the parieto-temporal-preoccipital cortex that did not damage sensory projection areas, it appears that this part of the cortex contains separate foci concerned with discriminative hearing dependent upon vision and somesthetic sense and with the formation of complex habits. It is also probable that several functions may be shared by common neuronal pools (Blum, Chow, and Pribram, 1950).

Speech and the Cerebral Cortex. The neural mechanism possessed by man which allows him speech sets him far apart from the lower animals. With uprightness of posture and freedom of his hands from use in ordinary locomotion, and speech, man has been able to produce all the artifacts of civilization. With spoken words an individual man can communicate ideas, however elaborate, to his fellows about him, and they can transmit these to others at

as a song previously memorized. Such memories were complete and specific and resembled dreams, and, though they lasted only as long as the stimulus was applied, could be repeated by reapplication of the stimulus. Furthermore, there accompanied the evoked memory the emotional pattern attending an original incident remembered. This was particularly true of fear, which emotion at times was produced alone from cortical stimulation without attendant hallucination. It is of interest that the patients showed a doubling of conscious experience, in that there was not only awareness of the elicited memory but of the environment in the operating room. Penfield offers evidence that the integration of memories is not dependent on association systems of the cerebral cortex alone but perhaps also on central ("centrencephalic") connections in the higher brain stem as was assumed by Hughlings Jackson (Penfield, 1950, 1955).

Memory seems to require time to become fixed in the nervous system. Animals learning a maze did not recall it subsequently if electric shocks were applied within a few minutes after the trial runs, though they did learn and recall it if the shocks were delayed as long as four hours afterwards (Gerard, 1955).

Such significant observations lead into enticing trails of speculation as to the mechanism of voluntary recall of past experiences; or that of conditioned responses; or that of emotions and their "cortical control." Does the frontal pole of the depressed patient, which by lobotomy is disconnected from the thalamus in cases of severe anxiety, abnormally stir up memories from the temporal cortex with the attendant emotion, or perhaps the emotion alone, and is the relief from anxiety based on the destruction of the influence of such an agitator? Does the memory of remote events persist in the senile individual and that of recent events disappear because the scattered cortical destruction that occurs with senile vascular sclerosis limits the receptivity of current experience, while dismissing the censor that normally represses continuous recall of past memories?

As has been intimated elsewhere, it is chiefly those nervous impulses, which are aroused by stimuli acting upon the body from without, that rise above the subconscious level and produce clear-cut sensations. The importance of these sensations in our conscious experience is no doubt correlated with the fact that it is through the reactions, called forth by such external stimuli, that the organism is enabled to respond appropriately to the various situations in its constantly changing environment. To meet these complex and variable situations correctly requires the nicest correlation of sensory impulses from the various sources as well as their integration with vestiges of past experience, and it is in connection with these higher correlations and adjustments that consciousness appears. The responses initiated by interoceptive and proprioceptive afferent impulses are more stereotyped and invariable in character; and these reactions are for the most part carried out without the individual being aware of the stimulus or the response.

The more elaborate the development of the nervous system the greater its capacity to react with discrimination to stimuli. To put it in other terms:

the more intercalary neurons in the nervous system the more possible internuncial paths are there between the incoming sensory stimulus and the outgoing
motor ones and the less sterotyped the response may be. Man with his most
highly developed nervous system has the greatest opportunity for variation
in response to stimuli. With more internuncial neurons between the receptor
and effector, there is delay in response to a stimulus, and so it is possible to
state that the cerebral cortex must affect action in at least three ways: by
delaying the response to stimulus, allowing for choice in the response, and
aiding in integrating the action involved. The time of conduction being relatively
brief, the advantages in choice and integration of the response more than
compensate for the implied danger of the delay.

CHAPTER XIX

The Great Afferent
and Efferent Systems

EXTEROCEPTIVE PATHWAYS TO THE CEREBRAL CORTEX

This chapter repeats items that have been given in various parts of the text but it seems desirable to sum up the main facts about the sensory and motor pathways here. Other specific details may be found in the appropriate sections.

The outer world has for the most part a crossed representation in the cerebral cortex. Cutaneous stimuli received from objects touching the right side of the body, and optic stimuli produced by light waves coming from the right half of the field of vision, are propagated to the cortex of the left hemi-

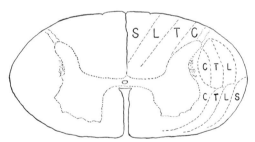

FIGURE 263. Diagram of the cervical spinal cord (after Walker) to show the relative position of fibers associated with different regions of the body in the tracts of the spinal cord. The dividing lines are arbitrary as there is much overlapping and intermingling of fibers. *C*, Cervical; *T*, thoracic; *L*, lumbar; *S*, sacral.

sphere. The crossed representation in the case of hearing is less complete, partly because every sound wave reaches both ears, but also because the crossing of the central auditory pathway seems to be incomplete.

The **grouping of the afferent fibers** in the peripheral nerves differs from that in the spinal cord. In each of the *spinal nerves* several varieties of sensory fibers are freely mingled. In the cutaneous branches are found conductors of thermal, tactile, and painful sensibility, while the deeper nerves contain fibers for pain and sensations of pressure-touch as well as for muscle, joint, and

383

tendon sensibility. Because of the intermingling of the various kinds of fibers a lesion of a spinal nerve results in a loss of all modalities of sensation in the area supplied exclusively by that nerve. At the margin of any such area there is a distinct overlap by nerves supplying adjacent areas, so marked that a small nerve may not be missed if its fibers are cut, or the loss of it may be detected only by a diminution of sensitivity from an area.

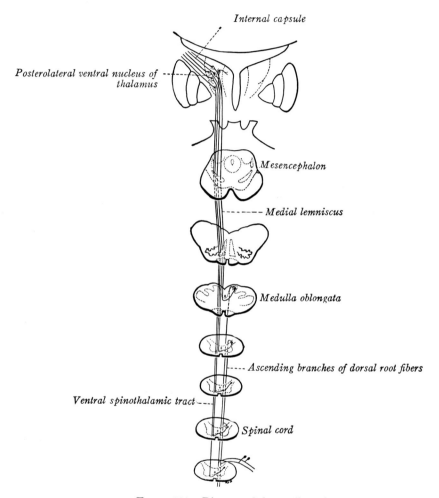

FIGURE 264.   Diagram of the tactile path.

In the *spinal cord* a regrouping of the afferent impulses occurs, such that all of a given modality travel in a path by themselves. All those of touch and pressure, whether originally conveyed by the superficial or deep nerves, find their way into a common path in the cord. In the same way all painful impulses, whether arising in the skin or deeper parts, follow a special course through the cord. Another intramedullary path conveys impulses from the muscles, joints, and tendons. These various lines of conduction within the cord are so distinct from each other that a localized spinal lesion may interrupt one without affecting the others. A striking illustration of this is the loss of sensibility to pain and temperature over part of the body surface without any impairment of tactile sensibility as a result of a disease of the spinal cord, known as syringomyelia.

While we shall here confine our attention to the afferent channels leading directly toward the cerebral cortex, it should not be forgotten that these are in communication with the reflex apparatus pertaining to all levels of the spinal cord and brain stem.

The Spinal Path for Sensations of Touch and Pressure.   Tactile impulses which reach the central nervous system by way of the spinal nerves are relayed to the cerebral cortex by a series of at least three units.

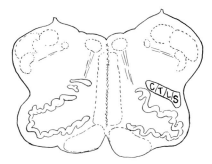

FIGURE 265.   Diagram of the medulla at the level of the inferior olivary nucleus to show the relative position in the lateral spinothalamic tract of fibers from the cervical (*C*), thoracic (*T*), lumbar (*L*), and sacral (*S*) regions of the spinal cord (after Schwartz and O'Leary).

NEURON I.   The first of this conduction system has its cell body, which typically is unipolar, located in the spinal ganglion, and its axon divides in the manner of a **T** or **Y** into a central and a peripheral branch. The peripheral branch runs through the corresponding spinal nerve to the skin, or in the case of those fibers subserving the tactile functions of deep sensibility, to the underlying tissues. The central branch from the stem process of the spinal ganglion cell enters the spinal cord by way of the dorsal roots. The touch fibers are myelinated and enter the posterior funiculus through the medial division of the dorsal root, and, like all other dorsal root fibers, they divide into ascending and descending branches. The ascending branches run for varying distances in the posterior funiculus, giving off collaterals before they terminate in the gray matter of the spinal cord, some few at least even reaching the nucleus gracilis and cuneatus in the medulla oblongata. At varying levels the collaterals enter the gray substance of the columna posterior and form synapses with the neurons of the second order (Fig. 264).

Neuron II with its cell body located in the posterior gray column, sends its axon across the median plane into the ventral spinothalamic tract in the opposite anterior funiculus. In this the fiber ascends through the spinal cord and brain stem to the thalamus. This tract gives off fibers, either collateral or terminal, to the recticular formation of the brain stem.

Other neurons of the second order in the tactile path are located in the gracile and cuneate nuclei of the medulla oblongata, and their axons after crossing the median plane ascend in the medial lemniscus of the opposite side to end in the thalamus. All of these secondary tactile fibers end within the posterolateral ventral nucleus.

The course of the ventral spinothalamic tract through the medulla oblongata and pons is not accurately known. It has generally been figured as joining the lateral spinothalamic tract dorso-lateral to the olive. But, since lesions in the lateral area of the medulla oblongata may cause a loss of pain and temperature sensation over the opposite half of the body without affecting tactile sensibility, it is not improbable that Déjerine (1914) is correct in supposing that it follows a median course, its fibers accompanying those of the medial lemniscus (Figs. 264, 268; Economo, 1911; Spiller, 1915).

There is reason to believe that the ventral as well as the lateral spinothalamic tract consists in part of short relays with synaptic interruptions in the gray matter of the spinal cord and brain stem, and the two tracts are sometimes designated as the spino-reticulo-thalamic path.

Thus in the spinal cord there appear to be two tracts which convey tactile impulses toward the brain, an uncrossed one in the posterior funiculus and another that crosses into the opposite anterior funiculus. Since these overlap each other for many segments, this arrangement would account for the fact that contact sensibility is usually unaffected by a purely unilateral lesion (Head and Thompson, 1906; Rothmann, 1906; Petrén, 1902).

Among the fibers of contact sensibility, which ascend in the posterior funiculus to the cuneate and gracile nuclei of the same side, are those that subserve the function of tactile discrimination, or, in other words, the ability to recognize the duality of two closely juxtaposed points of contact, as when the two points of the compasses or dividers are applied simultaneously to the skin. Furthermore, those elements of tactile sensibility, which underlie the appreciation of the form of objects or stereognosis, ascend uncrossed in the posterior funiculus to the gracile and cuneate nuclei.

NEURON III. The neurons located in the posterolateral ventral nucleus of the thalamus, with which the tactile fibers of the second order enter into synaptic relations, send their axons by way of the thalamic radiation through the posterior limb of the internal capsule and the corona radiata to the somes-thetic area of the cerebral cortex in the posterior central gyrus (Figs. 205, 259).

The Spinal Path for Pain and Temperature Sensations. Pain and temperature sensations are mediated by closely associated though not identical paths, and it is convenient to consider them at the same time.

NEURON I. The first neuron of this system has its cell of origin located in the spinal ganglion. Its axon divides into a peripheral branch, directed through the peripheral nerve to the skin, or in the case of the pain fibers also to the deeper tissues, and a central branch, which enters the spinal cord through the dorsal root and *almost at once* terminates in the gray matter of the posterior gray column (Fig. 266).

NEURON II. From these dorsal root fibers the impulses are transmitted (perhaps through the intermediation of one or more intercalated neurons) to the neurons of the second order. These have their cell bodies located in the posterior gray column, and their axons promptly cross the median plane and ascend in the lateral spinothalamic tract to end in the posterolateral ventral nucleus of the thalamus. In addition to this long uninterrupted path there probably also exists a chain of short neurons with frequent interruptions in the

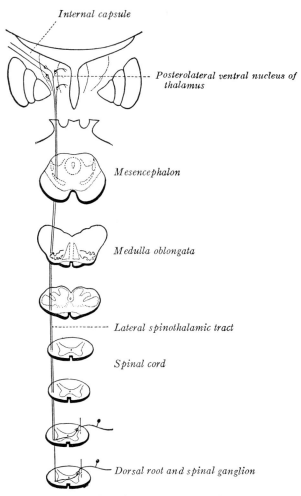

FIGURE 266. Diagram of the path for pain and temperature sensations.

gray matter of the spinal cord, which serves as an accessory path to the same end station. In the medulla oblongata the spinothalamic tract lies dorsolateral to the inferior olivary nucleus; in the pons it approaches the lateral border of the medial lemniscus which it accompanies through the mesencephalon to the thalamus (Figs. 265, 268); while it is situated quite superficially in the mesencephalon and is more closely associated at this level with the lateral than with the medial lemniscus.

The spinothalamic tract can be reached by operation in three general regions and cut without appreciable disturbance of motor paths. It is not uncommonly cut in cases of intractable pain in the spinal cord where it may be reached by a shallow incision ventrolaterally; it may be cut in the lateral portion of the medulla oblongata just ventral to the spinal tract of the trigeminal nerve; and it can be reached surgically and severed at a level slightly caudal to the exit of the trochlear nerve (Rasmussen and Peyton, 1941). The "tickling" sensation produced by repeated light contact is abolished by severance of the lateral spinothalamic tract in the medulla for intractable pain, even though the medial lemniscus is left intact.

NEURON III.   Fibers arising from nerve cells located in the posterolateral ventral nucleus of the thalamus convey thermal and painful impulses to the somesthetic area of the cerebral cortex in the posterior central gyrus by way of the thalamic radiation and the posterior limb of the internal capsule.

The Exteroceptive Paths Associated with the Trigeminal Nerve.   The trigeminal nerve mediates tactile, thermal, and painful sensations from a large part of the cutaneous and mucous surfaces of the head. While there is reason to believe that the tactile impulses mediated by this nerve follow a central course distinct from that of thermal and painful sensibility (Gerard, 1923), we shall for the sake of simplicity consider the exteroceptive connections of this nerve as a unit.

NEURON I.   The axon of a unipolar cell in the semilunar ganglion divides into a peripheral branch, distributed to the skin or mucous membrane of the head, and a central branch, which runs through the sensory root (pars major) of the trigeminal nerve into the pons. Here it divides into a short ascending and a long descending branch. The former terminates in the main sensory nucleus, and the latter in the spinal nucleus of that nerve (Fig. 267).

NEURON II.   The fibers of the second order in the sensory paths of the trigeminal nerve arise from cells located in the main sensory and the spinal nucleus of that nerve, and after crossing the raphe they run in two tracts to the posteromedial ventral nucleus of the thalamus. The *ventral* secondary afferent path is located in the ventral part of the reticular formation, close to the lateral spinothalamic tract in the medulla oblongata and dorsal to the medial lemniscus in the pons and mesencephalon (Figs. 185, 268). The *dorsal* tract lies not far from the floor of the fourth ventricle and the central gray matter of the cerebral aqueduct. It consists in considerable part of uncrossed fibers and of fibers having a short course (Wallenberg, 1905; von Economo, 1911; Déjerine, 1914).

NEURON III.   The afferent impulses are relayed from the thalamus to the cortex of the posterior central gyrus by fibers of the third order, which run through the posterior limb of the internal capsule. Their cells of origin are located in the posteromedial ventral nucleus of the thalamus (Fig. 205).

The Neural Mechanism for Hearing.   The spiral organ of Corti within the cochlea is connected with the auditory center in the cerebral cortex by a chain of three or more units.

NEURON I.   The bipolar cells of the spiral ganglion within the cochlea each

A. BY WAY OF THE DORSAL EXTERNAL ARCUATE FIBERS:

NEURON I of this chain is the same as in the path to the cerebral cortex just described, the fibers from the dorsal root reaching the lateral cuneate nuclei.

NEURON II. From cells located in these nuclei axons run as dorsal external arcuate fibers to the restiform body of the same side, and thence through the white center of the cerebellum, to end in the cerebellar cortex (Fig. 269, red).

B. BY WAY OF THE VENTRAL SPINOCEREBELLAR TRACT:

NEURON I. The first neuron in this chain is similar to the primary neuron in the two preceding paths. The impulses, however, travel over collateral and terminal branches of the dorsal root fibers to reach the posterior gray column and intermediate gray matter of the spinal cord.

NEURON II. From cells located in the posterior gray column and inter-mediate gray matter fibers run in the ventral spinocerebellar tracts of the same or opposite side through the spinal cord, medulla oblongata, and pons, bend around the brachium conjuctivum, and then course back along the anterior medullary velum to the cortex of the rostral part of the vermis and the declive, pyramis and uvula (Yoss, 1953) (Fig. 269, blue).

C. BY WAY OF THE DORSAL SPINOCEREBELLAR TRACT:

NEURON I. The first neuron of this chain is similar to the primary neuron in the three preceding paths. The impulses, however, travel over those collateral and terminal branches of the dorsal root fibers which ramify about the cells of the nucleus dorsalis.

NEURON II. From cells in the nucleus dorsalis fibers run to the dorsal spino-cerebellar tract and through the restiform body to the cortex of both the rostral and the caudal portions of the vermis (Fig. 269, red).

Cerebellar Connections of the Vestibular Nerve. The vestibular nerve conducts impulses from specialized sense organs in the semicircular canals, saccule, and utricle, which are stimulated by movements and changes in posture of the head.

NEURON I. From the bipolar cells of the vestibular ganglion (of Scarpa), located within the internal auditory meatus, peripheral processes run to the maculae of the utricle and saccule and to the cristae of the semicircular canals. The central processes are directed through the vestibular nerve toward the floor of the fourth ventricle and divide into ascending and descending branches. While the descending and many of the ascending branches terminate in the vestibular nuclei, many other ascending branches pass without interruption to end in the cortex of the flocculonodular lobe and the lingula of the cerebellum (Figs. 188, 189).

NEURON II. Some of the cells situated in the vestibular nuclei send their axons, along with the ascending branches mentioned above in the vestibulo-cerebellar tract, to the cortex of the vermis, and to a less extent to the cortex of the cerebellar hemisphere also.

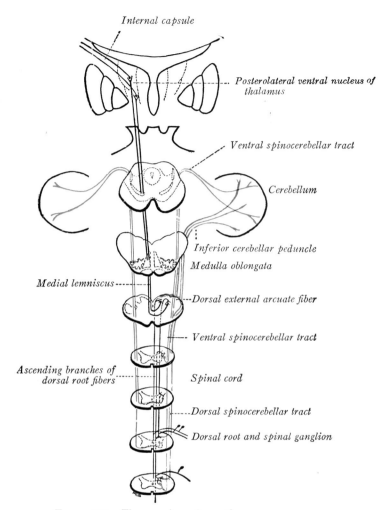

FIGURE 269. The proprioceptive paths.

EFFERENT PATHS

The **motor apparatus** is a complex mechanism into which the pyramidal system enters as a single factor. The primary motor neurons of the brain stem and spinal cord are also under the influence of other motor centers than those found in the cerebral cortex. They receive impulses from the corpora quadrigemina through the tectospinal tract, from the lateral vestibular nucleus by way of the vestibulospinal tract, from the large motor cells of the reticular formation through the reticulospinal path, and from the cerebellum by way of the red nucleus and rubrospinal fasciculus, etc. (Fig. 275).

The individual parts of this complex mechanism do not function separately. Each of the motor centers contributes its share to the control of the primary motor neuron, upon which as the "final common path" all efferent pathways converge. Only by keeping this fact constantly in mind can the motor functions be properly understood. The same idea has been well stated by Walshe (1919): "In stimulation experiments on the motor cortex we see a complex motor mechanism at work under the influence of an abnormally induced, crude form of hyperactivity of the predominant partner in this mechanism. Conversely, after destructive lesions, we observe it at work liberated from the control of this predominant partner and deprived of its actual cooperation."

On the other hand, the grave motor disturbances resulting from lesions in the basal ganglia and especially the corpus striatum with little or no involvement of the corticospinal tracts (paralysis agitans; bilateral athetosis, and progressive lenticular degeneration, Wilson, 1912, 1914) have called attention to the clinical importance of the corpus striatum and the extrapyramidal motor paths. In these diseases voluntary movements are impeded by tremor, rigidity, and athetosis, and in all probability these disturbances arise because the pyramidal system is deprived of the cooperation of one of the subordinate "partners" in the motor combine.

Even after cerebral control has been entirely eliminated in the cat by removal of the cerebral hemispheres, corpus striatum, and thalamus, leaving only the hypothalamus and subthalamus in connection with the brain stem, this animal is able to stand and walk. Subordinate motor centers situated in the sub-thalamus and rostral portion of the mesencephalon play a very important part in the reflexes involved in standing and walking (Hinsey, Ranson, and McNat-tin, 1930). If all of the brain is removed, many spinal reflexes can still be elicited; and we know that somewhat similar independent reflex activity may occur in the spinal cord of man after total transverse lesions.

In the cat with spinal cord transected in the thoracic region the hind limbs will support the body in a standing position for a while if the animal's hindquarters are not allowed to topple sidewise. An interesting observation on rhythmic action in such a preparation can also be made. If a sensory nerve is stimulated in the portion connected with isolated spinal cord, the homolateral limb is flexed and the contralateral one is extended. Simultaneous stimulation of sensory nerves on each side results in alternate flexion and extension of a limb when the body is suspended. The mechanisms for standing and the basis of rhythm are thus within the spinal gray matter, but are under regulation by higher centers in the intact animal.

THE GREAT MOTOR PATH

The great motor path from the cerebral cortex to the skeletal musculature, through which the bodily activities are placed directly under voluntary control, is in all mammals but especially in man the dominant factor in the motor mechanism. Afferent channels from the various exteroceptors reach the cerebral cortex; and through correlation of olfactory, auditory, visual, tactile, thermal, and painful afferent impulses which pour into it, there is built up within the cortex a representation of the outer world and its constantly changing conditions. The responses appropriate to meet the entire situation in which the individual finds himself from moment to moment are in large part at least initiated in the cerebral cortex and are executed through the motor mechanism. In these responses the great motor path is the dominant factor, although other parts of the mechanism are secondarily called into action, especially the proprioceptive reflexes arcs, including the coordinating mechanism of the cerebellum.

This great motor path consists of a chain of at least two neurons, extending from cortex to muscle. The cell body of the cortical neuron is a pyramidal cell (though not a desirable term it is often called an "upper motor neuron"), the axon of which extends from the motor cortex to the motor nuclei of the cerebral nerves or to the anterior gray columns of the spinal cord. In the spinal gray matter one or more anterior horn cells are in connection with the long corticospinal fibers, either directly or through the intervention of locally placed internuncial neurons. The anterior horn cells or primary motor neurons (frequently called "lower" motor neurons) send their axons through appropriate motor cells to skeletal muscles where each axon branches and supplies endings to a hundred

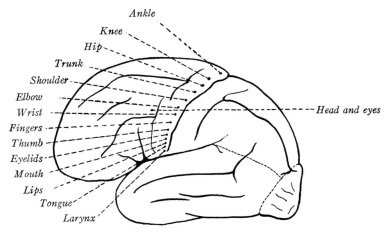

FIGURE 270. Cortical localization upon the lateral aspect of the human cerebral hemisphere.

or more muscle fibers. It is possible that another and much shorter element is intercalated between the two chief units of this conduction system.

The motor cortex occupies the rostral lip of the central sulcus and the adjacent portion of the anterior central gyrus, extending over the medial border of the hemisphere into the paracentral lobule. Within this area the skeletal musculature of the body is represented in an inverted pattern, that moving the feet lying superiorly in the precentral gyrus and on the medial border of the hemisphere. The area from which the corticobulbar tract arises is situated near the lateral cerebral fissure (the region marked Eyelids, Mouth, Lips, Tongue, Larynx in Fig. 270). From all the rest of the motor cortex arise the fibers of the corticospinal tract supplying the remainder of the body musculature. From different parts of the motor area fibers descend to the appropriate collection of primary motor neurons supplying the muscles. In this arrangement, however, there is not a strict limitation of descending fibers to corresponding segments of the cord. Some fibers from the hand area in the monkey's cortex, for example, reach as far caudalward as the lumbar region of the spinal cord.

The **motor path for the spinal nerves** includes the corticospinal tract and the spinal primary motor neurons.

Neuron I, or upper motor neuron. The giant pyramidal cells and certain other smaller cells of the motor cortex and other cerebral areas give rise to the

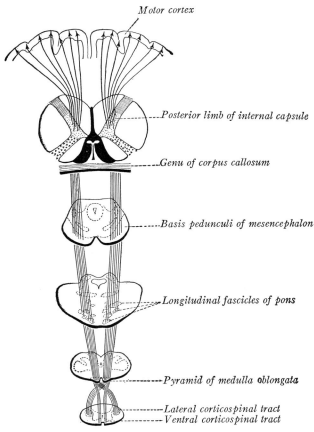

Motor cortex

Posterior limb of internal capsule

Genu of corpus callosum

Basis pedunculi of mesencephalon

Longitudinal fascicles of pons

Pyramid of medulla oblongata

Lateral corticospinal tract
Ventral corticospinal tract

Figure 271. The corticospinal path.

fibers of the corticospinal tract, which is also known as the cerebrospinal fasciculus or pyramidal tract. These fibers traverse the rostral half of the posterior limb of the internal capsule, the intermediate three-fifths of the basis pedunculi, the basilar portion of the pons, and the pyramid of the medulla oblongata, and after undergoing a partial decussation are continued into the spinal cord (Figs. 271, 272). At the pyramidal decussation in the caudal part of the medulla oblongata, the greater part of the tract crosses to the opposite side of the spinal cord and is continued as the lateral corticospinal tract in the lateral funiculus. The smaller part is continued directly into the ventral funiculus of the same side, as the ventral corticospinal tract. The fibers of the ventral tract cross the median plane a few at a time and terminate, as do those of the lateral tract, directly or indirectly in synaptic relations with the primary motor neurons within the anterior gray column (Fig. 273). The ventral tract is not evident as a well marked bundle below the level of the midthoracic

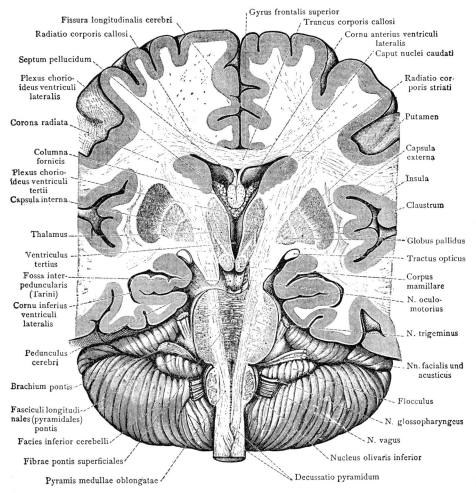

Figure 272. Section through the brain in the axis of the brain stem, showing the entire extent of the corticospinal tract. (Toldt.)

region. In a small percentage of human cases there is no uncrossed pyramidal tract.

It has long been known that in the higher mammals the lateral pyramidal tract, although consisting predominatingly of crossed fibers, contains a few homolateral fibers also, and according to the observations of Déjerine (1914) and other investigators this holds true for man. Déjerine speaks of these uncrossed fibers in the lateral corticospinal tract as a third bundle arising out of the motor decussation, and calls it the "homolateral" corticospinal fasciculus.

Neuron II. The large multipolar cells of the anterior gray column of the spinal cord are the primary motor neurons. They give rise to the motor fibers that leave the spinal cord through the ventral roots to be distributed through the spinal nerves to the skeletal musculature.

The **motor path for the cranial nerves** includes the corticonuclear (cortico-bulbar) tract and those fibers of the cranial nerves which innervate striated musculature.

Neuron I. The corticobulbar fibers arise from the giant pyramidal cells of the part of the motor cortex near the lateral fissure. These fibers run through the genu of the internal capsule and the basis pedunculi to end, directly or indirectly by way of internuncial neurons, in synaptic relation to the primary

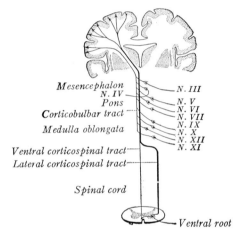

FIGURE 273.   The corticobulbar and corticospinal tracts.

motor neurons of the somatic motor and special visceral motor nuclei of the brain stem. Before terminating, the majority cross the median plane, but some end in the motor nuclei of the same side (Fig. 273).

Neuron II, primary motor neuron. From the large multipolar cells of the somatic motor and special visceral motor nuclei arise fibers, which run through the cranial nerves to end in striated musculature.

The Corticonuclear Tract. According to Déjerine (1914), who, because of the careful study which he and his associates made of this efferent system, was most entitled to speak authoritatively on the subject, the corticonuclear fibers occupy chiefly the medial part of the basis pedunculi and its deeper layer. The fibers separate into two major groups. One part follows the course of the corticospinal tract and descends in the basilar portion of the pons and the pyramids of the medulla oblongata. Another part, which he designates as the system of *aberrant pyramidal fibers*, detaches itself from the preceding in small bundles at successive levels of the brain stem. These enter the reticular formation and descend within the region occupied by the medial lemniscus, giving off fibers to the motor nuclei of the cranial nerves (Fig. 274). The fibers undergo an incomplete decussation in the raphe and go chiefly to the nuclei of the opposite side. The decussating fibers are grouped in very small bundles, those for a given nucleus crossing at the level of that nucleus. There is great variation in the course of the bundles of aberrant pyramidal fibers in different brains.

The *chief aberrant bundles* which can be traced dorsalward into the reticular formation (indicated in solid red in Fig. 268) are as follows:

1. The aberrant fibers of the peduncle (Fig. 274, *F. A. Pd.*) form two bundles, which have been called by some authors the median and lateral

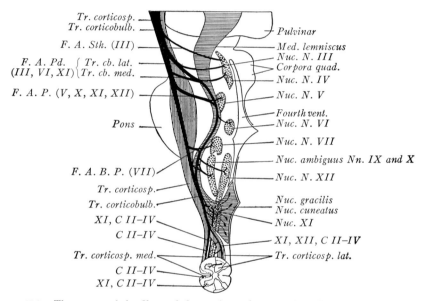

FIGURE 274. The course of the fibers of the corticonuclear (corticobulbar) tract. Redrawn from Déjerine. Corticobulbar tract, solid black; corticospinal tract, vertical lines; the medial lemniscus, horizontal lines. *F. A. B. P.*, Bulbopontile aberrant fibers; *F. A. P.*, aberrant fibers of the pons; *F. A. Pd.*, aberrant fibers of the peduncle; *F. A. Sth.*, subthalamic aberrant fibers; *Tr. cb. lat.*, tractus corticobulbaris lateralis; *Tr. cb. med.*, tractus corticobulbaris medialis. The Roman numerals indicate the nuclei of the cranial and cervical nerves which are supplied by the various bundles.

corticobulbar tracts. These descend in the territory of the medial lemniscus (Figs. 265, 274) and give off fibers to the nuclei of the third, sixth, and eleventh cranial nerves. With these two bundles run some fibers destined for the upper cervical segments of the spinal cord. This group of aberrant fibers, therefore, controls the movements of the eyes and the associated movements of the head.

2. The aberrant fibers of the pons (Fig. 274, *F. A. P.*) which join the preceding in the medial lemniscus run to the motor nuclei of the trigeminal and hypoglossal nerves and to the nucleus ambiguus.

3. The bulbopontile aberrant fibers (Fig. 274, *F. A. B. P.*) leave the main trunk of the pyramidal system near the level of the sulcus between the pons and medulla. They reinforce the preceding groups, supply the motor nucleus

of the facial nerve, and send fibers to the nucleus ambiguus and to that of the hypoglossal nerve.

These facts are of the greatest importance for the clinical neurologist. Lesions restricted to the basilar portion of the pons are likely to destroy at the same time the corticospinal fibers and those of the corticobulbar tract which end in the facial nucleus. A lesion confined to the reticular formation and

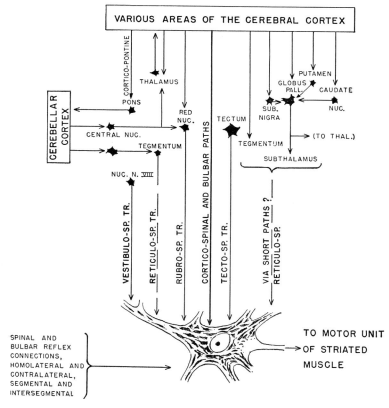

FIGURE 275. A diagram showing many of the routes by which impulses reach the primary motor neuron, the final common path to skeletal muscle.

involving the medial lemniscus may, according to its level, sever the cortico-bulbar fibers for the motor nuclei of the eye-muscle nerves or those for the motor nuclei of the trigeminal, accessory, and hypoglossal nerves without involvement of the corticospinal tracts. Conjugate deviation of the head and eyes, not often seen as a result of damage to the basilar portion of the pons, may result from tegmental lesions involving the aberrant fibers of the peduncle.

The Extrapyramidal Motor Paths. In recent years it has become increasingly evident that the pyramidal system is not the only channel through which volitional impulses are able to reach the primary motor neurons of the brain stem and spinal cord. After the motor cortex of Area 4 has been removed, strong faradic stimulations of Areas 6, 5, and 22 evoke mass movements of the opposite side of the body (Fig. 256). The impulses initiating these movements travel to the spinal cord over extrapyramidal motor paths, concerning which surprisingly little is known. After removal of Area 4 volitional acts can still be performed to some extent, and, in higher primates, increase in ability to use a paralyzed forelimb can be obtained when the use of the normal hand is restricted. Other information concerning extrapyramidal motor functions is given on pp. 317, 361–363.

THE CORTICOPONTOCEREBELLAR PATH

The corticopontocerebellar path is an important descending conduction system which places the cerebellum under the influence of the cerebral cortex.

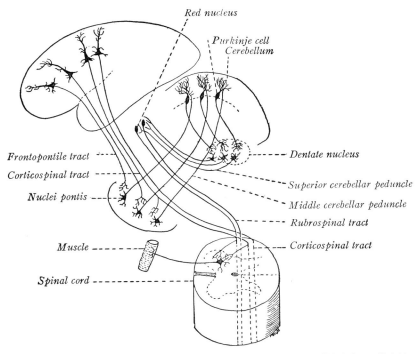

FIGURE 276.   The corticopontocerebellar and cerebellorubrospinal paths. (Modified from Cajal.)

Since a part of the corticopontile fibers are collaterals given off to the nuclei of the pons by the corticospinal fibers, and since in many mammals practically all of the corticopontile fibers are represented by such collaterals (Cajal, 1909), one can scarcely avoid the conclusion that through this system the coordinating mechanism of the cerebellum is brought into play for the regulation of movements initiated from the cerebral cortex (Fig. 276).

NEURON I.   From pyramidal cells in the frontal lobe of the cerebral cortex fibers pass through the anterior limb of the internal capsule and the medial one-fifth of the basis pedunculi, and similar fibers from the temporal lobe descend through the sublenticular part of the internal capsule and the lateral one-fifth of the basis pedunculi. These fibers, together with corticopontine fibers from the parietal lobe and the corticospinal tract, form the longitudinal fasciculi of the pons, and, along with collaterals from the pyramidal tract, they end within the nuclei pontis in synaptic relations with the neurons of the second order (Figs. 161, 276).

NEURON II.   Arising from cells in the nuclei pontis, the transverse fibers of the pons cross the median plane and run by way of the middle cerebellar peduncle and white substance of the cerebellum to the cerebellar cortex of the opposite side.

The corticopontocerebellar system appears to play an important part in the coordination of large movement complexes. According to Turner and German (1941), section of the brachium pontis in monkeys caused a serious disturbance in the coordination of the lower with the upper extremities in locomotion but did not significantly affect the execution of precise manual functions or learned behavior. Section of the frontopontine path in man results in no apparent deficit. It is likely that more precise quantitative measurement of the effects would be necessary to disclose the effects of such a lesion.

THE CEREBELLORUBROSPINAL PATH

The cerebellorubrospinal path is the conduction system through which the cerebellum contributes part of its important share to the control of the primary motor neurons of the spinal cord for the regulation of muscular tone and the production of motor synergy. Other efferent connections of the cerebellum have been discussed on page 281.

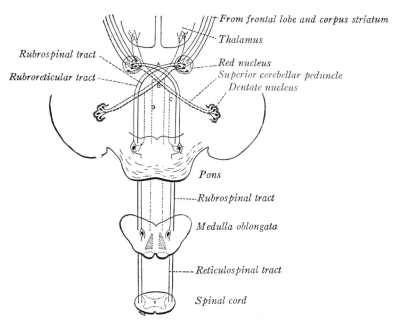

FIGURE 277.   Diagram showing the connections of the red nucleus: *A*, Ventral tegmental decussation; *B*, decussation of the superior cerebellar peduncle; *C* and *D*, descending fibers from superior cerebellar peduncle, before and after its decussation respectively.

NEURON I. From the Purkinje cells of the cerebellar cortex fibers run to terminate in the central nuclei of the cerebellum, especially the dentate nucleus (Fig. 276).

NEURON II. Arising chiefly from the cells of the dentate nucleus, fibers run through the superior cerebellar peduncle, undergo decussation in the tegmentum of the midbrain ventral to the inferior colliculi, and end in the red nucleus and in the nucleus ventralis lateralis of the thalamus (this thalamic nucleus projects fibers to the precentral motor areas of the cerebral cortex) (Figs. 276, 277).

NEURON III. From the cells in the red nucleus arise the fibers of the rubrospinal tract, which cross the median plane in the ventral tegmental decussation, and descend through the reticular formation of the brain stem and the lateral funiculus of the spinal cord. Here this tract occupies a position just ventral to the lateral corticospinal tract, and its fibers end in the anterior gray column in relation to the primary motor neurons. The fibers that reach lumbosacral segments of the cord come from ventral and ventrolateral portions of the red nucleus, while cervical and thoracic segments are supplied by fibers from the dorsal and dorsomedial portions (Pompeiano and Brodal, 1957) (Fig. 169).

RETICULAR FORMATION

Running through the brain stem, forming a good proportion of the background in the medulla and higher levels, are a number of fibers belonging to the reticular pathways, which have been studied increasingly in recent years. More or less paralleling the named motor and sensory pathways, and involving phylogenetically old and new connections, the reticular system has basically important effects on nervous mechanisms. It contains both *inhibitory* and *excitatory* elements in terms of the effect on other structures. Toward the caudal position of the nervous system, the effects are shown in contributions to proper motor performance. In higher levels the work of the reticular system appears to be fundamental to the state of "wakefulness" and so of most cerebral functions (Magoun, 1950). Various connections of the reticular mechanism, though by no means all of them, have been considered. It is not feasible to arrange them in the order of a sequence of neurons.

CHAPTER XX

Reflexes and Reflex Arcs

We have considered the afferent paths leading to the cerebral cortex and to the cerebellum as well as the efferent channels which conduct impulses from these centers to the skeletal musculature. But there are many paths by which impulses may travel more directly from receptor to effector; these are known as reflex arcs. The ascending or descending fibers may be quite long: some reflexes, for example placing reactions of lower animals, are dependent upon the integrity of the motor area of the cerebral cortex. It will be worth while to review briefly a few of the more important of these rather direct receptor to effector circuits.

Reflex Arcs of the Spinal Cord. NEURON I. Primary sensory neurons, with cell bodies in the spinal ganglia, convey impulses from the sensory endings to the spinal cord, then along the ascending and descending branches resulting from the bifurcation of the dorsal root fibers within the cord, and along the collaterals of these branches to the primary motor neurons, either directly or through an intercalated central unit (Figs. 96, 138, 139).

NEURON II. The central neurons have their cell bodies in the posterior gray column and may belong to Golgi's Type II, having short axons restricted to the gray matter; or their axons may be long, running through the fasciculi proprii to the ventral horn cells at other levels of the cord. Some of these central axons cross the median plane in the anterior commissure.

NEURON III. Primary motor neurons, with cell bodies in the anterior gray column, send their axons through the ventral roots and spinal nerves to the skeletal musculature. In the case of visceral reflexes, the motor neuron has its cell body located in the intermediolateral cell column, and its axon runs as a preganglionic fiber to an autonomic ganglion, whence the impulses are relayed by a fourth or postganglionic neuron to involuntary muscle or glandular tissue.

The **reflex paths of the cranial nerves** are similarly constituted. Rarely if ever do the sensory fibers form synapses directly with the motor cells. The central neuron, which has its cell located in the sensory nucleus of a given nerve, sends its axon through the reticular formation to the motor nucleus of the same or of some other nerve (Figs. 151, 165). Two of the reflex circuits connected with the vestibular nerve require special attention.

405

Vestibular Reflex Arc through the Medial Longitudinal Bundle. NEURON
I. The bipolar cells of the vestibular ganglion in the internal auditory meatus
send peripheral processes to the cristae of the semicircular canals and maculae
of the saccule and utricle. Their central processes run through the vestibular
nerve to the vestibular nuclei (Figs. 188, 278).

NEURON II. Cells in the medial, spinal, and superior vestibular nuclei
send their axons into the medial longitudinal fasciculus of the same or the
opposite side, within which they run giving off branches to the nuclei of the

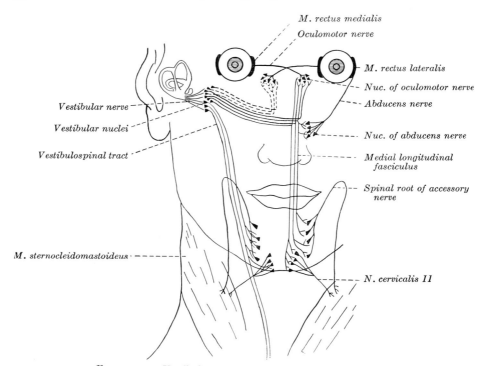

FIGURE 278. Vestibular reflex arcs. (Modified after Edinger.)

oculomotor,, trochlear, and abducens nerves and to the motor cells of the
cervical portion of the spinal cord (Fig. 278).

NEURON III. Primary motor neurons of the oculomotor, trochlear, abducens, accessory, and cervical spinal nerves send their axons to the muscles that
move the head and eyes.

This arc is concerned with the reflex regulation of the combined movements
of the head and eyes in response to the vestibular stimulation which results
from every movement and change of posture of the head. Strong stimulation
of the semicircular canals, vestibular nerve, or Deiters' nucleus causes an
oscillatory side-to-side movement of the eyes, known as nystagmus, a reflex
response of an abnormal character mediated through this arc (Wilson and
Pike, 1915).

A *vestibulospinal reflex arc* is established between the vestibular sense

organs and the skeletal musculature and consists of the following parts: the
vestibular nerve; the vestibulospinal tract, which has its origin in the lateral
vestibular nucleus, and descends in the ventral funiculus of the same side
of the spinal cord; and the primary motor neurons of the spinal cord (Fig. 278).

The afferent impulses reaching the medulla oblongata by way of the *vagus*
give rise to a great variety of reflexes. While these are for the most part purely
visceral, some are executed by the somatic musculature.

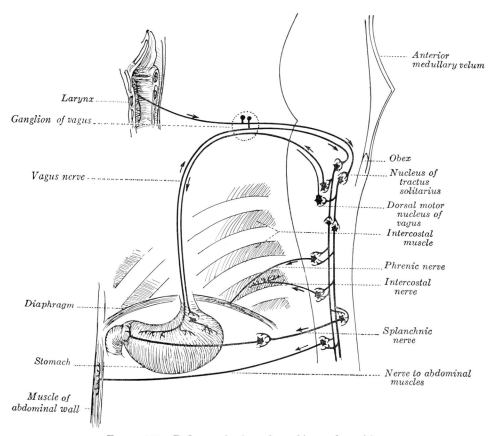

FIGURE 279.   Reflex mechanism of coughing and vomiting.

The **reflex mechanism for vomiting and coughing** is illustrated in Fig. 279.
As the result of an irritation of the stomach, gallbladder, or duodenum, and
other viscera, nerve impulses pass along splanchnic nerves and on through
dorsal roots to the spinal cord as well as along afferent fibers of the vagus nerve
to the tractus solitarius (Borison, 1957). After passing through synapses in the
nucleus of that tract and probably through other synapses in the reticular
formation, the impulses travel down the spinal cord to the primary motor
neurons which give rise to the fibers innervating the diaphragm and abdominal
muscles. At the same time the musculature, surrounding the cardiac orifice

of the stomach, relaxes owing to inhibitory impulses reaching the cardia from the dorsal motor nucleus of the vagus over the visceral efferent fibers of that nerve and an intercalated postganglionic neuron. Closure of the pylorus is caused by impulses leaving the spinal cord over the splanchnic nerves.

Vomiting is elicited in animals by electrical stimulation of the region about the nucleus solitarius and adjacent lateral reticular formation. Near this region are zones related to the other phenomena accompanying emesis: salivation, forced respiratory control, vasomotor changes (Borison and Wang, 1949).

A similar neural circuit is probably responsible for reflex coughing. From the irritated respiratory mucous membrane, as, for example, of the larynx, a disturbance is propagated along the afferent fibers of the vagus, through the nucleus of the tractus solitarius and the descending fibers arising in it to the spinal primary motor neurons, which innervate the diaphragm and the intercostal and abdominal muscles. It is of interest that the epiglottis is innervated profusely on the side toward the larynx and rather sparsely on the lingual side. Touching the laryngeal side results in closure of the glottis, though this does not normally follow stimulation of the lingual side (Feindel, 1956).

The **corpora quadrigemina** are important reflex centers. The path for *reflexes in response to sound* begins in the spiral organ of Corti and follows the cochlear nerve and its central connections, including the lateral lemniscus, to the inferior colliculus of the opposite side, and to a less extent of the same side also. Connections here presumably are made with the large cells of the tectum that give rise to tectospinal and tectobulbar fibers reaching primary motor neurons of the cerebrospinal nerves. The *visual reflex arc* begins in the retina, follows the optic nerve and optic tract with partial decussation in the chiasma, to the superior colliculus of the corpora quadrigemina; thence it is continued by way of the tectospinal and tectobulbar paths to the primary motor neurons of the cerebrospinal nerves (Fig. 191).

Pupillary Reactions. The iris is innervated by two sets of autonomic nerve-fibers derived from the ciliary and the superior cervical sympathetic ganglia, respectively. Impulses reaching the iris through the latter ganglion induce dilatation of the pupil; those through the ciliary ganglion cause constriction. The latter reaction always accompanies accommodation. The preganglionic outflow for pupillary dilatation has been shown to leave the spinal cord by spinal nerves in man between the 8th cervical and the 4th thoracic spinal segments (Ray, Hinsey, and Geohegan, 1943). The preganglionic outflow for pupillary constriction is by way of the oculomotor nerve. When vision is focused on a near object, contraction of the ciliary muscle results in accommodation; at the same time contraction of the two internal rectus muscles brings about a convergence of the visual axes. These two movements are always associated with a third, the contraction of the sphincter pupillae. In addition to this constriction of the pupil, which accompanies accommodation, two other pupillary reactions require attention (Fig. 280).

THE PUPILLARY REFLEX (LIGHT REFLEX). When light impinges on the retina, there results a contraction of the sphincter pupillae and a corresponding constriction of the pupil. The reflex circuit, which is traversed by the impulses bringing about this reaction, begins in the retina and includes the following elements: the fibers of the optic nerve and tract, with a partial decussation in the optic chiasma; synapses in the pretectal region, the zone of transition between the thalamus and superior colliculus; fibers arising in the pretectal region and, after a partial crossing in the posterior commissure, arching ventrally around the gray matter surrounding the rostral end of the cerebral aqueduct to end in or near the nucleus of Edinger-Westphal (visceral efferent portion of the oculomotor nucleus); the visceral efferent fibers of the oculomotor

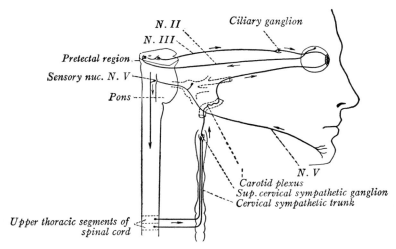

FIGURE 280.   Pupillary reflex arcs.

nerve, ending in the ciliary ganglion; and the postganglionic fibers extending from the ciliary ganglion to the iris.

In tabes dorsalis the reaction of the pupil to light is lost while the reaction to accommodation remains unimpaired. This condition is known as the Argyll Robertson pupil. Wilkinson (1927) has suggested that the contraction of the pupil during accommodation is really associated with the accompanying convergence and is a reflex initiated through the proprioceptive endings in the extrinsic muscles of the eye. An Argyll Robertson pupil is produced by a lesion interrupting the afferent limb of the arc for the pupillary reflex to light while the optic fibers ending in the lateral geniculate body remain intact (Fig. 280). Such a lesion does not affect the pathways involved in the reaction of accommodation.

The *pupillary-skin reflex* is a dilatation of the pupil following scratching of the skin of the cheek or chin. This is but one example of the fact that dilatation of the pupil can be induced by strong stimulation of many sensory nerves and constantly occurs in severe pain. The path, as it has usually been described, includes the following parts: the fibers of these sensory nerves and their central connections in the brain stem and spinal cord; preganglionic visceral efferent fibers, which arise from the cells of the intermediolateral column of the spinal cord and run through the upper white rami and the sympathetic trunk to the superior cervical sympathetic ganglion; and post-ganglionic fibers, which arise in that ganglion and run through the plexus on the internal carotid artery and then through the ophthalmic division of the fifth nerve, its nasociliary branch, and the ciliary nerves to the radial bundles of the iris. Some of the fibers pass through the ciliary ganglion but are not interrupted there. Impulses traveling this path cause dilatation of the pupil. However, inhibition of the tonic activity of the Edinger-Westphal nucleus (or neighboring cells) can also cause dilatation of the pupils. In the cat this is the most important factor in pupillo-dilatation, and is the mechanism of the pupillary-pain reflex. Furthermore this reaction is not impaired by section of the cervical sympathetic trunk (Ury and Gellhorn, 1939). But in the monkey and probably also in man, reflex dilatation of the pupil may be evoked by activation of its sympathetic innervation as well as by inhibition of its parasympathetic innervation. According to Harris, Hodes, and Magoun (1943), the path for impulses resulting in pupillary dilatation following sciatic, splanchnic, or trigeminal stimulation is still complete after the brain is transected above the mesencephalon. The pathway is in the lateral funiculus in the cord and reticular formation of the medulla but is distinct from the pain path in the lateral spinothalamic tract.

When dealing with reflexes involving somatic receptors and effectors it is often easy to define a single reflex arc and its components. But even when this is done, it is usually only an example of a special instance since most efferent paths may be excited by sensory stimuli from a number of sources. For visceral effectors it is often more difficult to select a customary afferent path, but the efferent paths are naturally constant. In some of the following examples details of locations of portions of reflex arcs are omitted but the student can easily fill in these to suit the needs of a special case. It should be emphasized that reflexes do not adhere to strictly functional classifications of fibers, both visceral or somatic afferents being able to set off reflex responses through either visceral or somatic efferent paths and effectors in a single reflex.

Respiration and Blood Pressure. *Receptors* of great importance for the regulation of respiration and blood pressure are situated in the *carotid sinus* and *aortic arch* and in the *aortic* and *carotid bodies* (Heymans et al., 1933). The carotid sinus is an enlargement of the carotid artery at its bifurcation; in contact with it is the carotid body which has the appearance of a gland with thin-walled sinusoidal vessels. The aortic body with a similar structure lies in contact with the aortic arch. The glossopharyngeal nerve sends a branch to the carotid body and carotid sinus (Fig. 281). The vagus nerve supplies the aortic arch and aortic body. The fibers for the arch form a branch of the vagus, known as the depressor nerve, which in the rabbit runs a separate course through the neck from the level of the superior laryngeal nerve.

Tension on the arterial wall due to pressure of the contained blood is the stimulus activating the nerve endings in the carotid sinus and aortic arch. As the pressure rises, stimulation increases and reflexly causes a fall in blood pressure and a slowing of the heart. On the other hand, section of the branches of the glossopharyngeal and vagus nerves supplying these receptors removes this source of inhibition, allowing vasoconstriction and cardiac acceleration to cause a rise in blood pressure. The inhibitory effect of impulses from the carotid sinus and aortic arch is exerted through the vasomotor center in the reticular formation of the medulla.

The chemoreceptors of the carotid and aortic bodies are stimulated by the changes in the blood which occur during asphyxia, i. e., by decreases in oxygen and by increases in carbon dioxide and in hydrogen ion concentration. Impulses arising in these receptors reach the respiratory center by way of the glossopharyngeal and vagus nerves, and, since these receptors are relatively

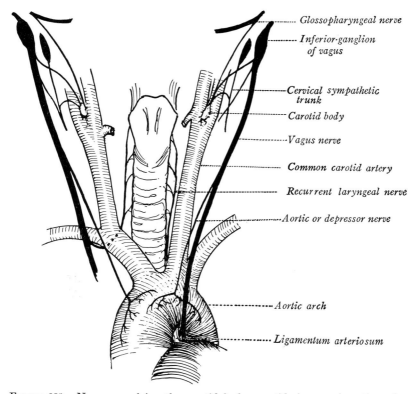

FIGURE 281. Nerves supplying the carotid body, carotid sinus, and aortic arch.

resistant to asphyxia, they are able to drive that center when its activity is so impaired that it does not respond directly to the altered condition of the blood flowing through it.

The **vasomotor center** is situated in the reticular formation of the medulla and perhaps extends upward into the pons. In an animal decerebrated by transection through the mesencephalon, blood pressure and vascular reflexes are normal, but after a section through the lower part of the medulla blood pressure falls to a low level and the usual vascular reflexes are abolished.

The **respiratory center** is located in the reticular formation and extends from slightly below the pons to the level of the calamus scriptorius. Transection of the brain stem below the latter level stops respiration. When the interior of the medulla is explored in cats or monkeys with a needle electrode, through which stimulation is applied to one point after another in the reticular formation, either inspiration or expiration can be produced depending on the location of the point stimulated (Pitts et al., 1939, 1940; Beaton and Magoun, 1941). The points in the reticular formation which cause expiration (circles in Fig. 282) tend to lie dorsal to those that cause inspiration (represented by triangles).

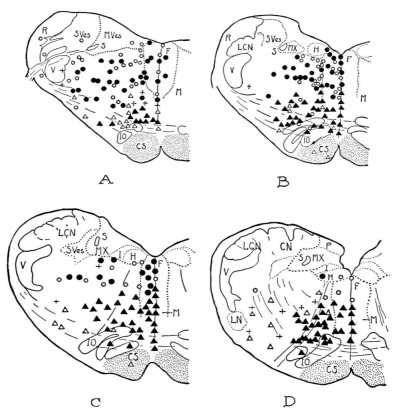

FIGURE 282. Sections of the medulla of the cat showing the location of the respiratory center and its separation into a ventrally situated inspiratory subdivision, marked by triangles, and a dorsally situated expiratory subdivision, marked by circles. (Pitts and Magoun.) *CN*, cuneate nucleus; *CS*, corticospinal tract; *F*, medial longitudinal fasciculus; *H*, hypoglossal nucleus; *I*, intercalate nucleus; *IO*, inferior olive; *LCN*, lateral cuneate nucleus; *LN*, lateral reticular nucleus; *M*, medial lemniscus; *MX*, motor nucleus of vagus; *M ves*, medial vestibular nucleus; *P*, area postrema; *R*, restiform body; *S*, tractus solitarius; *S ves*, spinal vestibular nucleus; *V*, spinal tract of trigeminal nerve. The dark symbols represent the more intense responses.

By this method it has been possible to determine the extent and outline of the respiratory center and to show that it includes a dorsal expiratory division, corresponding to the dorsal part of the reticular formation, and a ventral inspiratory division, corresponding to the ventral part of the reticular formation. The outline and extent of each of these is shown for the cat in Fig. 283, in which to avoid overlapping the expiratory division is represented only

on the left, the inspiratory division only on the right. It was formerly supposed
that the respiratory center possessed an inherent rhythmicity of its own, but,
whether or not this is true, its activity is controlled by the condition of the
blood in its capillaries and by impulses reaching it from various sources,
especially from the lungs by way of the vagi. The dorsal boundary of the
expiratory center extends along the tractus solitarius and its lateral limits along
the spinal tract of the trigeminal nerve.

The activity of the respiratory center can be augmented by a small increase
in the *carbon dioxide tension of the blood* flowing through it. Changes in the
oxygen tension and hydrogen ion concentration are less effective.

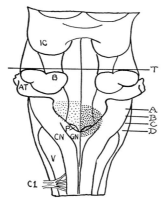

FIGURE 283.   Dorsal view of brain stem of cat with cerebellum removed. Location of the respiratory center as projected on the floor of the fourth ventricle. To avoid overlapping, the expiratory
subdivision is indicated only on the left, inspiratory only on the right. The lines on the right side
of the figure show the levels of sections *A, B, C,* and *D* in Fig. 282. The line *T* shows the level of
a transection of the brain stem, which, combined with bilateral section of the vagi causes a continuous inspiratory spasm. (Pitts and Magoun.) *AT,* Acoustic tubercle; *B,* superior cerebellar
peduncle; *C1,* first cervical root; *CN,* cuneate nucleus; *GN,* gracile nucleus; *IC,* inferior colliculus;
P, area postrema; *V,* tuberculum cinereum.

Afferent impulses aroused in the lungs by their alternate inflation and
deflation reach the respiratory center by way of the vagus (Fig. 284). They
are essential factors in the regulation of breathing. The impulses set up by
inflation inhibit inspiration, those resulting from deflation excite it. The
receptors from which these vagal impulses arise are located in the most dis-
tensible part of the lungs, probably in the alveolar ducts. Impulses reaching
the respiratory center by way of the glossopharyngeal nerves from the carotid
sinuses and carotid bodies and by way of the vagus from the aortic arch and
aortic bodies (Fig. 281) are not important factors under ordinary conditions;
but, when the sensitivity of the respiratory center has been impaired, as for
instance under deep anesthesia, the chemoreceptors of the carotid and aortic
bodies are stimulated by the decrease in oxygen and increase in carbon dioxide
and in hydrogen ion concentration in the blood and drive the respiratory center
when it would otherwise fail. Afferent impulses reach the respiratory center
from other sources such as the trigeminal nerve and the nerves of the thoracic

wall, but while such impulses can affect the respiratory rhythm they are not essential factors in normal breathing.

After section of both vagi, the respiration becomes deep and slow because impulses set up by stretching the lungs no longer act on the respiratory center to limit inspiration. A somewhat similar type of slow deep breathing is caused by transection of the pons at level *T*, Fig. 283. When such a transection is combined with section of both vagi, breathing is arrested in a state of deep

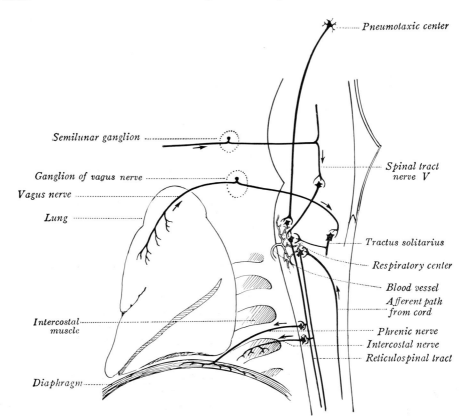

FIGURE 284. Reflex mechanism of respiration.

inspiration. This has been explained on the assumption that a *pneumotaxic center* exists in the upper pons or mesencephalon which is able to act like the vagi in limiting inspiration and allowing expiration to begin. If either one of these limiting mechanisms remains, breathing continues although it is deep and slow; if both are removed the chest may be held in a fixed state of inspiration interrupted only by the death of the animal (Stella, 1938; Pitts et al., 1939).

Descending fibers from the respiratory center run to the anterior gray columns of the thoracic and third, fourth, and fifth cervical segments of the spinal cord through the anterior funiculus and the anterior part of the lateral funiculus, and give impulses to anterior horn cells, which lie in the most medial group of the ventromedial group of cells in the ventral horn (Keswani and Hollinshead, 1956) and whose axons pass through the phrenic nerve to the musculature of the diaphragm. Other respiratory muscles also receive such impulses.

There are a number of neural pathways to **viscera** that are of interest. The receptors and afferent paths which can set off visceral responses are numerous. For example, acceleration of the heart may be reflexly produced by exercise, by

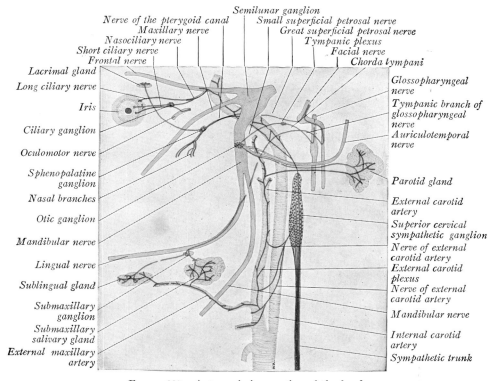

FIGURE 285. Autonomic innervation of the head.

alterations in blood pressure with hemorrhage, by a disturbing sound or situation, by painful stimulation in any part of the body, and so on. As has been mentioned before, visceral reflexes may be set off by stimuli coursing over somatic or visceral afferent paths. In the account of the following significant reflex mechanisms efferent paths are chiefly stressed.

The **submaxillary and sublingual salivary glands** receive their *parasympathetic* innervation through preganglionic fibers which arise in the salivatory nucleus and run through the nervus intermedius, facial nerve, chorda tympani, and lingual nerve to end in the submaxillary ganglion (for the sublingual gland) and in relation to scattered cells of this ganglion which lie along the submaxillary duct (for the submaxillary gland). From cells in these locations postganglionic fibers are distributed to the glands (Fig. 285). Stimulation of the chorda tympani causes dilation of the vessels supplying the glands and an abundant secretion of saliva. These glands receive their *sympathetic* supply through preganglionic fibers from the upper white rami that end in the superior cervical ganglion. From cells in this ganglion postganglionic fibers run through the plexuses on the external carotid and external maxillary arteries to the submaxillary and sublingual glands. Impulses traveling this path cause vasoconstriction and a small amount of secretion. The antagonism of the two divisions of the autonomic system is evident in the blood vessels but both cause secretion.

The **parotid gland** receives *parasympathetic* innervation through preganglionic fibers, which arise in the salivatory nucleus and run through the glossopharyngeal nerve, its tympanic branch, the tympanic plexus, and the small superficial petrosal nerve to the otic ganglion. Postganglionic fibers, arising in this ganglion, reach the parotid gland by way of the auriculotemporal nerve (Fig. 285). *Sympathetic* preganglionic fibers from the upper thoracic white rami end in the superior cervical sympathetic ganglion. Postganglionic fibers arising here run to the gland along with its arterial supply. The action of the two systems on the parotid is the same as on the submaxillary and sublingual glands.

The **heart** receives its *parasympathetic* innervation from the dorsal motor nucleus of the vagus by way of that nerve and its cardiac branches. These preganglionic fibers end in the cardiac ganglia on the auricles. The postganglionic fibers arising from cells in these ganglia end in the sino-auricular and auriculoventricular nodes, the auriculoventricular bundle, and the auricular musculature. The *sympathetic* preganglionic fibers run through the upper white rami to the sympathetic trunk and end in the lower cervical and upper thoracic ganglia (chiefly in the stellate ganglion). Postganglionic fibers run through the sympathetic cardiac nerves to the heart, and many of them are distributed to the ventricles. They probably supply muscle cells as well as the nodes and auriculoventricular bundle. The vagus slows the heart and weakens the contraction of the auricles; the sympathetic accelerates the heart rate and increases the force of the auricular and ventricular contraction.

The **bronchioles** receive their innervation through the pulmonary plexuses. *Parasympathetic* impulses from the dorsal motor nucleus, mediated through the vagus, cause constriction of the bronchi. *Sympathetic* impulses cause inhibition of the bronchial musculature and dilation of these air passages.

The **stomach and small intestines** receive their *parasympathetic* innervation from the dorsal motor nucleus of the vagus by way of the vagus nerve. The preganglionic fibers reach the gut wall and end in the small ganglia of the enteric plexuses. The postganglionic neurons are located entirely within the gut wall and the fibers are thought to end directly on the muscle cells. The intestines are supplied mainly by the right vagus which sends a branch to the celiac plexus (Fig. 286). *Sympathetic* preganglionic fibers from the lower thoracic white rami run through the thoracic sympathetic chain without interruption and through the splanchnic nerves to the celiac plexus. They end in the celiac and mesenteric ganglia. Postganglionic fibers, arising in these

Not only do the procedures used in the physical examination test the function of the peripheral nerves, they bring to light the state of functioning of cell bodies with which the axons in the nerves are connected, and the internuncial neurons ("centers," nuclei, and pathways) between the point of entrance of the sensory nerve used on the side of the stimulus and the motor nerve giving the response. The testing stimulus and response may bring out at the same time the state of functioning of additional central nuclei and pathways, including every level from the reflex centers in spinal cord and brain stem to the cerebellum, the tectum, the larger gray masses in the cerebrum, and the cerebral cortex. Finally, the same type of testing allows the examiner to make comments upon the speech, the state of consciousness, the memory, the intelligence, and other phenomena representing the activity of the whole individual.

In the physical examination a neurologic defect may be discovered that may or may not have been evident to the patient. The patient comes presenting a symptom and it is the examiner's problem to interpret it in terms of physiology and anatomy. Whatever the symptom, the examiner's problem is to think of it in terms of the primary cause, and, if it can be shown to be due to an involvement of the nervous system, it must be interpreted in terms of individual neurons or groups of them.

To search out the location of the underlying cause of a particular neurologic deficit, the examiner needs to consider the possible locations of lesions which *could* produce the symptoms by damage to particular neurons. He must then search for specific circumstances which would allow the location of the lesions in a particular one of the several possible places.

Deficits in sensation can appear from lesions at various points; for example, in the case of general sensibility, destruction of the peripheral endings (as in destructive skin lesions) or their severance from their connections (as in a skin graft) results in loss of sensory perception of stimuli to that area. Interference with the anatomic integrity or physiology of the fibers in a nerve trunk or root from any cause (pressure on the nerve, mechanical interruption of its fibers, peripheral neuritis) will prevent the passage of an impulse over that nerve to the central nervous system. Likewise, destruction of cell bodies of cerebrospinal ganglion cells (tabes, herpes), or of association or intercalary neurons in various central gray masses is followed by loss of the fibers extending from them, and comparable disturbance of function. Interruption of pathways by lesions (cutting injury, tumors, abscesses, syringomyelia, hemorrhage) within the central nervous system permanently eliminates the fibers involved, while pressure upon the nervous tissue (from edema, hemorrhage, tumors, fractures) may only temporarily block function.

Small local sensory losses in cutaneous innervation from any of the above causes may be overlooked because of the possibility of overlapping function from adjacent nerves, or because the deficit is relatively slight in terms of the normal behavior of the person involved. In the case of special senses, on the other hand, there is usually a more conspicuous effect from small lesions. In the eye, for example, blocking in any way the impulses from the macula lutea, a relatively small area of the retina, may abolish the function of that eye in reading and other detailed vision, even though its vision still aids in a stereoscopic way in reflex guidance of visually directed motion.

Just as the sensory neurologic mechanism may be attacked at any point, **abnormality in motor responses** may appear from lesions in various locations. Disturbance of function may be the result of anoxia, atrophy, inflammation, or edema in the effector (muscle or gland cells). Defective responses may also appear as the result of interference with the function of the nerve ending (curare poisoning, myasthenia gravis) or interruption of the peripheral nerve fibers (neuritis) or cell bodies in central nervous system (poliomyelitis). In the case of the visceral supply, the pre- or postganglionic autonomic neurons may be affected. Centrally there may be damage to the large motor paths and their multiple connections at higher levels.

As the examiner applies the various tests in the form of stimuli with observation of the responses he may eliminate certain structures as being involved in pathology because the result of the test demonstrates their normality of function. At the same time he may find other structures abnormal by whatever test he applies. The ingenuity of the neurologist lies in applying the right tests so that the structures not functioning properly may be conspicuously indicated. Then with the total picture of the symptoms he may discover the part of the nervous system that has been selectively affected by the underlying pathology. From previous experience the clinician may know that certain structures in the nervous system are susceptible to types of disease, and this knowledge improves his capacity to select the most probable explanation of the symptoms for a particular patient out of several possibilities.

Abnormalities of Motion.　　Among the most conspicuous effects from lesions of the central nervous system are those following damage to the great motor pathways, the *corticospinal* and *corticobulbar tracts*. The accompanying symptoms aid in the diagnosis and location of the lesion, especially when there are additional symptoms of localizing value.

The *physiologic* and *clinical significance* of the course of the corticospinal and corticobulbar tracts is obvious: It is because of the decussation of these fibers that the muscular contractions produced by cortical stimulation occur chiefly on the opposite side of the body, and that the paralyses resulting from lesions in the pyramidal system above the decussation are contralateral. If the primary motor neuron is injured, the associated muscle atrophies and a flaccid paralysis results. Injury to the motor cortex or to the pyramidal tract leads to a loss of function without atrophy, but with an increased tonicity of the affected muscle, i.e., to a spastic paralysis. By means of such differential characteristics as these it is possible to tell which of the two parts of the motor path has been broken.

In order to understand the combination of symptoms which result from damage to the motor path at different levels, it is necessary to have in mind the topography of its constituent parts. Some of these relations are indicated in Fig. 287. Since the motor cortex is spread out over a rather extensive area, it is usually not entirely destroyed by injury or disease. A restricted cortical lesion may cause a *monoplegia*, i.e., paralysis of a single part, such as the arm or leg (Fig. 287, *A*). But in the internal capsule the motor fibers are grouped within a small area and are frequently all destroyed together. This causes paralysis of the opposite half of the body or *hemiplegia* (Fig. 287, *B*). Damage to the pyramidal system in the cerebral peduncle, pons, or upper part of the medulla oblongata may also cause hemiplegia; in such cases those corticobulbar fibers which leave the main strand of pyramidal fibers above the level of the

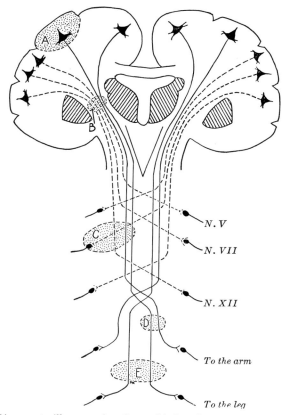

FIGURE 287.   Diagram to illustrate the effects of lesions in various parts of the motor path.

lesion may escape injury and the corresponding cranial nerves need not be involved (Fig. 287, *C*). Furthermore, in lesions of the brain stem the motor nucleus or emergent fibers of one of the cranial nerves may be destroyed along with the pyramidal fibers, in which case there would result a paralysis of the muscles supplied by that nerve as well as a paralysis of the opposite half of the body below that level—*a crossed paralysis* (Fig. 287, *C*). While damage to the spinal cord may affect only one lateral half and cause a homolateral paralysis below the lesion (Fig. 287, *D*), it is common for both lateral halves to be involved and for the resulting paralysis to be bilateral (Fig. 287, *E*).

It is of interest that Lassek (1944) stated after studying the fibers in the pyramids from 90 cases that came to autopsy that complete destruction of the pyramidal tract was the exception and not the rule after hemiplegia or hemiparesis. He further observed that some cases showed no *observable* diminution in number of fibers and that it was common to find more fibers preserved than destroyed.

Bucy (1944) has summed up the evidence based on clinical and physiologic observations for the mechanism of such abnormal movements as athetosis, chorea, and tremor. Impulses for activity in voluntary muscle are known to pass directly to spinal centers from the cerebral cortex (corticospinal tract) and less directly by way of extrapyramidal paths which bring the influences of other centers (basal ganglia, and other cellular accumulations in the cerebrum, cerebellum and its connections) to play upon the spinal centers. The final common path (anterior horn cells), being activated by the total effect of all these centers, sends impulses to muscles that produce well coordinated activity. Interruptions on the various paths result in abnormality of movements which have since Hughlings Jackson's time been interpreted as "release phenomena," that is, the abnormality occurs from the activity of the remaining normal centers acting without the controlling effects of those mechanisms that have been eliminated by lesions. The interaction of the suppressor areas recently described (see p. 365) and the motor areas of the brain are believed to be involved not only in these abnormal motions but normal ones as well.

Though the exact causes of abnormal movements are not known, some fairly definite statements are made about them. Following is a brief summary of present day interpretations of the most common abnormal movements found in neurologic disease.

Choreo-athetoid movements are involuntary, coarse, irregular, at times jerky movements, especially of distal portions of the extremities, which appear most commonly after lesions in the caudate nucleus alone, or caudate and putamen. They are probably conducted by fibers other than the pyramidal tract which arise presumably from Areas 4 and 6. Such movements have been abolished by anterior chordotomy without injury to the lateral corticospinal tract.

Hemiballismus is a condition which shows movements of more violence than those called choreo-athetoid and involves proximal portions of the extremity more than the distal. It has been found to be associated with lesions in the subthalamic nucleus of Luys though similar disturbances of motion can occur with lesions in its connections and without obvious damage to the subthalamic nucleus (Martin, 1957). In monkeys similar symptoms from experimentally placed lesions have been abolished by removal of cortical Areas 4 and 6 contralateral to the symptoms with resultant paresis without spasticity.

Intention tremor is a coarse oscillation of a part of the body which occurs during volitional but not reflex movements. It appears after lesions of the cerebellum that include the dentate nucleus or its efferent fibers to the red nucleus and ventrolateral nucleus of the thalamus, and has been abolished by removal of precentral areas, especially Area 4. The tremor is presumably carried by impulses over the pyramidal tract.

Tremor at "rest" of Parkinsonism is a coarse tremor, which is abolished during sleep as well as during ordinary movement. It is said to result from lesions of the substantia nigra and globus pallidus. It is not abolished by anterior chordotomy but has been abolished by cutting the lateral corticospinal tract which is presumably its route of transmission. Partial relief from symptoms has resulted from removal of precentral cortical areas, or sectioning the anterior limb of the internal capsule and removal of the head of the caudate nucleus, or sectioning the fibers leaving the globus pallidus in the ansa and fasciculus lenticularis (Carpenter and Mettler, 1951).

It seems probable that the abnormal movements just described may depend on lesions of both cortex and basal ganglia (Kennard and Fulton, 1941), but tremor has been seen following purely cortical lesions in Area 6 (Welch and Kennard, 1944).

For discussion of symptoms of cerebellar lesions see page 289.

Pain. Pain as a stimulus is closely related to the normal pattern of behavior, and is considered protective as it warns of injury; furthermore, it has great significance in the phenomenon of disease. It is perhaps the symptom most commonly responsible for directing attention to disease, and careful consideration of the distribution and character of pain often reveals the site of a pathologic process.

It has been demonstrated by various means that the nerve endings responsive to pain-producing stimuli are bare, branching fibers, unencapsulated. Such endings are more numerous in the skin than in deeper structures, and some areas of skin appear more plentifully supplied with them than others. In the cornea this is the only type of ending found. It has been definitely demonstrated that the smaller nerve fibers, mostly unmyelinated but also small myelinated fibers with slow velocity of conduction, convey pain impulses. There is evidence, however, that some larger fibers also carry impulses of pain. Subjectively, pain from a pin-prick can be recognized to have an immediate bright sharp quality followed after a short interval by another peak of intensity. It appears likely that the first report of pain is conveyed over larger fast conducting fibers, while the second peak is the result of impulses arriving over smaller fibers which conduct more slowly. The latter is the burning type of pain in the skin (see p. 148).

Within the skin pain terminals end in an overlapping mosaic, and a pin-prick usually stimulates more than one terminal. In scarred areas, or in regions of skin being reinnervated after nerve damage, where there is a reduction of the normal complement of nerve endings, pin-prick may cause pain of an unpleasant quality, different from that following the same stimulus in normal skin. Not only is the response unpleasant, but there may be a delay in perception, reminding one of the slower or second pain response from normal skin. Such unpleasant response to pin-prick has been related by experiment to stimulation of pain endings which were isolated from their neighbors. It has been suggested that the over-reaction to pain associated with various clinical pictures has as its basis a reduction in the pattern of afferent impulses. Such reduction could be due to either peripheral or central disturbance of the pain-perceiving mechanism.

Pain itself is a subjective experience, though reaction to what would be painful stimuli occurs in the absence of consciousness. The appreciation of pain varies with the state of the individual experiencing it, and apparently differs in individuals. There is a central factor in pain, and the exaggeration of its quality, as in causalgia, may at times be dependent upon abnormal activity of internuncial neurons in reverberating circuits. The phenomenon of phantom limb, in which after amputation the patient experiences discomfort apparently in the part amputated, has been relieved not only by removal of terminal neuromata but by suggestion (as the cremation of the amputated extremity), and also by operative methods designed to diminish internuncial activity which would maintain or facilitate any sensory impressions coming from the stump.

Characterization of sensation, even touch, as disagreeable, with exaggeration of pain sensation is found in many individuals following lesions in the brain, such as a hemorrhage in the internal capsule, that interrupts connections between the thalamus and the somesthetic area. This has been studied experimentally and may depend upon a sensitization of neurons that have had part of their afferent supply cut off (Spiegel and Szekely, 1955), somewhat like the sensitization of postganglionic neurons by preganglionic sympathectomy.

The pain threshold as measured in various individuals is uniform, even though the reaction to a standard stimulus may vary from one person to another (Wolf and Hardy, 1947). Pain is localizable readily in most cutaneous areas and the mucous membranes closely related to the skin. It is fairly well localized from slightly deeper structures as fasciae, ligaments, and tendons, while pain from viscera tends to be diffuse and poorly localized. Normal viscera as such are not sensitive to many stimuli that provoke pain in other regions. Mesenteries and parietal serous layers are more sensitive than viscera. Stretching these structures is an adequate stimulus for pain. Knowledge of the various areas to which visceral pain may be "referred" is extremely useful in locating specific pathology.

Pain of visceral origin is of two types. One is dull, somewhat vague, and poorly localized, but occurs in the general area of the diseased viscus; the other type may be aching or sharp, and is commonly localized superficially within the dermatomes supplied by the spinal segments which supply the diseased viscus. The second type is referred pain and may at times be relieved by local anesthetic in the skin area affected. Referred pain may be dependent upon more than one mechanism for its explanation. Facilitation of internuncial neurons within the gray matter of the cord by normal impulses of touch and temperature and pressure from the area to which the pain is referred may play a part. On some such basis the effect of local anesthetics on referred pain could be explained. An interesting commentary on this may be found in the observation that pinching of superficial or deep structures in an area of anesthesia following unilateral anterior cordotomy can result in pain coming apparently from the opposite side but in a diffuse manner (Wolff, 1943; Wolff and Wolf, 1948).

Through the efforts of a number of clinical investigators direct stimulation of various deep structures in patients has revealed the character and location of pain referred from specific parts. Such observations have special value in that they are made on normal as well as diseased areas. When an area is inflamed or engorged, the pain is greater in response to a given stimulus than when the tissue is normal. Pain arising from one structure may be mingled with that from another source, as for example when the lesion in an organ encroaches on an adjacent area, or the adjacent area is mechanically involved from distention of a hollow organ or traction through attached structures.

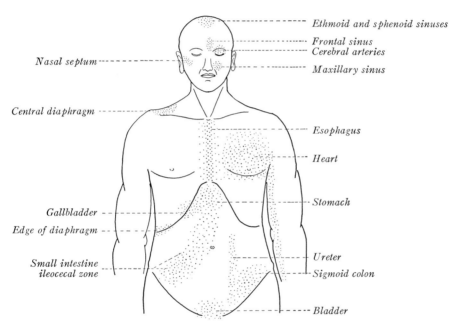

FIGURE 288.   Diagram to show some examples of sites of reference of visceral pain as determined by artificial stimulation and clinical observations. The areas may be larger and more diffuse, dependent upon conditions.

Because of the overlap of referred pain areas from different organs and the vagueness of the boundaries of some of these areas, the observer needs additional data to associate a particular pain with the proper source. A careful history and examination are indispensable aids to interpretation.

PAIN IN THE HEAD.   Pains in and about the head have different origins. Headache occurs in normal persons when standing erect after removal of 20 cc. of cerebrospinal fluid (about 1 per cent of the intracranial contents). The pain may be relieved by lying down or at times by movement of the head. The cause appears to be altered tension on the structures anchoring the brain to the cranium. Headache may result from traction, tension, inflammation, or distention of pain-sensitive structures. The location of the headache may give a clue as to its site of origin (Ray and Wolff, 1941).

Pain is felt within, behind, or over the homolateral eye when the first portions of the anterior, middle, or posterior cerebral arteries are electrically stimulated. Following stimulation of the basilar and vertebral arteries, pain is felt in the occipital and suboccipital region. The pathway for pain from dilatation of supratentorial vessels is the trigeminal nerve, while for the vessels in the infratentorial region the pathway is through the 9th and 10th cranial nerves and the upper cervical.

The paranasal sinuses in disease are the source of pains about the head and the pain is referred to nearby regions; from the frontal sinus the pain is diffuse over the frontal region; from the maxillary sinus to the maxillary region; from the sphenoidal sinus and ethmoid cells the pain occurs back of the eyes and over the vertex.

In cooperative normal subjects it is shown that punching the nasal septum near its middle causes pain over the zygoma and toward the ear; from the ethmoid portion the pain is at the outer and inner canthus of the homolateral eye. Punching the turbinates causes local pain and some spread to teeth and region of the zygoma, and eye. Punching the eardrum gives local sharp pain, not referred, and punching the pharyngeal region causes local pain plus at times reference toward the ear.

THORACIC PAIN. Pains in the chest from diaphragm and pleura illustrate well the principle of reference. Punching the diaphragm along its margin causes pain in the chest wall near the costal margin and near the point punched. Punching the diaphragm in its central portion gives distinct pain over the ridge of the trapezius muscle in the shoulder. These differences illustrate the sensory innervation of the diaphragm by the lower intercostal nerves at the margin and the phrenic nerve centrally, and recall the embryologic origin of the diaphragm from the septum transversum in the cervical region, with its acquisition of muscle masses and a nerve supply as it migrates past the region of the 3rd and 4th (and 5th) cervical segments. Pain from lesions affecting the central and peripheral portions of the diaphragm is located as that described for mechanical stimulation of these parts. While the parietal pleura when inflamed or punched causes local pain, the visceral pleura may be cut or punched without pain.

Sensory impulses from the *lungs* are apparently entirely carried by the vagus nerves, and not by way of the sympathetic trunks. The cough reflex from tickling the tracheal bifurcation has its afferent path over the vagus. Pain as such is not characteristic of involvement of the deeper portions of the lung or bronchial tree.

Pain from the region of the *heart* is of especial interest in relation to heart disease. Touching the parietal pericardium with a probe above the 5th and 6th intercostal space causes pain over the trapezius in the shoulder. Touching the visceral pericardium or the heart produces no pain but some discomfort. Areas of referred pain from the heart are over the upper thoracic and lower cervical segments. The pain of angina pectoris is characteristically in a band about the chest and down the inner side of the left arm, following approximately the distribution of the medial cutaneous nerves of the arm and forearm, and the ulnar nerve. Section of the upper five thoracic dorsal roots has given complete relief from the constricting type of pain from the heart in patients with angina, though there may remain a sense of substernal discomfort on exertion. This is interpreted as sensation by way of the vagus nerves. In experimental animals the signs of pain from occlusion of coronary arteries are abolished by section of thoracic dorsal roots one through five, or removal of the stellate and upper three thoracic sympathetic ganglia, which interrupts the same sensory nerve fibers on their way from the heart to the dorsal roots.

ABDOMINAL PAIN. Referred pain from the intestinal tract has been studied by inflating balloons at different points along the tract in cooperative patients and comparing this with the pain of localized disease (Jones, 1942). The *esophagus* is supplied largely by the vagus nerves and the pain from distention is substernal at the approximate level of distention, and is like that described as "heart burn." It is present after high cordotomy.

The *stomach* also is supplied with sensory fibers by the vagus, and sensations of gastric fullness or hunger are felt after transection of the cervical spinal cord. Referred pain from the stomach is felt in the epigastric region. Electrical stimulation of duodenum and stomach from within, by means of an electrode on a stomach tube, in normal subjects (Boyden and Rigler, 1934) caused a deep pain that was localized definitely by the subject. The stimulation was usually followed by ring contraction of the gut accompanied by some abdominal rigidity and the accompanying pain might be slight or severe and colicky. Each region stimulated was localized by the subject in a small area over the upper abdomen. Anesthetization of the spot of skin under which the pain was localized resulted in a shift of the pain to an adjacent area. With change of position of the subject there was some shifting in the site of pain. Pain from distention of the *small intestine* beginning with the duodenum and progressing along the intestine is felt from the midline or right epigastric region and through the umbilical zone to the right lower quadrant of the abdomen where pain of distention of the ileocecal valve is found. Pain from distention of the *colon* is less well localized, being mostly near the midline in the hypogastric region, though the flexures give local signs and pain from the sigmoid is localized in the left lower quadrant. Pain from the *rectum* or lower sigmoid is felt in the suprapubic or sacral region.

Pain from the *gallbladder* is referred to the epigastric region anteriorly and to the point just beneath the inferior angle of the scapula posteriorly. Pain from the stomach is abolished by blocking the splanchnic nerves or by spinal block to the 7th thoracic segment. Pain from mesenteries and small intestine is relieved by block of the splanchnic nerves, that from lower colon and rectum by block of sacral nerves 2, 3, and 4.

Pain from the fundus of the *uterus* is referred to thoracic segments 11 and 12, while from the cervix pain impulses pass to sacral segments 2, 3, and 4 as is also true of pain from the *prostate* and *neck of the bladder*. Consistent with the high embryologic origin of the structures, pain from the *fallopian tubes* and *ovaries* reaches as high as the 10th thoracic segment. Pain from the *testis* is referred as high as the 10th thoracic level but also to lumbar segments 1 and 2 and to sacral segments 2, 3, and 4. The descent of the testis to its scrotal position explains this spread of pain reference.

The *bladder* is supplied by sacral nerves 2, 3, and 4, but its upper peritoneal covering may be supplied by fibers from the lower thoracic and upper lumbar segments by way of the hypogastric plexus. The usual reference of pain from bladder distention is in the suprapubic region and in the urethra. Pain from the trigone or ureteral openings is referred to the urethra. Pain from the ureter appears generally along the margin of the homolateral rectus abdominis; from the kidney pelvis it is referred to the costovertebral angle in the back and not to the abdomen.

Observations on the bladder with the aid of the cystoscope show that punching or pulling the normal mucosa produces sensation akin to touch, while the same stimulus to an inflamed mucosa is painful. It is also of interest that pain from the bladder is lost by bilateral cordotomy, but sensations of fullness of the rectum and bladder are not significantly altered by bilateral section of the anterolateral columns of the cord. On the other hand, in patients having posterior column disease (pernicious anemia, tabes) there is impairment in the sensation produced by fullness of the bladder and colon. It thus appears probable that the stretch reflex of these viscera may be dependent upon fibers in the posterior columns, which raises the question of the upper connections of such fibers. Demonstration by Chambers of increase in intravesical pressure and of bladder emptying following stimulation of the interior of the cerebellum near the fastigial nucleus is suggestive of a relationship here.

Certain types of headaches are often associated with pelvic pathology although the method of reference is not clear. Sir Henry Head pointed out relationship between the sites of pelvic disease and specific points of pain in the head. The observation that fullness in the bladder in patients with transverse lesions of the spinal cord is signalled by pain in the back of the head is of interest in this connection. The explanation of the phenomenon is obscure.

Abnormalities of Vision. Loss of vision for one half of the visual field is known as hemianopsia. In Fig. 289 there is illustrated the effect upon the fields of vision produced by lesions at various points along the optic pathway. Complete blindness in the left eye is caused by interruption of the left optic nerve (A). Bitemporal hemianopsia, blindness in the temporal halves of the fields of vision of both eyes, results from interruption of the fibers crossing in the optic chiasma and is sometimes caused by pituitary tumors (B). Blindness in the nasal half of the field of vision (nasal hemianopsia) can be produced in one eye by damage to the corresponding side of the chiasma (C). Right homonymous hemianopsia, blindness in the right halves of both visual fields, results from interruption of the left optic tract or left geniculocalcarine fasciculus (D). A lesion in the lower part of the left geniculocalcarine tract produces blindness in both right upper quadrants (E), and one in the upper part of the same tract causes blindness in both right lower quadrants (F). Right homonymous hemianopsia with preservation of macular vision may result from large cortical lesions in the striate area of the left hemisphere (G).

For some reason, not well understood, in hemianopsia from cortical lesions macular vision is often spared. Lesions in the temporal lobe often involve the geniculocalcarine tract as they bend around the inferior horn of the lateral ventricle (Fig. 192).

An excellent review of anatomic neurology can be obtained by a study of a series of neurologic patients and an attempt to interpret their symptoms in terms of damaged cell masses and fiber tracts. The following brief case

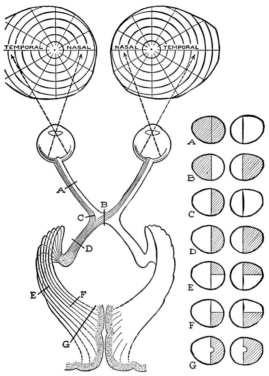

FIGURE 289. Diagram showing the effects on the fields of vision produced by lesions at various points along the optic pathway. *A*, Complete blindness in left eye; *B*, bitemporal hemianopsia; *C*, nasal hemianopsia of left eye; *D*, right homonymous hemianopsia; *E* and *F*, right upper and lower quadrant hemianopsias; *G*, right homonymous hemianopsia with preservation of central vision. (Homans: A Textbook of Surgery. Charles C Thomas.)

histories may serve in lieu of actual patients. Each will be found to illustrate some important facts concerning the organization of the nervous system.

CASE 1

A boy, five years old, complained of pain in the back and legs and had a fever of 102° F. The following morning he was unable to get out of bed and he could not move his right leg. Examination showed no disturbance in the movements of the head and neck, arms, or left leg, but there was complete paralysis of the right thigh, leg, and foot. Muscular tone was greatly reduced and the tendon reflexes (knee jerk and Achilles' tendon reflex) were abolished

in the right lower extremity. After three weeks he was able to flex and adduct
the right thigh and extend the knee, but no other movements returned in that
extremity, and at the end of a month the muscles of the foot and leg and of
the back of the thigh were relaxed and showed the reaction of degeneration
and marked atrophy. Aside from the pain suffered at the time of the onset
there were no sensory disturbances.

The initial pain indicates that the dorsal nerve roots or their connections
within the spinal cord were irritated to some extent by the inflammatory

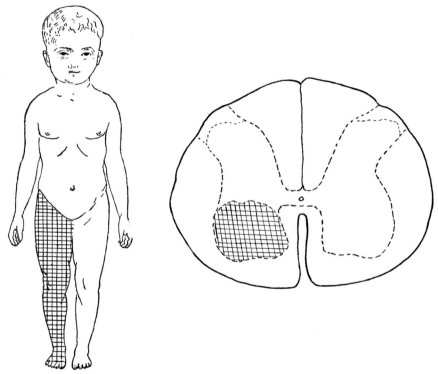

FIGURE 290.   Case 1.

reaction, but the absence of any permanent sensory disturbances shows that
these parts suffered no serious damage.

The lesion obviously involved the somatic motor apparatus for the right
lower extremity. The path for impulses initiating voluntary movements consists
of two sets of neurons (1) cortical neurons with cells in the motor center of the
cerebral cortex and axons in the pyramidal tracts; and (2) primary motor
neurons with their axons running through the peripheral nerves to the muscles.
When the cortical set is destroyed there is paralysis without atrophy of the
muscles and their electrical reactions are normal. The paralyzed muscles show
an increased tone; there is increased resistance to passive movement, and the
tendon reflexes, including the knee jerk and Achilles' tendon reflex, are ex-

aggerated. In spite of the fact that in man such a spastic paralysis is quite regularly associated with lesions of the pyramidal system, many physiologists now believe that the spasticity is due to associated damage to the extra-pyramidal system. When the primary motor neurons are destroyed, the result-ing paralysis is of the flaccid type. The muscles are relaxed, shrink in size, and become atrophic. The tendon reflexes are abolished.

The muscles can no longer be stimulated by the faradic current, but respond to galvanic stimulation with a slow contraction, and the anodal con-traction on closure is greater than the cathodal (ACC > CCC). This sort of response is characteristic of muscles which have been deprived of their motor innervation and is called the reaction of degeneration.

In the case under consideration was it the upper or lower motor neuron which was affected, and why? If the lesion had been in the peripheral nerves where sensory and motor fibers are mingled together, there would have been more or less loss of sensation in the affected limb. Where, then, must the lesion have been located? What nerve fibers would be found degenerated? Which segments of the cord were involved at the onset, and in which of these did the inflammation subside without causing a complete destruction of the motor elements? (See Fig. 26).

DIAGNOSIS. Acute anterior poliomyelitis, an infectious disease of children with inflammation affecting chiefly the anterior gray columns of the spinal cord.

CASE 2

A man of forty-two years noticed an increasing stiffness in the legs. The feet could not be lifted from the ground, but were dragged along, the entire

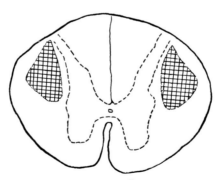

FIGURE 291. Case 2.

leg moving as one piece from the hip. No sensory disturbances were noted. Examination showed loss of voluntary control of the muscles of the legs, which were rigid and offered marked resistance to passive movements. The knee jerk and Achilles' tendon reflexes were markedly exaggerated. There was no atrophy of the affected muscles. Sensation was normal throughout.

Obviously the somatic motor apparatus was at fault in this case. Did the lesion involve the cortical or primary neurons, and why? What tracts were involved?

DIAGNOSIS. Lateral sclerosis, a selective degeneration of the lateral pyramidal tracts. Primary lateral sclerosis is thought by some to be a rare form of amyotrophic lateral sclerosis, in which there is degeneration of the giant Betz cells and other pyramidal cells of the third and fifth laminae in the precentral cortex especially, but also of other areas both anterior and posterior to the central sulcus. Some anterior horn cells of the spinal cord may also undergo degeneration.

CASE 3

A blacksmith, aged forty-eight, presented himself for treatment of a burn on his right hand caused by his having picked up a hot iron. He did not feel

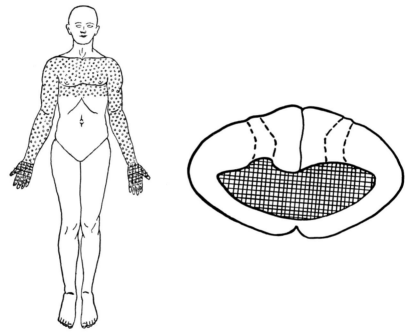

FIGURE 292. Case 3.

either heat or pain at the time, nor had the burn since caused him any pain. Examination showed a loss of pain and temperature sensibility over the thorax and both upper extremities. There was no disturbance of tactile sensibility, no ataxia or loss of the sense of posture or of passive movement. The knee jerk was normal and there was no disturbance of motor functions except that there was weakness and atrophy of the small muscles of both hands.

Does this paralysis with atrophy of the intrinsic muscles of the hand indicate a cortical or a primary motor neuron lesion? Why would you locate this lesion in the 8th cervical and 1st thoracic segments of the cord? What structures in these segments must have been destroyed?

The lesion also extended for some distance up and down the cord, but except in the two segments just mentioned it was confined to the gray matter around the central canal and to the commissures of the cord. Assuming that the centrally placed lesion extended from the 4th cervical to the 6th thoracic segment, how would you account for the loss of pain and temperature sensation in the thorax and upper extremities? Why were the proprioceptive impulses not interrupted? Why was not tactile sensibility disturbed?

DIAGNOSIS. Syringomyelia, a disease of the spinal cord, characterized by cavity formation within the central gray matter disrupting the fibers of the spinothalamic tracts as they cross in the ventral white commissure. The cavity usually enlarges and involves other parts of the gray matter and even the white substance of the spinal cord. In this case it invaded the anterior gray column in the last cervical and first thoracic segments.

CASE 4

A man, aged thirty-four, noticed a tingling sensation in his feet and later suffered from shooting pains in his legs. After several months he experienced

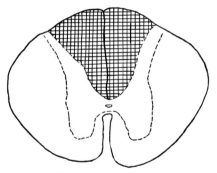

FIGURE 293. Case 4.

difficulty in walking in the dark, and when walking in the light it was necessary to watch the ground to keep from falling. Although his legs were as strong as ever, he would stagger and sway from side to side as he walked. Examination disclosed no weakness or atrophy of the muscles, but when relaxed they did not exhibit the normal tone. The knee jerk was abolished. There was a complete loss of the sense of posture and passive movement and of the vibratory sense in the legs. When the skin of the leg was touched with the two points of a compass he could not recognize the duality of the contact or accurately locate the area stimulated. Except for this loss of tactile localization and tactile discrimination there was not much disturbance of exteroceptive sensibility. A delayed sense of pain to pin-prick might have been found.

What evidence is there in this case of damage to the nerve fibers in the posterior funiculus? How would you account for: (1) the incoordination of the movements of the legs in walking and (2) the loss of the sense of posture and passive movement? The afferent impulses from the muscles, joints, and tendons act through spinal and cerebellar reflex arcs to maintain the normal muscular tone, and the cutting off of these impulses accounts for the atonic condition of the muscles. The knee jerk was missing because the tendon reflexes could not be elicited from atonic muscles and because the afferent limb of this reflex arc was damaged. The shooting pains early in the course of the disease were due to an irritation of the dorsal roots.

DIAGNOSIS.   Tabes dorsalis, a disease of the dorsal roots resulting in a degeneration of the posterior funiculi of the spinal cord. The proprioceptive fibers suffer more serious damage than those of the exteroceptive group. Cells in the dorsal root ganglia show damage.

CASE 5

A bartender, aged forty-six, received a stab wound in the back. Two years after the injury there still remained evidences of a lesion of the spinal cord.

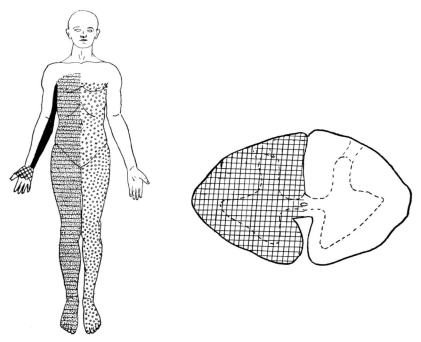

FIGURE 294.   Case 5.

There was a wasting of the small muscles of the right hand. In the right leg there was spastic paralysis with an increase of the knee jerk together with a loss of the sense of posture and of passive movement. On the left side there was no paralysis or muscular wasting, and the reflexes were normal. There was a loss of sensibility to pain, heat, and cold over the entire left half of the body as high as the level of the third rib, but no disturbance of proprioceptive sensibility. All cutaneous sensibility was abolished over a strip along the ulnar side of the right arm, but except for this area tactile sensibility was normal over the entire body.

What does the atrophy of the small muscles of the right hand indicate? What kind of paralysis? What neurons must have been involved? Compare with Case 3. What side of the cord was the lesion on? What segments of the cord must have been involved? Could the spastic paralysis of the right leg have been produced by the same lesion, assuming that the lesion was large enough to involve the entire lateral half of the cord at that level? Give your reasons.

What does the loss of sensibility to pain, heat, and cold on the left and of proprioceptive sensibility on the right indicate as to the side of the cord on which the lesion was located? Taking into consideration the fact that in unilateral lesions of the cord the upper limit of analgesia is usually one or two segments below the lesion, at approximately what level was the lesion situated? How does this level correspond with that deduced from the atrophic paralysis in the hand? Can all the symptoms be explained on the basis of a unilateral lesion? If so, how do you account for the loss of proprioceptive sensibility on one side of the body and of pain and temperature sensibility on the opposite side? What tracts must have been involved? Compare Fig. 294 with Fig. 102 and explain the loss of all cutaneous sensibility along the ulnar side of the right arm. Why was tactile sensibility normal over all the rest of the body?

Which tracts would you expect to find degenerated above this lesion and which would degenerate below?

DIAGNOSIS. A unilateral lesion involving the eighth cervical and first thoracic segments of the spinal cord on the right side (Brown-Séquard syndrome).

CASE 6

A woman of sixty-three years while working about the house suddenly fell to the floor and was unable to rise. She had difficulty in speaking and her left arm and leg were paralyzed. An examination made two months after the onset of the symptoms showed a spastic paralysis of the left arm and leg. The tone of the muscles in these limbs was much increased and there was an exaggeration of the tendon reflexes. When the tongue was protruded it turned to the right because of paralysis of its musculature on that side. The right half of the tongue was much atrophied.

The involvement of both the arm and the leg on one side speaks for a brain lesion. What type of paralysis was exhibited by the arm and leg, and what neurons must have been involved? On which side of the brain was the lesion located? What evidence is there as to the level of the lesion? What type of paralysis was exhibited by the right half of the tongue, and what nerve was affected? How does this help to locate the lesion? How could you explain the symptoms from a lesion occupying the area outlined in Fig. 295? What nerve fibers underwent degeneration, and in what direction?

DIAGNOSIS. Crossed hypoglossal paralysis due to a vascular lesion in the right side of the medulla oblongata involving the pyramid and the emerging fibers of the hypoglossal nerve. The tongue deviates toward the side of its paralysis. Since the movement in protrusion is performed by contraction of the genioglossus muscle, the active muscle pulls the root of the tongue toward the anterior point of the jaw and the paralyzed side lags behind.

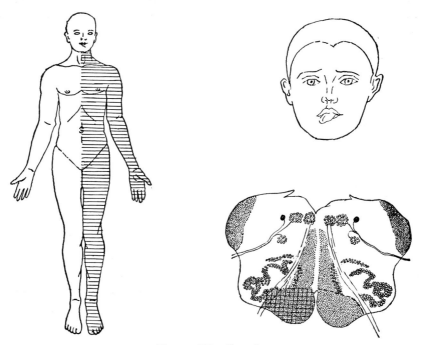

FIGURE 295.   Case 6.

CASE 7

A man, sixty-seven years old, suffered an apoplectic stroke and was unconscious for several hours. After recovering consciousness he could not speak and his right arm and leg were paralyzed. After a few days his speech returned, though he had considerable difficulty in using his tongue. An examination made six weeks after the seizure showed a spastic paralysis of the right arm and leg with increased muscle tone and exaggerated tendon reflexes. When protruded the tongue turned to the left and the musculature of its left side showed atrophy. There was no paralysis of the soft palate, pharynx, or larynx. Pain and temperature sensibility were normal over the entire body, but there was a loss of the sense of posture and of passive movement (sensations from the muscles, joints, and tendons) and an impairment of tactile sensibility over all of the right side of the body except the head.

What can you deduce from the impairment of motor functions as to the location of the lesion? What tract in the medulla oblongata must have been included in the lesion to give rise to the sensory symptoms? On which side was the lesion located? What parts of the medulla oblongata can you be sure

Sections of the Brain

This division is composed of illustrations accompanied by a brief descriptive text and contains the following seven subdivisions:

1. Transverse sections of the brain stem at twenty levels.
2. The nuclei of the brain stem as seen in transverse sections at twenty-five levels.
3. Oblique sections through the region of transition between midbrain and thalamus at five levels.
4. Horizontal sections through the internal capsule at three levels.
5. Frontal sections through the cerebrum representing twelve planes.
6. Parasagittal sections through the brain stem at fifteen positions.
7. The brain of the sheep.

Transverse Sections of the Brain Stem. The illustrations which follow have been drawn from selected transverse sections of the brain stem of a child prepared by the Pal-Weigert method. They are sufficiently numerous to show the gradual rearrangement of fiber tracts which is seen when a series of sections is followed rostrally from the spinal cord through the brain stem. It is hoped that the descriptions which accompany the drawings will aid the student in his first study of such sections, but no effort should be made to remember the content of these paragraphs. After the first survey of the sections has been made, the student should turn at once to the text.

While this series of sections is arranged so that the various tracts are followed rostrally, it is well to keep in mind which of the tracts are being followed toward their terminations in nuclei of the higher centers, proceeding in the direction an impulse would take, and which ones are being traced toward their origins and in a direction opposite to that which an impulse would travel.

For purposes of orientation a key figure showing the location of the plane of section accompanies each drawing. Further assistance in visualizing the plane of these sections can be obtained by comparing these key figures with a drawing of the brain *in situ* (Fig. 28). The structures which are seen in transverse sections all extend for longer or shorter distances parallel to the long axis of the brain stem. If careful attention is paid to these planes of section

449

the student should have little difficulty in determining approximately the longitudinal extent of each structure and should be able to build up a tridimensional conception of the brain stem. Figures 303 and 304 have been inserted as aids to the interpretation of the key figures.

Nuclei of the Brain Stem. Along with the sections drawn from Weigert preparations, the nuclei of the brain stem as seen in transverse sections are illustrated in a series of figures reproduced from Jacobsohn's (1909) monograph. The drawings are from preparations stained with toluidin blue. While the figures have not been altered to any considerable extent the designation of the nuclei has been changed in many instances. Details as to the shape and structure of the cells in these nuclei can be found along with good illustrations in articles by Gagel and Bodechtel (1930), and Stern (1936).

In general the dorsal aspect of the sections showing nerve cell groups lies at a position slightly cranial to the Weigert-stained sections at the corresponding level. It is rare that series of sections from two brain stems will coincide in plane, so the variation in the two series illustrated may be advantageous in the study of other series available to the student.

Since the nuclei of the brain stem may extend craniocaudally through several of the illustrated transverse sections, a brief description of the chief nuclei encountered in the entire series precedes the illustrations. Additional details appear in the description of the separate levels in the Weigert series which accompanies the appropriate level, and in the earlier chapters in the text.

It is suggested that this series showing the groups of cell bodies of neurons has its chief value in the outlining of specific nuclei through some distance. The student may, for example, find it valuable to follow single nuclei through the several sections in which they appear and thus gain appreciation of them in three dimensions. Furthermore, small cell groups, as the nucleus ambiguus, may be easier to visualize than they are in Weigert-stained series.

The abbreviations listed below have been used throughout the series:

abd	nucleus of abducens nerve	fr	formatio reticularis
ac	nucleus of spinal root of accessory nerve	fr a	nuclei of formatio reticularis alba
		grac	nucleus gracilis
ac fac	accessory facial nucleus	h	nucleus of hypoglossal nerve
amb	nucleus ambiguus	if h	nucleus interfascicularis hypoglossi
a post	area postrema	if h′	rostral continuation of the nucleus interfascicularis hypoglossi
arc	arcuate nucleus		
cen sup	nucleus centralis superior	in	nucleus intercalatus
c g	central gray matter	inf col	nucleus of inferior colliculus
com	commissural nucleus	inf ol	inferior olivary nucleus
cun	nucleus cuneatus	infratri	infratrigeminal portion of lateral reticular nucleus
d ac ol	dorsal accessory olivary nucleus		
d c	dorsal cochlear nucleus	i pe	interpeduncular nucleus
den	dentate nucleus	l cun	lateral cuneate nucleus
d mo vg	dorsal motor nucleus of vagus	l lem	nucleus of lateral lemniscus
d r	dorsal nucleus of the raphe	l ret	lateral reticular nucleus
d tg	dorsal tegmental nucleus	l tg pr	lateral tegmental process of pontile nuclei
E W	Edinger-Westphal nucleus		
fac	nucleus of facial nerve	l ve	lateral vestibular nucleus
fast	fastigial nucleus	m ac ol	medial accessory olivary nucleus

mag fr	magnocellular nucleus of reticular formation	pi tg p	nucleus pigmentosus tegmentopontilis
mes V	mesencephalic nucleus of trigeminal nerve	pm d	nucleus paramedianus dorsalis
m gen	medial geniculate body	prae	nucleus praepositus
mo fr	motor cells of formatio reticularis	r	nucleus of the raphe
mo tec	motor cells of tectum	R	nucleus of Roller
mo tg pe	motor tegmentopeduncular nucleus	red	red nucleus
mo V	motor nucleus of trigeminal nerve	retrofac	retrofacial nucleus
m tg pr	medial tegmental process of pontile nuclei	retrotri	retrotrigeminal motor nucleus
		ret tg	reticular tegmental nucleus
m ve	medial vestibular nucleus	sen V	main sensory nucleus of trigeminal nerve
oc	oculomotor nucleus	sol	nucleus of tractus solitarius
p	nuclei pontis	sp V	nucleus of the spinal tract of the trigeminal nerve
pa r	nucleus pallidus of raphe		
p b	pontobulbar nucleus	sp ve	spinal vestibular nucleus
pe p tg	pedunculopontile tegmental nucleus	st gr	stratum griseum
periped	peripeduncular nucleus	st lem	stratum lemnisci
peri vg	perivagal portion of lateral reticular nucleus	st op	stratum opticum
		sub n	substantia nigra
p fr a	perpendicular nucleus of formatio reticularis alba	sup ol	superior olive
		suprasp	supraspinal nucleus
pi c	pigmented cells	sup ve	superior vestibular nucleus
pi med o	nucleus pigmentosus of medulla oblongata	tr b	nucleus of trapezoid body
		tro	nucleus of trochlear nerve
pi p	nucleus pigmentosus pontis	v c	ventral cochlear nucleus
pi tg cbl	nucleus pigmentosus tegmentocerebellaris	v tg	ventral tegmental nucleus

The nerve cells of the brain stem may be grouped into four classes according to size, but the function of the cell is not indicated by its size. In general the larger cells give rise to larger axons, which run for long distances. Smaller cells, however, may have long axons, but they are small in diameter. Very large cells with an average diameter of 40μ or more are found in the lateral vestibular nucleus, the magnocellular portion of the red nucleus, and in the reticular formation dorsal to the dorsal accessory olive. Large cells with average measurements of 27 to 40μ are found in the lateral cuneate nucleus, ventral cochlear nucleus, mesencephalic nucleus of the trigeminal, and in the motor nuclei supplying skeletal muscle (Fig. 180, hypoglossal nucleus). Medium sized cells averaging 16 to 22μ in diameter are found in the olivary, arcuate, and pontile nuclei, the parvocellular portion of the red nucleus, the nucleus gracilis and cuneatus, the lateral reticular nucleus, and in the visceromotor nuclei such as the dorsal motor nucleus of the vagus (Fig. 180). Small cells with diameters less than 15μ are characteristic of the main sensory and spinal nuclei of the trigeminal nerve, the interpeduncular nucleus and the nucleus of the tractus solitarius (Fig. 180).

The column of large motor cells found in the anterior horn of the spinal cord is continued into the medulla oblongata forming the supraspinal, accessory, and hypoglossal nuclei. In the lower levels of the medulla, where the decussation of the pyramids occurs, these large cells of the anterior horn are numerous and may be divided into two groups. The more lateral of the two is the *nucleus of the spinal root of the accessory nerve* (Fig. 308), which can be followed caudally into the lateral part of the anterior horn of the cervical spinal cord. The medial group is the *nucleus supraspinalis* (Figs. 308–317) which sends fibers into the ventral root of the first cervical nerve. It decreases in size as it is followed rostrally and ends where the hypoglossal nucleus begins. The cells within this column are of the large multipolar type with conspicuous dendrites. As seen in the cresyl violet preparations, their abundant cytoplasm is lightly stained and contains large discrete tigroid masses. Such cells are typical of nuclei supplying skeletal muscle (Fig. 179).

The substantia gelatinosa Rolandi of the spinal cord is continuous without change of structure with the *nucleus of the spinal tract of the fifth nerve* (Figs. 308–317). In sections caudal to the olive it is composed of closely packed small cells with little cytoplasm. On its outer surface and infiltrating the spinal tract of the trigeminal nerve are medium sized cells (nucleus marginalis). On its medial surface in the position occupied by the head of the posterior horn in the spinal cord is another scattered group of medium sized cells. At the level of the olive the nucleus becomes less well defined and irregularly triangular or oval in cross-section and is broken up into islands by longitudinal and transverse fiber bundles. Its histologic appearance also changes. The small cells are less numerous and the medium sized cells are scattered indiscriminately or in small groups throughout its cross-section.

A few scattered cells of the *nucleus of the funiculus gracilis* (Figs. 308–320) are found in that funiculus at the level of the lower end of the pyramidal decussation. These very gradually increase in number as the serial sections are followed rostrally. At the level of the middle of the decussation the *cuneate nucleus* makes its appearance in the form of a wedge projecting into the cuneate fasciculus from the ventral side (Figs. 308–311).

In sharp contrast with the two preceding, the *lateral or accessory cuneate nucleus* (Figs. 314–327) is composed of large rounded or polygonal cells with deeply stained cytoplasm and small, not very sharply defined Nissl bodies. These cells resemble those found in the nucleus dorsalis of the spinal cord. They send their fibers by way of the restiform body to the cerebellum. This nucleus, which occupies a position superficial to the cuneate nucleus, begins at the level of the caudal end of the olive and increases in size rostrally. Enlarging rapidly as the cuneate nucleus decreases in size, it underlies the developing restiform body. In Fig. 323 it forms a large triangular field dorsal to the nucleus of the spinal tract of the fifth nerve, and at certain points, as in Figs. 323 and 324, it projects as a column of cells through the restiform body and comes into relation with the pontobulbar nucleus.

The cells of the *lateral reticular nucleus* (Figs. 314–323) are scattered among the longitudinal fibers of the lateral funiculus between the nucleus of the spinal tract of the fifth nerve and the olive. It is largest near its beginning at the lower border of the olive where it has in cross-section a triangular outline with apex directed medialward. A few detached cells may lie in front of the inferior olivary nucleus (Fig. 317). More rostrally it decreases in size and lies deeper in the medulla on the dorsal side of the olive. In its upper part the nucleus is broken up into smaller parts and changes form repeatedly due to the shifting relations of the fiber bundles of the reticular formation. Jacobsohn distinguishes as separate nuclei belonging to this group the nucleus infratrigeminalis (Fig. 324) and nucleus perivagalis (Fig. 323), the cells of which are said to differ from those of the main group. In its lower part where the nucleus is largest it is composed of medium sized cells of various forms—triangular, fusiform, polygonal, or pear-shaped.

The *nuclei of the olive* are conspicuous features in sections through the upper part of the medulla. They are composed of medium sized cells, deeply stained, and rounded or polygonal in shape. These cells are rather closely grouped and the nuclei are sharply outlined. The *inferior olivary nucleus* (Figs. 317–335) is the largest gray mass in the medulla. It consists of a very extensive lamina of gray matter bent and folded on itself in the form of a crumpled sac with the mouth or hilus directed medially. The *medial accessory olivary nucleus* extends the farthest caudally. It appears first as a ventrodorsally directed plate on the medial side of the supraspinal nucleus (Fig. 311). At a little higher level this plate becomes bent on itself at a right angle and extends laterally under the lateral reticular nucleus (Fig. 314). Still higher it lies medial to the hilus of the inferior olivary nucleus (Figs. 317–324). At this point it is sometimes split into two parallel plates lying close together. The *dorsal accessory olive,* smaller than the preceding, forms a curved plate lying dorsal to the rostral part of the inferior olivary nucleus (Figs. 323–328).

The *arcuate nuclei* are irregular masses of gray matter lying on the surface of the pyramids from the caudal border of the olive to the pons (Figs. 314–335). They do not form a continuous sheet but rather a series of plaques. They are largest at the rostral end of the medulla, where, at least in some specimens, they are continuous along the medial surface of the pyramids with the pontile nuclei which are composed of the same type of cells. The cells are of medium size, rounded or polygonal in outline, and closely packed together.

The *nucleus ambiguus* (Figs. 308–332), which sends fibers into the ninth, tenth, and eleventh nerves, is a slender column of cells extending the entire length of the medulla oblongata. It begins at the lower end of the medulla as scattered cells in the lateral part of the reticular formation ventromedial to the nucleus of the spinal tract of the trigeminal nerve. In some of the more caudal sections only one or two of these cells can be seen. In other sections larger clumps are visible in close proximity to bundles of fibers belonging to the roots of the vagus or bulbar portion of the accessory nerve. Toward the rostral end of the medulla the nucleus increases in size, shifts dorsomedially and, becoming smaller again, comes to lie close to the ventromedial side of the tractus solitarius (Fig. 331). It ends at the level of the cochlear nuclei where it is situated close to the dorsal motor nucleus of the vagus (Fig. 332). The cells are similar to those of the other motor nuclei supplying skeletal musculature—large multipolar cells with conspicuous dendrites, abundant lightly staining cytoplasm, and large discrete Nissl bodies.

The *dorsal motor nucleus of the vagus* (Figs. 308–331) contains the cells of origin of general visceral efferent fibers, many of which reach that nerve through the bulbar rootlets of the accessory and its internal ramus. Like other general visceral efferent nuclei it is composed of medium sized cells with rather lightly stained cytoplasm and small but fairly discrete Nissl bodies (Fig. 179). Many of the cells are fusiform in shape. This nucleus begins at the level of the lower part of the sensory decussation as a few cells in the lateral part of the central gray matter. At the level of the caudal part of the hypoglossal nucleus these vagal cells become more numerous and the nucleus shifts dorsally with the central canal and finally comes to lie beneath the ala cinerea in the floor of the fourth ventricle. Here it has in cross-section the shape of an elongated oval with long axis directed ventrolaterally from the ventricular floor. Its dorsal border lies close to the floor of the fourth ventricle and its ventral border intervenes between the nucleus of the tractus solitarius and the hypoglossal nucleus. In sections through the rostral end of the medulla it leaves the floor of the fourth ventricle and, greatly reduced in size, comes to lie close to the nucleus ambiguus and the nucleus of the tractus solitarius (Figs. 331, 332).

The *nucleus of the tractus solitarius* begins dorsal to the central canal at the level of the lower border of the olive. Here the nuclei of the two sides meet forming Cajal's commissural nucleus (Fig. 317). More rostrally the two nuclei form an inverted V with the apex at the posterior median fissure and then move ventrolaterally and become associated on each side with the tractus solitarius forming the nucleus of this tract (Figs. 331, 388). A few cells infiltrate this tract. At their upper end where the cochlear nucleus begins to appear, the tract and nucleus lie very close to the spinal nucleus of the fifth nerve (Fig. 331). Fibers from the tractus solitarius are distributed to all parts of its nucleus including the commissural portion. The taste fibers of the facial and glosso-pharyngeal nerves end in the rostral portion; only vagal fibers reach the caudal portion of the nucleus. The cells of the nucleus of the tractus solitarius are small, their cytoplasm is scanty and lightly stained, and the Nissl bodies are small and poorly defined. These cells resemble those seen in the nucleus of the spinal fifth tract. In association with this and other vagal nuclei are found a few pigmented cells (nucleus pigmentosus of the medulla oblongata).

The *nuclei salivatorii* cannot be recognized in sections of the normal brain stem and there is good reason to question the work of Kohnstamm (1902, 1903), since according to him these nuclei contain large cells and since all nuclei which are known to give rise to general visceral efferent fibers contain medium sized cells of the type seen in the dorsal motor nucleus of the vagus.

The *hypoglossal nucleus* (Figs. 317–328) represents the rostral continuation of the somatic motor column to which the supraspinal and accessory nuclei also belong. It begins at the level of the lower border of the olive in the ventral part of the central gray substance (Fig. 317) and extends to a point just caudal to the beginning of the cochlear nuclei, lying in the floor of the fourth ventricle close to the midline (Fig. 328). It is smaller at its two ends than in the middle part of its course. Its cells are of the same type as those of other nuclei supplying skeletal muscle, large multipolar cells with abundant lightly staining cytoplasm and large discrete Nissl bodies. Somewhat smaller cells are also present and lie predominantly in the medial part of the nucleus.

The *nucleus intercalatus* lies in the floor of the fourth ventricle between the hypoglossal nucleus and the dorsal motor nucleus of the vagus (Figs. 323–327). Its constituent cells vary in size and appearance. Most of the cells are small, but medium sized cells are found in clumps near its deep surface and in smaller numbers throughout the nucleus. The rostral end of the nucleus intercalatus is not well defined. It passes without sharp line of demarcation into the *nucleus praepositus* which Jacobsohn calls the nucleus of the funiculus teres. This nucleus begins where the hypoglossal ends and extends to a point near the abducens nucleus (Figs. 331–339). The field occupied by the nucleus praepositus is often considered a part of the medial vestibular nucleus and is not marked off from that nucleus in Figs. 162, 330 and 334. The cells vary considerably in size and shape. They are mostly of medium size and stain rather lightly.

The *nucleus paramedianus dorsalis* (Figs. 320–340) is situated on either side of the midline ventral to the central canal and in the floor of the fourth ventricle. At the level of the cochlear nuclei and in the caudal part of the pons it is relatively large (Figs. 331–335) and is commonly known as the nucleus of the eminentia teres (Figs. 162 and 330). More rostrally it decreases in size and disappears at about the level of the facial nucleus. This column is interrupted at places and sometimes it is absent for a short distance on one side and present on the other. The cells are closely packed and of small size. They are rounded or fusiform in shape and are rather deeply stained with small poorly defined Nissl bodies. This nucleus projects to the cerebellum and receives fibers from higher levels of the brain stem and from the spinal cord.

Nuclei of the Formatio Reticularis Grisea. Nerve cells are scattered throughout the reticular formation but in certain regions they are much more numerous than in others. Several such accumulations of reticular cells are recognized. Some of these are located along the course of the root fibers of the hypoglossal nerve (nuclei interfasciculares hypoglossi, Figs. 323, 324). At the level of the caudal border of the cochlear nuclei cells are found forming an arch over the median longitudinal fasciculus and joining the cells along the hypoglossal root with the nucleus of the raphe (Fig. 331). Ventral to the hypoglossal nucleus there is an accumulation of closely packed small cells forming the *nucleus of Roller* (also known as the small-celled hypoglossal nucleus and as the nucleus sublingualis, Figs. 323–327). These cells send their axons into the reticular formation, not into the hypoglossal nerve. Isolated large cells of the motor type are scattered through the reticular formation (nucleus motorius dissipatus formationis reticularis or motor cells of the formatio reticularis, Figs. 327, 328, 336–349). In the rostral part of the medulla there is an accumulation of very large cells situated dorsal to the olive, the magnocellular nucleus of the reticular formation (Figs. 323–335). These giant cells are larger than the cells of the motor nuclei and have smaller, less discrete Nissl bodies.

Nucleus of the Raphe and Formatio Reticularis Alba. Cells are found along the raphe and in lines extending lateralward into the formatio reticularis alba (Figs. 323, 324). A prominent group of these lies behind the pyramids and corresponds to Cajal's postpyramidal nuclei. Another prominent group is seen dorsal to the medial accessory olive at about the middle of the medulla (perpendicular nucleus of formatio reticularis alba, Fig. 324). At the upper end of the medulla cells accumulate in large numbers along the raphe (nucleus of the raphe, Figs. 324–331). At the level of the cochlear nuclei an aggregation of pale cells along the raphe bulges laterally into the reticular formation (nucleus pallidus of the raphe, Figs. 332–336).

The *area postrema* (Fig. 320) is an accumulation of glial cells, pigmented nerve cells, and venous sinusoids along the lateral border of the caudal end of the fourth ventricle extending into and producing a thickening of the lateral margin of the roof of the ventricle. It has been torn away from the section represented in Fig. 323 but is partly responsible for the thickening in the ventricular roof shown in Fig. 324.

NUCLEUS PONTOBULBARIS. Part of the thickening in the roof of the fourth ventricle shown in Fig. 324 is composed of medium sized nerve cells. Similar cells form a band that can be followed laterally and then ventrally and rostrally along the surface of the restiform body (Figs. 324–328). This band of cells lies under the caudal border of the ventral cochlear nucleus (Fig. 331) and joins a much larger accumulation of cells of the same type ventral to the restiform body (Figs. 332–339). The pontobulbar nucleus which, as indicated above, partly encircles the restiform body consists of closely packed medium sized cells similar to those of the pontile nuclei with which it appears to be continuous. The nucleus with its accompanying fibers forms the corpus pontobulbare (Figs. 32 and 159). The part which rests upon the dorsolateral surface of the restiform body has been called by Jacobsohn the nucleus marginalis corpus restiformis. The pontobulbar body may represent an outlying part of the pons.

The *cochlear nuclei* are the nuclei of reception of the cochlear nerve. The ventral cochlear nucleus (Figs. 331–335) lies lateral to the ventral part of the restiform body in close relation to the pontobulbar nucleus; and at a slightly more rostral level it is covered by the cerebellum forming a buried mass of gray matter which in cross-section has a triangular shape (Figs. 336, 339 and right side of Fig. 334). It is composed of closely arranged large round cells with darkly staining cytoplasm and small Nissl granules. The unstained spaces occupied by these cells give the nucleus its characteristic lacy appearance in Weigert preparations (Fig. 162). The dorsal cochlear nucleus rests upon the dorsolateral aspect of the restiform body (Figs. 328–335). Its cells are of an entirely different type than those in the ventral nucleus. They are much smaller and fusiform in shape. They lie among and with their long axes parallel to the bundles of auditory fibers of the second order which curve around the restiform body. Among these are some medium sized polygonal cells which stain less heavily than the cells of the ventral cochlear nucleus.

Vestibular nuclei, four in number, are arranged as shown in Fig. 189. At the point where the vestibular nerve reaches the gray matter beneath the floor of the fourth ventricle many large cells are seen. These constitute the *lateral vestibular nucleus* (Fig. 335). Along the course of the vestibular nerve as it penetrates the brain stem, small groups of similar cells are scattered (Figs. 336, 339). This nucleus extends rostrally to the level of the nucleus of the abducens nerve (Fig. 340). The cells are multipolar and very large. They differ from those found in the motor nuclei in that they are larger, their cytoplasm is more heavily stained, and the Nissl bodies are less sharply defined.

Throughout its extent the descending vestibular root contains a meshwork of gray matter in which are found small and medium sized cells in a loose arrangement. These cells vary greatly in shape and their cytoplasm stains rather deeply. They constitute the *spinal vestibular nucleus* (Figs. 331, 332).

The *medial vestibular nucleus* (Figs. 324–336) lies in the floor of the fourth ventricle, medial to the lateral and spinal vestibular nuclei and lateral to the nucleus praepositus. At lower levels it lies lateral to the nuclei of the vagus nerve. It is composed of small and medium sized cells of various shapes. At its rostral end it becomes reduced in size and is continuous with the superior nucleus.

The *superior vestibular or angular nucleus* lies in the angle between the pons and cerebellum (Figs. 339–346). It is continued rostrally as far as the caudal border of the motor nucleus of the trigeminal nerve. It is composed of cells which resemble those found in the spinal nucleus—small and medium sized cells of various shapes.

NUCLEI OF THE TRAPEZOID BODY. According to Jacobsohn there are two trapezoid nuclei, one directly ventral to the facial nucleus and the other somewhat more lateral (Fig. 336). The cells are small and polygonal and embedded in a dense glial feltwork.

The *superior olivary nucleus* (Figs. 339–352) extends from the level of the facial nucleus to that of the motor nucleus of the trigeminal. It is largest at its caudal end where it lies ventromedial to the facial nucleus. Here it is composed of two groups of cells. Medially there is a very compact group forming a thin flat plate directed dorsoventrally, indicated by a dark line in the figures. This is surrounded by a dense feltwork of glia which gives this mass its oval form. More laterally there is a curved plate of more diffusely arranged cells which partly surrounds the preceding. The cells are of medium size and contain very large sharply defined tigroid masses. In the flat plate of the medial group the cells are fusiform in shape and densely packed together. This characteristic group of cells can be followed rostrally, decreasing in size, to the level of the motor nuclei of the trigeminal nerve.

The *facial nucleus* is situated ventromedial to the nucleus of the spinal tract of the fifth nerve and is found in the most rostral level of the medulla oblongata and in the caudal part of the pons (Figs. 335–343). It is composed of large multipolar cells with lightly staining cytoplasm and large sharply defined Nissl bodies, similar to the cells found in the other nuclei supplying skeletal muscle. Small isolated groups of similar cells are found somewhat farther dorsally (accessory facial, Figs. 339, 340; retrotrigeminal, Fig. 343), and these seem to represent a bridge between the facial and motor trigeminal nuclei. Caudal to the facial nucleus in the medulla is a small group of large cells which differ in size and appearance from those of the nucleus ambiguus, which at this level is deeply situated near the tractus solitarius. This group has been called by Jacobsohn the nucleus retrofacialis (Fig. 331).

The *abducens nucleus* (Fig. 340) helps to form the facial colliculus in the floor of the fourth ventricle. It is a large spherical mass of cells not far from the midline but separated from it by the genu of the facial nerve. It is composed of cells of the type usually found in nuclei supplying skeletal muscle.

The *nuclei of the trigeminal nerve* are shown diagrammatically in Fig. 165.

The *nucleus of the spinal tract* of the fifth nerve has already been described. It can be followed rostrally to the point where the more caudal fibers of the fifth nerve join the spinal fifth tract. Here (Fig. 343) it becomes reduced in size and broken up into small islands which form the transition between the spinal and the main sensory nucleus. Along the dorsomedial border of this transitional zone and extending rostrally in a similar relation to the main sensory nucleus, there is a nuclear column characterized by a dense feltwork of fine myelinated fibers and a paucity of cells which forms, in Weigert sections, a very characteristic feature of this zone of transition (Fig. 342, three light spots dorsomedial to the spinal fifth tract).

At the level where the motor fifth nucleus begins to appear, the sensory column increases in size and becomes more compact and forms on the dorsolateral side of the motor fifth nucleus the *main sensory nucleus of the trigeminal nerve* (Figs. 324–352). It may be questioned whether the cell groups shown by Jacobsohn close to the floor and lateral wall of the fourth ventricle (Fig. 346) actually belong to the trigeminal nerve. The main sensory nucleus is closely packed with small cells.

The *motor nucleus of the trigeminal nerve* forms a well defined oval mass situated on the ventromedial side of the main sensory nucleus (Figs. 346–352). It is composed of large multipolar cells of the skeletal motor type.

The *mesencephalic nucleus of the trigeminal nerve* is composed of large oval or round cells devoid of dendrites with deeply staining cytoplasm and fine, not very discrete Nissl bodies. It begins at the upper border of the motor and main sensory nuclei and is continued rostrally as a very slender, frequently interrupted column close to the lateral angle of the rostral part of the fourth ventricle (Figs. 349–353) and in the lateral part of the central gray surrounding the cerebral aqueduct (Figs. 356–368) to the level of the superior colliculus. It lies dorsal to the nucleus pigmentosus pontis of the locus coeruleus.

The *pontile nuclei* are large accumulations of medium sized rounded or polygonal, deeply staining, finely granular cells which are closely packed together. Near the caudal border of the pons these nuclei form a ring around the pyramid (Fig. 339). More rostrally they are separated into islands by the longitudinal and transverse fibers of the pons (Fig. 356). In Figs. 343–353 only those cells which lie close to the tegmentum are shown.

According to Jacobsohn, nuclear masses continuous with the pontile nuclei project into the tegmental portion of the upper part of the pons. He distinguishes two of these projections on each side, one near the midline and the other extending into the lateral part of the tegmentum. The medial tegmental process (Figs. 346–353) includes what are usually known as the reticular tegmental nucleus, the superior central nucleus, and possibly the ventral tegmental nucleus. Papez (1926) has shown that fibers from the reticular tegmental nucleus and perhaps also from the superior central nucleus run by way of the deep transverse fibers of the pons to the cerebellum. The lateral tegmental process (Figs. 346–353) projects dorsalward into the lateral part of the tegmentum.

TEGMENTAL AND RETICULAR NUCLEI. The *reticulotegmental nucleus* (Figs. 349, 352) resembles the pontile nuclei. It lies near the midline medial and dorsal to the medial lemniscus. Dorsal to it and spreading laterally into the reticular formation is the superior central nucleus (Figs. 349, 352). It is composed of medium sized cells. Ventral to the medial longitudinal fasciculus is a group of cells of medium size which is known as the *ventral tegmental nucleus*. In the caudal part of the mesencephalon there is found within the central gray matter a group of cells upon the dorsal surface of the medial longitudinal fasciculus. This is known as the *dorsal tegmental nucleus* (Fig. 357). The area designated by this name in Figs. 357–363 was labeled supratrochlear nucleus by Jacobsohn. It includes in addition to the dorsal tegmental nucleus other cell groups such as that designated by Marburg as the lateral nucleus of the aqueduct. At the level of the dorsal tegmental nucleus and more caudally in the region of transition between the fourth ventricle and aqueduct a lamina of cells is found within the central gray matter on each side of the midline. This is the *dorsal nucleus of the raphe* (Fig. 356).

At the junction of the pons and mesencephalon the cells of the reticular formation are displaced laterally by the decussation of the brachium conjunctivum, producing at this level a rather dense accumulation of medium sized cells, the *pedunculopontile tegmental nucleus* (Figs. 356, 357). In the mesencephalon small groups of large multipolar cells are found in the tegmentum between the midline and the red nucleus, the *motor tegmentopeduncular nucleus* (Figs. 360, 363).

Nucleus of the Lateral Lemniscus. At about the level of the decussation of the trochlear nerve there is found in the course of the lateral lemniscus a meshwork of gray matter which is known as the *nucleus of the lateral lemniscus* (Fig. 356). Within the strands of this gray mesh are seen medium sized cells, many of which are fusiform in shape.

The *nucleus pigmentosus pontis* consists of polymorphous cells whose cytoplasm contains brown pigment. These cells are too large to be described as medium sized but not as large as some of those of the adjacent mesencephalic nucleus of the fifth nerve. The main mass of these cells forms the pigmented nucleus of the locus coeruleus (Figs. 352–360). It lies at the lateral angle of the rostral part of the fourth ventricle and in the mesencephalon along the lateral border of the medial longitudinal fasciculus. The nucleus decreases in size as it is followed rostrally. Scattered pigmented cells which appear to form extensions of this nucleus are found in the lateral part of the tegmentum of the pons (Figs. 343–349, nucleus pigmentosus tegmentopontilis) and in the cerebellum close to the lateral part of the roof of the fourth ventricle (Figs. 343–349, nucleus pigmentosus tegmentocerebellaris).

The *red nucleus* (Figs. 360–363) consists of two parts. The *magnocellular portion*, not represented in these drawings, is small and rudimentary in man and represented by very large multipolar cells in the brachium conjunctivum at the level where this is penetrated by the most caudal fibers of the third nerve, i.e., just caudal to the level where the red nucleus becomes clearly evident. What is ordinarily known as the red nucleus in the human brain is the *parvocellular portion*, a large cylindrical column of gray matter extending rostrally into the subthalamus. It is composed of medium sized cells. In lower forms, the cat for instance, the magnocellular part constitutes almost the entire red nucleus and the parvocellular portion is difficult to find.

The *substantia nigra* (Figs. 356–363) is a thick plate of gray matter resting upon the deep surface of the basis pedunculi and extending from the rostral border of the pons into the subthalamus. It contains an accumulation of large pigment cells which for the most part do not rest upon the deep surface of the basis pedunculi but form a compact but irregular and broken lamina that is separated from the basis by a thick layer of gray matter which contains scattered nerve cells. The layer of closely packed cells is known as the pars compacta. It is illustrated and labeled in Figs. 356–363 as if it constituted the entire substantia nigra. The scattered cells between the pars compacta and the basis pedunculi constitute the pars reticularis. It is represented by a few dots in Fig. 363 but is not represented at all in the other figures. As a result the basis pedunculi appears too massive. Some cells of the pars reticularis infiltrate the deep surface of the basis pedunculi. Pigmented cells are found not only in the substantia nigra but also scattered through the medial part of the tegmentum (Figs. 360, 363).

The *interpeduncular nucleus* lies in the floor of the interpeduncular fossa at the rostral border of the pons (Figs. 356, 360). It is composed of small pale cells.

In the inferior colliculus of the corpora quadrigemina there is a large gray mass composed of small cells among which there are also a few of medium size. This is the *nucleus of the inferior colliculus* (Figs. 357–360). Within the superior colliculus there are three not very well defined gray laminae composed for the most part of small cells. Scattered through the middle layer and to a much less extent through the other two are some large cells of the motor type. These three layers correspond from within outward to the *stratum lemnisci, stratum opticum, and stratum griseum,* respectively (Fig. 363). Superficial to these three layers and immediately beneath the tangential fibers of the stratum zonale there is a thin layer of small fusiform cells with long axes parallel to the surface of the colliculus.

The *trochlear nucleus* is embedded in the dorsal surface of the medial longitudinal fasciculus at the level of the inferior colliculus (Fig. 360). It is composed of large multipolar cells of the type which supplies skeletal muscle. At its rostral extremity it becomes reduced to two or three cells and then after a few sections becomes continuous with the oculomotor nucleus. The figures in Jacobsohn's monograph do not adequately represent the oculomotor nuclei or the nuclei associated with the rostral end of the medial longitudinal fasciculi.

The *oculomotor nuclei* lie in the trough formed by the medial longitudinal fasciculi. They are illustrated in Fig. 175.

The *nucleus of Darkschewitsch* lies at the edge of the central gray dorsomedial to the red nucleus at the point of transition between the third ventricle and aqueduct (Figs. 374, 377). Between it and the red nucleus lies the interstitial nucleus among the scattered fascicles representing the rostral end of the medial longitudinal fasciculus. The latter nucleus begins at a slightly lower level and extends downward a little farther than the nucleus of Darkschewitsch (Ingram and Ranson, 1935).

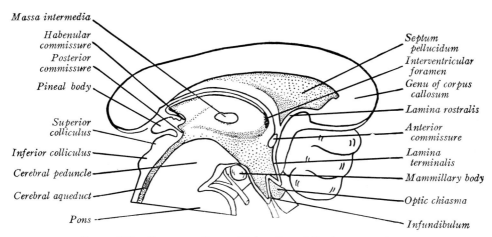

Massa intermedia
Habenular commissure
Posterior commissure
Pineal body
Superior colliculus
Inferior colliculus
Cerebral peduncle
Cerebral aqueduct
Pons

Septum pellucidum
Interventricular foramen
Genu of corpus callosum
Lamina rostralis
Anterior commissure
Lamina terminalis
Mammillary body
Optic chiasma
Infundibulum

FIGURE 303. From a median sagittal section of the human cerebrum.

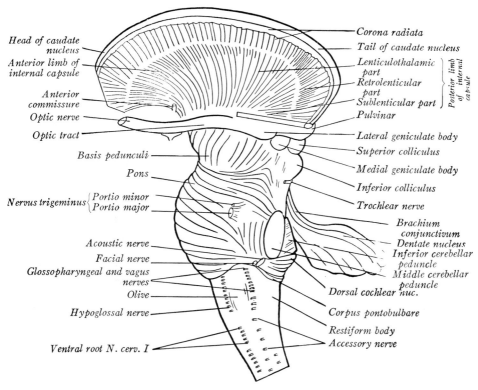

Head of caudate nucleus
Anterior limb of internal capsule
Anterior commissure
Optic nerve
Optic tract
Basis pedunculi
Pons
Nervus trigeminus { Portio minor / Portio major
Acoustic nerve
Facial nerve
Glossopharyngeal and vagus nerves
Olive
Hypoglossal nerve
Ventral root N. cerv. I

Corona radiata
Tail of caudate nucleus
Lenticulothalamic part
Retrolenticular part
Sublenticular part
} Posterior limb of internal capsule
Pulvinar
Lateral geniculate body
Superior colliculus
Medial geniculate body
Inferior colliculus
Trochlear nerve
Brachium conjunctivum
Dentate nucleus
Inferior cerebellar peduncle
Middle cerebellar peduncle
Dorsal cochlear nuc.
Corpus pontobulbare
Restiform body
Accessory nerve

FIGURE 304. Lateral view of human brain stem.

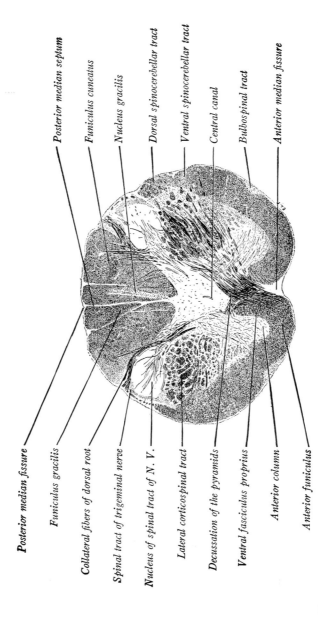

Posterior median septum

Funiculus cuneatus

Nucleus gracilis

Dorsal spinocerebellar tract

Ventral spinocerebellar tract

Central canal

Bulbospinal tract

Anterior median fissure

Posterior median fissure

Funiculus gracilis

Collateral fibers of dorsal root

Spinal tract of trigeminal nerve

Nucleus of spinal tract of N. V.

Lateral corticospinal tract

Decussation of the pyramids

Ventral fasciculus proprius

Anterior column

Anterior funiculus

FIGURE 305.   Section through the region of transition between the spinal cord and medulla oblongata in the plane indicated in Fig. 306.
Magnification 8½.

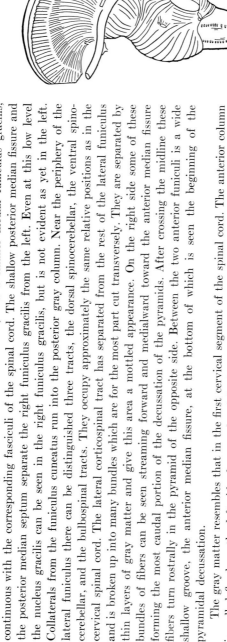

FIGURE 306.

Figure 305 represents a section passing through the line of transition between the spinal cord and medulla oblongata just rostral to the first cervical nerve. The posterior funiculi have the same appearance as in the upper cervical segments of the spinal cord. Each is divided by the posterior intermediate septum into two parts: a larger lateral funiculus cuneatus, and a smaller medial funiculus gracilis, continuous with the corresponding fasciculi of the spinal cord. The shallow posterior median fissure and the posterior median septum separate the right funiculus gracilis from the left. Even at this low level the nucleus gracilis can be seen in the right funiculus gracilis, but is not evident as yet in the left. Collaterals from the funiculus cuneatus run into the posterior gray column. Near the periphery of the lateral funiculus there can be distinguished three tracts, the dorsal spinocerebellar, the ventral spinocerebellar, and the bulbospinal tracts. They occupy approximately the same relative positions as in the cervical spinal cord. The lateral corticospinal tract has separated from the rest of the lateral funiculus and is broken up into many bundles which are for the most part cut transversely. They are separated by thin layers of gray matter and give this area a mottled appearance. On the right side some of these bundles of fibers can be seen streaming forward and medialward toward the anterior median fissure forming the most caudal portion of the decussation of the pyramids. After crossing the midline these fibers turn rostrally in the pyramid of the opposite side. Between the two anterior funiculi is a wide shallow groove, the anterior median fissure, at the bottom of which is seen the beginning of the pyramidal decussation.

The gray matter resembles that in the first cervical segment of the spinal cord. The anterior column is well defined on the left side, but on the right it has been partly cut off from the rest of the gray figure and broken up by bundles of pyramidal fibers. The gray matter surrounding the central canal is more abundant than in the spinal cord. The posterior gray columns are curved lateralward around the lateral corticospinal tracts. Each is capped by the substantia gelatinosa Rolandi which at this level becomes, without changing its appearance, the nucleus of the spinal tract of the trigeminal nerve. Between it and the surface of the cord is a lightly staining band of fibers designated as the spinal tract of the trigeminal nerve. At this level it is a mixed bundle composed of descending sensory fibers from the trigeminal nerve and ascending fibers from the tract of Lissauer. On the dorsomedial aspect of the posterior gray column is a prominent bundle of collaterals from the dorsal root of the first cervical nerve.

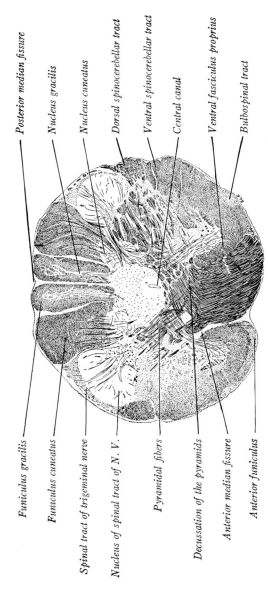

Posterior median fissure

Nucleus gracilis

Nucleus cuneatus

Dorsal spinocerebellar tract

Ventral spinocerebellar tract

Central canal

Ventral fasciculus proprius

Bulbospinal tract

Funiculus gracilis

Funiculus cuneatus

Spinal tract of trigeminal nerve

Nucleus of spinal tract of N. V.

Pyramidal fibers

Decussation of the pyramids

Anterior median fissure

Anterior funiculus

FIGURE 307. Section through the caudal end of the medulla oblongata in the plane indicated in Fig. 309. Magnification 8½.

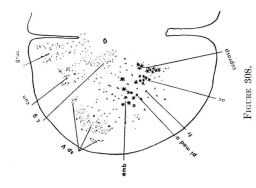

Figure 308.

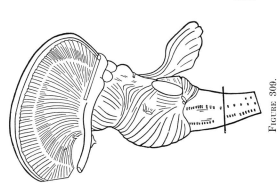

Figure 309.

In figure 307 the gracile and cuneate funiculi are more definitely separated from each other by a wider posterior intermediate septum. The nucleus gracilis is present bilaterally in this section and has become larger than in the preceding one. The cuneate nucleus is beginning to appear on the right side as a wedge-like invasion of the funiculus from the posterior gray matter, but there is only a suggestion of one on the left. Numerous fibers can still be seen coursing into the gray matter from the posterior funiculi. The lateral funiculi are little changed from the preceding level, except that the lateral corticospinal tracts have largely disappeared. The dorsal and ventral spinocerebellar tracts and the bulbospinal tract have retained the relative positions occupied in the preceding level and are still clearly delineated. At this level nearly all of the bundles of longitudinally coursing fibers making up the lateral corticospinal tract at the lower levels have changed their direction ventrorostrally to take part in the motor decussation. This motor or pyramidal decussation is very prominent, occupying the whole median ventral field. The fibers coursing ventralward across the midline from the left side are more prominent in this section, but some from the right side may be seen crossing over toward the left. The accumulation of these fibers on the ventral side of the medulla causes a displacement of the central canal dorsalward. The ventral fasciculus proprius stands out distinctly ventral to the anterior gray columns on both sides. The gray matter ventral to the central canal has been almost completely displaced by pyramidal fibers, but dorsal to the central canal there is an increase in the amount of gray substance. With the exception of this central gray substance and the tips of the four horns, the gray matter has been broken up by bundles of nerve fibers. The posterior gray columns are becoming indistinct except in the region of the nucleus of the spinal tract of the trigeminal nerve. This tract occupies the same relative position dorsolateral to its nucleus that it had at the lower level.

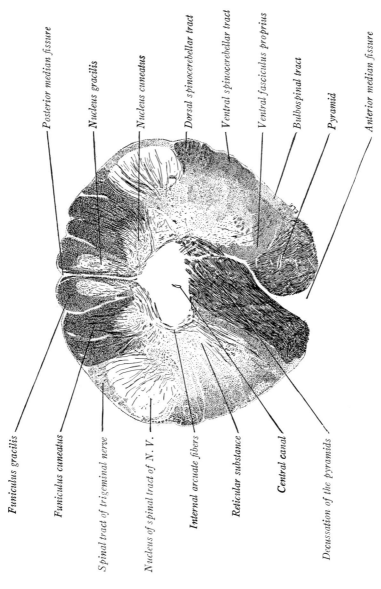

FIGURE 310. Section through the medulla oblongata near its caudal end in the plane indicated in Fig. 312. Magnification 8½.

Posterior median fissure

Nucleus gracilis

Nucleus cuneatus

Dorsal spinocerebellar tract

Ventral spinocerebellar tract

Ventral fasciculus proprius

Bulbospinal tract

Pyramid

Anterior median fissure

Funiculus gracilis

Funiculus cuneatus

Spinal tract of trigeminal nerve

Nucleus of spinal tract of N. V.

Internal arcuate fibers

Reticular substance

Central canal

Decussation of the pyramids

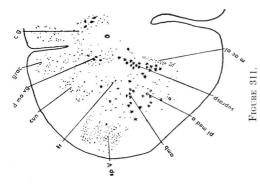

FIGURE 311.

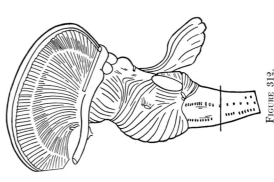

FIGURE 312.

In figure 310 the gracile and cuneate nuclei are prominent and cause enlargements of the corresponding funiculi which appear as elevations, the clava and tuberculum cuneatum, on the surface of the brain stem. As succeeding sections in a rostral direction will show, the fibers of the funiculus gracilis and cuneatus decrease in number with the increase in size of the corresponding nuclei, for these funiculi are made up of the long ascending branches of the sensory fibers of the dorsal roots which end in the nuclei. The cells of the cuneate and gracile nuclei then give rise to secondary fibers, here known as internal arcuate fibers, a few of which can be seen sweeping ventrally around the central gray matter toward the midline. The peripheral portion of the lateral area remains much the same. The lateral corticospinal tract has disappeared from this area and its place is taken by gray matter through which course many interlacing fibers. This is known as the reticular substance. The pyramid has a rounded outline on the right and a large bundle of crossing pyramidal fibers appears on the left. The ventral fasciculus proprius still lies close to the pyramid, and, on the left side, forms a flat band one edge of which almost reaches the central gray matter. It contains fibers of the medial longitudinal fasciculus and tectospinal tracts. The ⊢ shape of the gray matter characteristic of the cord is now entirely lost and both the anterior and posterior horns have disappeared, except that the apex of the posterior horn or substantia gelatinosa Rolandi is still recognizable in the form of the nucleus of the spinal tract of the trigeminal nerve. The remainder of the posterior horn and the anterior horn are represented by the reticular substance. The central gray matter has increased in extent and dorsal to it are the large gracile and cuneate nuclei. The spinal tract of the trigeminal nerve occupies a position at the periphery between the cuneate funiculus and the dorsal spinocerebellar tract.

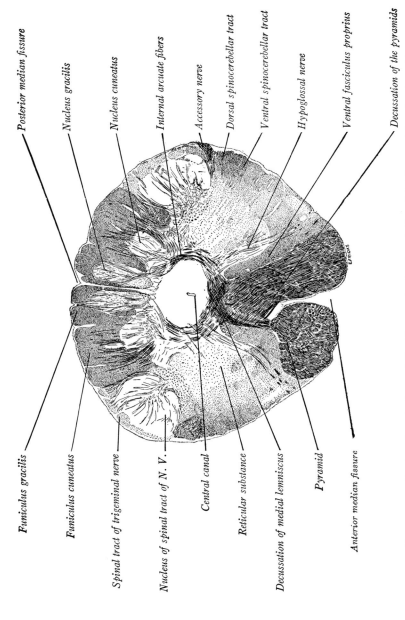

Posterior median fissure

Nucleus gracilis

Nucleus cuneatus

Internal arcuate fibers

Accessory nerve

Dorsal spinocerebellar tract

Ventral spinocerebellar tract

Hypoglossal nerve

Ventral fasciculus proprius

Decussation of the pyramids

Funiculus gracilis

Funiculus cuneatus

Spinal tract of trigeminal nerve

Nucleus of spinal tract of N. V.

Central canal

Reticular substance

Decussation of medial lemniscus

Pyramid

Anterior median fissure

FIGURE 313. Section through the medulla oblongata in the plane indicated in Fig. 315. Magnification 8½.

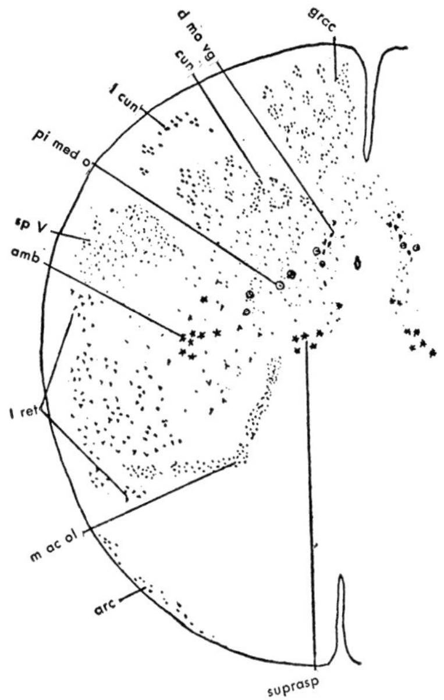

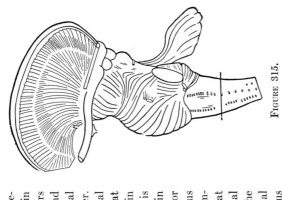

FIGURE 315.

FIGURE 314.

Figure 313 lies at the caudal end of the decussation of the medial lemniscus and the rostral end of the decussation of the pyramids. The number of fibers in the posterior funiculi decreases as the size of the nuclei increases. Arising from cells in the gracile and cuneate nuclei are the internal arcuate fibers which can be seen sweeping around the central gray matter and crossing in the midline to form the decussation of the medial lemniscus immediately ventral to the central gray matter. After these fibers cross they turn rostrally and form the medial lemniscus. The bundle of pyramidal fibers that is crossing at this level runs into the right instead of the left pyramid as in the preceding section. This will be understood when it is remembered that the pyramidal fibers cross the midline in large bundles and that these bundles interdigitate in the floor of the anterior median fissure (Fig. 272). The ventral fasciculus proprius continues to apply itself closely to the crossing pyramidal fibers on the right side and has been displaced somewhat dorsally by the fully formed pyramid on the left. The dorsal part of the fasciculus proprius near the decussation of the medial lemniscus contains the tectospinal tract and the medial longitudinal fasciculus. Just lateral to the fasciculus proprius the lowest fibers of the hypoglossal nerve are seen coursing ventrolaterally to make their exit from the medulla along the

lateral side of the pyramid. The peripheral portion of the lateral area is beginning to show a decrease in density because the reticular substance is encroaching upon it. The dorsal and ventral spinocerebellar tracts are still prominent just ventral to the spinal tract and nucleus of the trigeminal nerve, which appear much the same as in preceding sections. On the right side, one of the bulbar rootlets of the accessory nerve is seen leaving the medulla between the dorsal spinocerebellar tract and spinal tract of the trigeminal nerve.

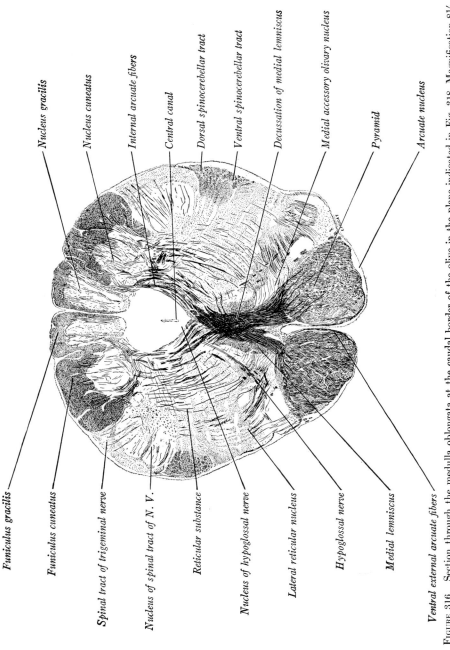

FIGURE 316. Section through the medulla oblongata at the caudal border of the olive in the plane indicated in Fig. 318. Magnification 8½.

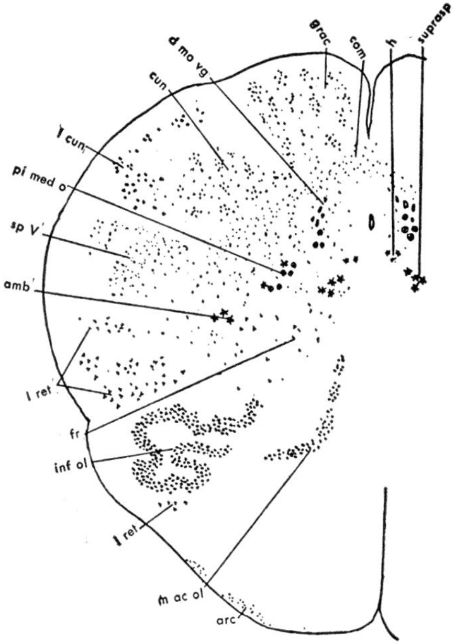

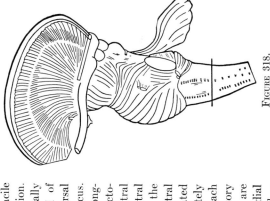

Figure 318.

Figure 317.

Figure 316 represents a section at the level of the decussation of the medial lemniscus. Numerous internal arcuate fibers emerge from the cuneate and gracile nuclei and cross the midline in the sensory decussation. Those that crossed at lower levels have turned rostrally and can be seen in cross-section forming a band of fibers situated on each side of the midline and dorsal to the pyramids. This is labeled the medial lemniscus. In the dorsal part of this same band are fibers belonging to the medial longitudinal fasciculus and the tectospinal tract. These are continued from the central fasciculus proprius of the preceding section. Ventral external arcuate fibers are seen coursing along the medial surfaces of the pyramids to reach the ventral surface of the medulla. The arcuate nuclei are situated upon the ventral aspects of the pyramids. Immediately adjacent and lateral to the medial lemniscus on each side are the lowest portions of the medial accessory olivary nuclei. Fibers of the hypoglossal nerve are seen coursing ventrally on the lateral side of the medial lemnisci and pyramids. In the central gray matter below the central canal and on each side of the midline is located a flattened nuclear mass applied closely to the curve formed by the internal arcuate fibers. This is the lowermost tip of the hypoglossal nucleus. The central gray matter is displaced further backward by the decussation of the medial lemniscus in front of it. The reticular substance has increased and extended further toward the periphery. It contains nerve cells scattered through it, and in its lateral part is an aggregation of cells known as the lateral reticular nucleus. The dorsal and ventral spinocerebellar tracts are still quite distinct in the same position as previously just ventral to the spinal tract of the trigeminal nerve. The nucleus of the spinal tract of the trigeminal nerve appears about the same as in the more caudal sections, but the tract is larger because at the more rostral level fewer of the descending fibers of which it is composed have terminated in the nucleus.

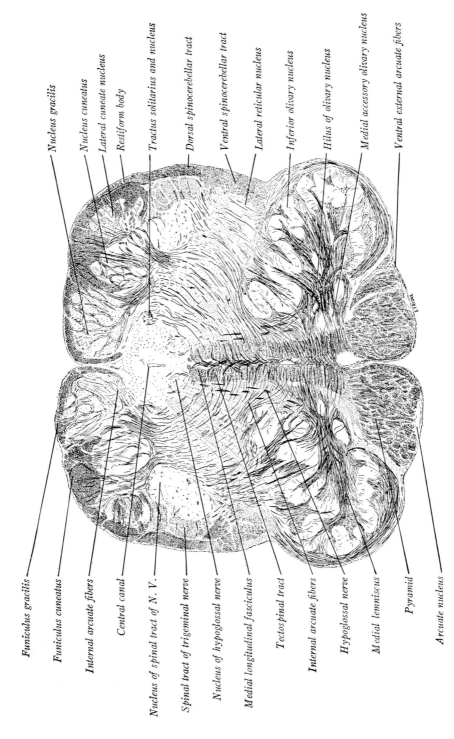

Nucleus gracilis

Nucleus cuneatus

Lateral cuneate nucleus

Restiform body

Tractus solitarius and nucleus

Dorsal spinocerebellar tract

Ventral spinocerebellar tract

Lateral reticular nucleus

Inferior olivary nucleus

Hilus of olivary nucleus

Medial accessory olivary nucleus

Ventral external arcuate fibers

Funiculus gracilis

Funiculus cuneatus

Internal arcuate fibers

Central canal

Nucleus of spinal tract of N. V.

Spinal tract of trigeminal nerve

Nucleus of hypoglossal nerve

Medial longitudinal fasciculus

Tectospinal tract

Internal arcuate fibers

Hypoglossal nerve

Medial lemniscus

Pyramid

Arcuate nucleus

FIGURE 319.   Section through the medulla oblongata near the caudal end of the olive in the plane indicated in Fig. 321. Magnification 8½.

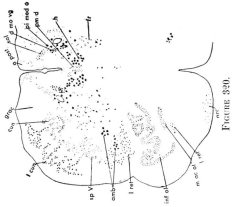

Figure 320.

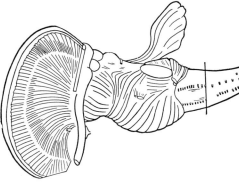

Figure 321.

Figure 319.   At this level the nucleus gracilis and nucleus cuneatus have attained their maximum extent and only a small number of the fibers from their respective funiculi are still coursing longitudinally. A few internal arcuate fibers can be seen leaving the gracile and cuneate nuclei and making their way in broad curves toward the median raphe to cross and turn rostrally in the medial lemniscus. The inferior cerebellar peduncle is just beginning to make its appearance at this level. It lies peripheral to the spinal tract of the trigeminal nerve and to the lateral part of the cuneate funiculus, within which is seen the lateral cuneate nucleus. The dorsal spinocerebellar tract has moved dorsally so that it occupies a position superficial to the spinal tract of the trigeminal nerve. The ventral spinocerebellar tract still occupies a superficial position ventral to the dorsal spinocerebellar tract. The spinal tract and nucleus of the trigeminal nerve lie ventral to the lateral part of the cuneate funiculus and are separated from the surface by the dorsal spinocerebellar tract which has displaced them medialward. The lateral reticular nucleus is an aggregation of cells in the reticular formation medial to the ventral spinocerebellar tract and dorsal to the inferior olivary nucleus. It appears as a broad irregularly folded band of gray matter having the general shape of a U, with the open part directed medially. This opening is called the "hilus," and through it stream the olivocerebellar fibers which arise from cells of the olivary nucleus. The arcuate nuclei are represented by a clear crescentic area ventral to each pyramid. A few fine fibers, the ventral external arcuate fibers from the raphe and arcuate nuclei, can be seen passing around the periphery of the pyramids and olives. The medial lemniscus is now well developed and can be seen as a flattened band of fibers on each side of the median raphe extending dorsally from the pyramids to the central gray matter. The dorsal third of this band contains the fibers of the tectospinal tract and the medial longitudinal fasciculus, the latter being the more dorsally located. The gray matter surrounding the central canal contains two prominent structures, the caudal part of the tractus solitarius and the nucleus of the hypoglossal nerve. The tractus solitarius, which is made up of the sensory components of the facial, glossopharyngeal, and vagus nerves, is located in the lateral part of the central gray matter ventral to the nucleus gracilis. Fibers of the hypoglossal nerve leave its nucleus and pass ventrally between the medial lemniscus and the olivary nucleus toward the lateral border of the pyramid.

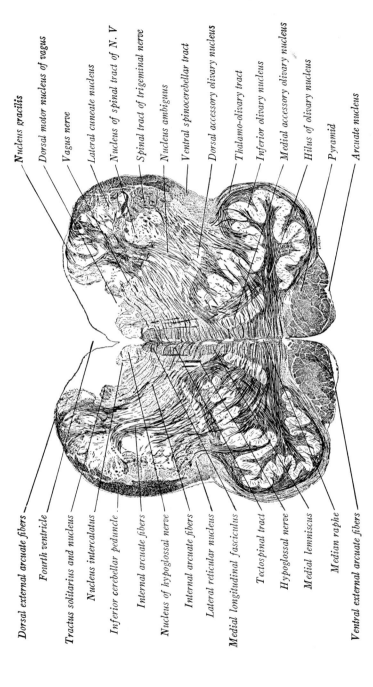

FIGURE 322. Section through the medulla oblongata at the level of the middle of the olive in the plane indicated in Fig. 325. Magnification 6½.

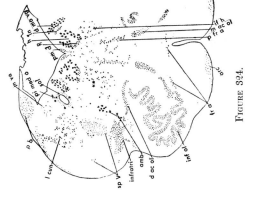

FIGURE 324.

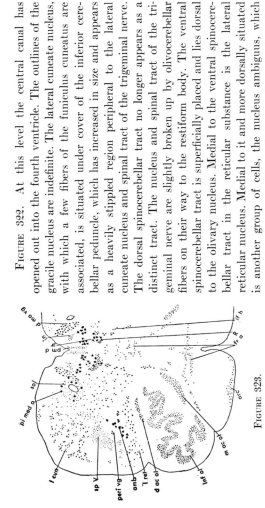

FIGURE 323.

FIGURE 322. At this level the central canal has opened out into the fourth ventricle. The outlines of the gracile nucleus are indefinite. The lateral cuneate nucleus, with which a few fibers of the funiculus cuneatus are associated, is situated under cover of the inferior cerebellar peduncle, which has increased in size and appears as a heavily stippled region peripheral to the lateral cuneate nucleus and spinal tract of the trigeminal nerve. The dorsal spinocerebellar tract no longer appears as a distinct tract. The nucleus and spinal tract of the trigeminal nerve are slightly broken up by olivocerebellar fibers on their way to the restiform body. The ventral spinocerebellar tract is superficially placed and lies dorsal to the olivary nucleus. Medial to the ventral spinocerebellar tract in the reticular substance is the lateral reticular nucleus. Medial to it and more dorsally situated is another group of cells, the nucleus ambiguus, which gives rise to motor fibers that run through the glossopharyngeal, vagus, and spinal accessory nerves. Dorsal to the inferior olivary nucleus is an elongated field of gray matter, the dorsal accessory olivary nucleus. The medial accessory olivary nucleus appears between the hilus of the inferior olivary nucleus and the medial lemniscus. The arcuate nuclei occupy small crescentic areas in the ventral part of the pyramids. The medial lemniscus, tectospinal tract, and medial longitudinal fasciculus occupy the same relative positions as in the preceding section. The hypoglossal nucleus is very prominent near the midline and is capped on its lateral aspect by the nucleus intercalatus. Fibers of the hypoglossal nerve run ventrally lateral to the medial lemniscus. The dorsal motor nucleus of the vagus occupies the region, in which no detail appears in this illustration, between the tractus solitarius laterally and the intercalate and hypoglossal nuclei medially. On the right side a few fibers of the vagus nerve run ventrolaterally from the nucleus, passing just beneath the tractus solitarius. The tractus solitarius is easily recognized close to the gray matter forming the floor of the fourth ventricle. It is surrounded by its nucleus.

FIGURE 325.

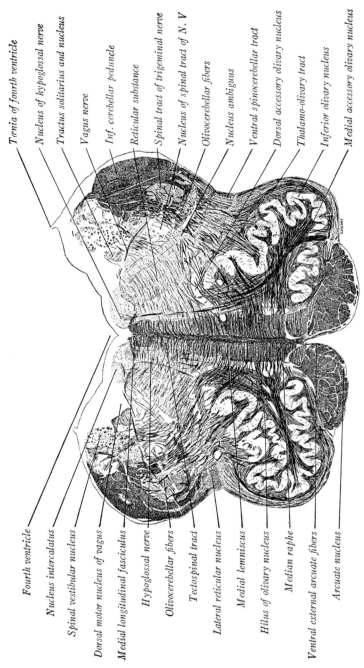

Tænia of fourth ventricle
Nucleus of hypoglossal nerve
Tractus solitarius and nucleus
Vagus nerve
Inf. cerebellar peduncle
Reticular substance
Spinal tract of trigeminal nerve
Nucleus of spinal tract of N. V
Olivocerebellar fibers
Nucleus ambiguus
Ventral spinocerebellar tract
Dorsal accessory olivary nucleus
Thalamo-olivary tract
Inferior olivary nucleus
Medial accessory olivary nucleus

Fourth ventricle
Nucleus intercalatus
Spinal vestibular nucleus
Dorsal motor nucleus of vagus
Medial longitudinal fasciculus
Hypoglossal nerve
Olivocerebellar fibers
Tectospinal tract
Lateral reticular nucleus
Medial lemniscus
Hilus of olivary nucleus
Median raphe
Ventral external arcuate fibers
Arcuate nucleus

Fɪɢᴜʀᴇ 326. Section through the medulla oblongata near the rostral end of the olive in the plane indicated in Fig. 329. Magnification 6½.

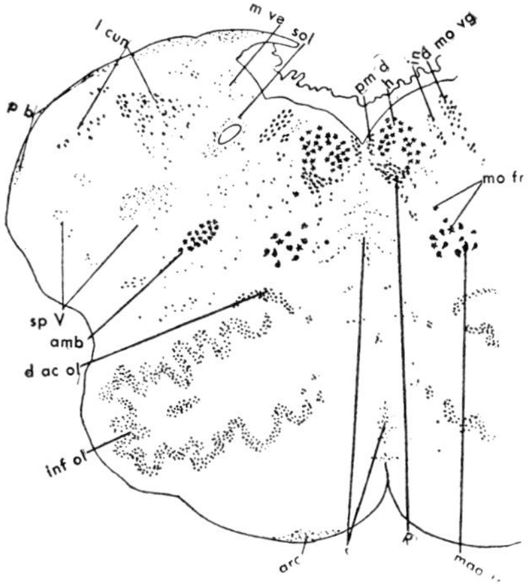

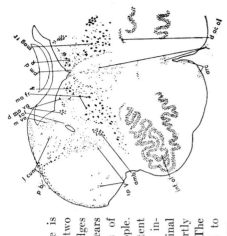

FIGURE 328.

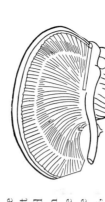

FIGURE 329.

FIGURE 326. The floor of the fourth ventricle is widened somewhat and its limits are shown by two small projections, the taenia, which are the torn edges of the thin roof. The spinal vestibular nucleus appears as a rounded light area with conspicuous bundles of fibers cut transversely and represented in coarse stipple. The inferior cerebellar peduncle has increased in extent and the dorsal spinocerebellar tract is completely incorporated within it. The spinal tract of the trigeminal nerve has been separated from its nucleus and partly broken up by heavy strands of olivocerebellar fibers. The nucleus ambiguus occupies the region ventromedial to the nucleus of the spinal tract of the trigeminal nerve. Likewise the lateral reticular nucleus is obscured by the network of fibers, but lies in the lateral part of the reticular substance. The ventral spinocerebellar tract remains at the periphery between the restiform body and the olive. Ventral external arcuate fibers can be seen

FIGURE 327.

running from the raphe around the medial borders of the pyramids. These continue around the periphery of the olive toward the restiform body. In close relation to these fibers are the arcuate nuclei which are located upon the ventral surface of the pyramids. The medial lemniscus, tectospinal tract, and medial longitudinal fasciculus form a broad band of transversely cut fibers on each side of the raphe. The medial longitudinal fasciculus is very prominent as a closely stippled region in the dorsal part of this band. The hypoglossal nucleus has attained its maximum extent at this level and together with the nucleus intercalatus, represented as a finely stippled ovoid area lateral to the hypoglossal nucleus, forms the elevation in the floor of the fourth ventricle on each side of the midline known as the trigonum hypoglossi. The dorsal motor nucleus of the vagus occupies the region in the gray matter of the floor of the fourth ventricle just lateral to the nucleus intercalatus. A few fibers of the vagus nerve are seen running ventrolaterally from the tractus solitarius which lies lateral to the dorsal motor nucleus of the vagus.

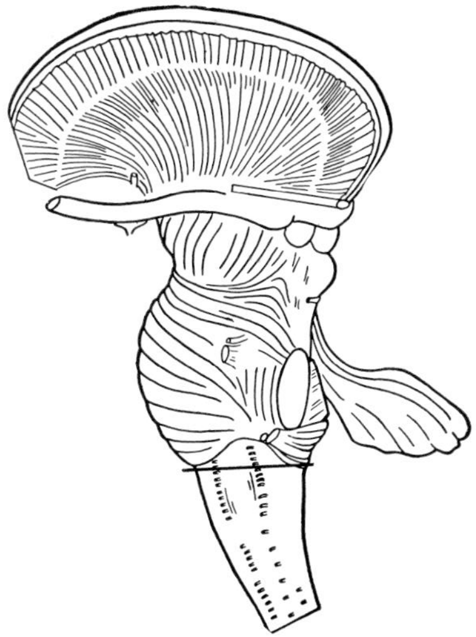

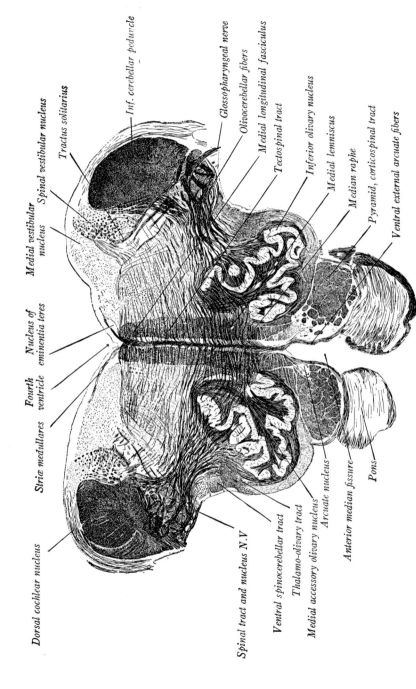

FIGURE 330. Section through the rostral end of the medulla oblongata and the caudal border of the pons in the plane indicated in Fig. 333. Magnification 6½.

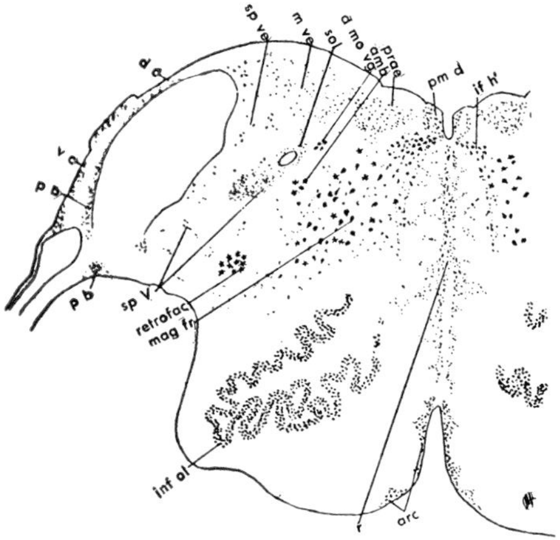

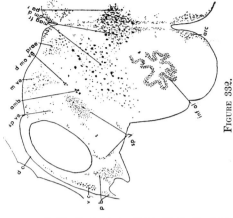

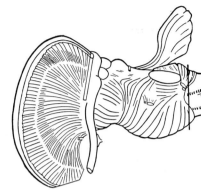

FIGURE 332.

FIGURE 333.

FIGURE 331.

FIGURE 330. At this level the floor of the fourth ventricle extends as far lateralward as the dorsal cochlear nucleus. The hypoglossal nucleus and nucleus intercalatus have been replaced at this level by a small group of cells on each side of the midline called the nucleus of the eminentia teres. A large lightly stippled area lateral to the nucleus of the eminentia teres represents the medial vestibular nucleus. Lateral to this is the spinal vestibular nucleus containing many small bundles of fibers cut transversely. These are the descending branches of the fibers of the vestibular nerve. The inferior cerebellar peduncle in the dorsolateral part of the section is large and definitely delineated. Upon its surface is seen the dorsal cochlear nucleus which has been cut near its caudal border. The spinal tract and nucleus of the trigeminal nerve have been broken up by olivocerebellar fibers. The glossopharyngeal nerve can be seen

entering the brain stem ventral to the restiform body and some of its fibers can be traced to the upper end of the tractus solitarius. The ventral spinocerebellar tract is located at the periphery dorsal to the inferior olive. The thalamo-olivary tract lies between the ventral spinocerebellar tract and the inferior olivary nucleus. It is composed of descending fibers which terminate in this nucleus. From the inferior olivary nuclei coarse bundles of olivocerebellar fibers run into the restiform body breaking up the spinal tract of the trigeminal nerve and separating it from its nucleus. The medial lemniscus, tectospinal tract, and medial longitudinal fasciculus are still represented by a long plate of fibers on each side of the raphe. Ventral external arcuate fibers are seen emerging from the raphe and coursing around the arcuate nuclei and the pyramids. The anterior median fissure is very wide at this point and the depression which it forms when covered by the caudal border of the pons is called the foramen cecum.

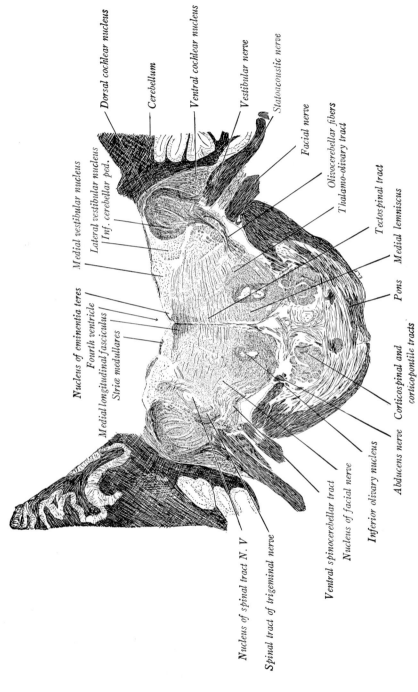

FIGURE 334. Section through the region of transition between the medulla and pons in the plane indicated in Fig. 337. Magnification 3¾.

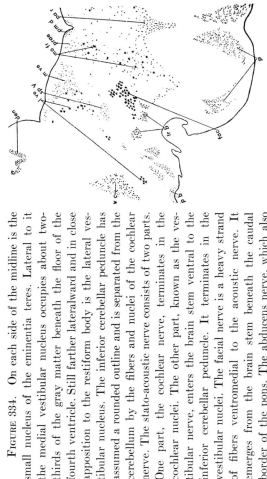

FIGURE 334.

FIGURE 336.

FIGURE 335.

FIGURE 337.

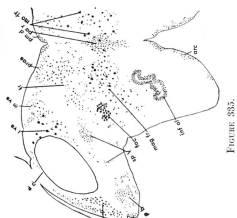

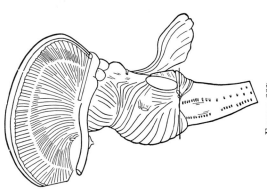

FIGURE 334. On each side of the midline is the small nucleus of the eminentia teres. Lateral to it the medial vestibular nucleus occupies about two-thirds of the gray matter beneath the floor of the fourth ventricle. Still farther lateralward and in close apposition to the restiform body is the lateral vestibular nucleus. The inferior cerebellar peduncle has assumed a rounded outline and is separated from the cerebellum by the fibers and nuclei of the cochlear nerve. The stato-acoustic nerve consists of two parts. One part, the cochlear nerve, terminates in the cochlear nuclei. The other part, known as the vestibular nerve, enters the brain stem ventral to the inferior cerebellar peduncle. It terminates in the vestibular nuclei. The facial nerve is a heavy strand of fibers ventromedial to the acoustic nerve. It emerges from the brain stem beneath the caudal border of the pons. The abducens nerve, which also has its superficial origin in the groove between the pons and the medulla, can be seen on the left. The ventral spinocerebellar tract maintains the same rela-tive position ventral to the spinal tract of the trigeminal nerve. The thalamo-olivary tract can be readily distinguished in the ventral part of the reticular substance dorsolateral to the rostral tip of the inferior olivary nucleus. The pyramids at this level have become embedded in the pons and the corticospinal fibers become intermingled with corticopontile fibers. The transverse fibers of the pons form a conspicuous band. The medial lemniscus is undergoing a change in shape, flattening dorsoventrally and spreading out laterally on the ventral side of the rostral tip of the inferior olivary nucleus. The tectospinal tract and the medial longitudinal fasciculus retain their positions near the midline. The medial longitudinal fasciculus stands out prominently, while the tectospinal fibers are not so compactly arranged.

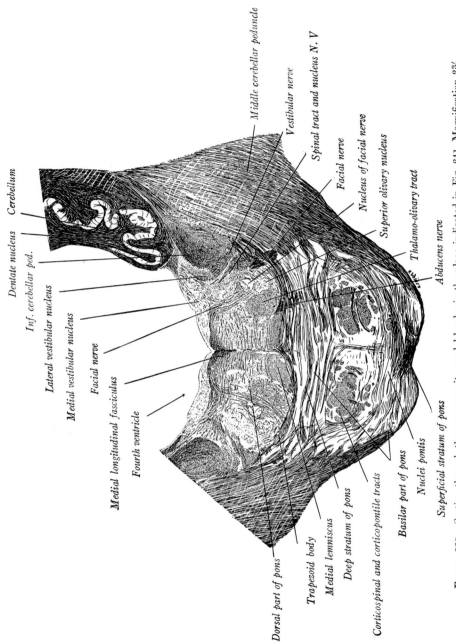

FIGURE 338. Section through the pons near its caudal border in the plane indicated in Fig. 341. Magnification 3¾.

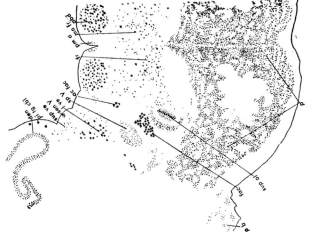

Figure 340.

Figure 339.

Figure 338 represents a section passing through the pons at the level of the nucleus of the facial nerve. The ventral or basilar part of the pons consists of transverse and longitudinal fiber separated by irregular masses of gray matter, the nuclei pontis. The longitudinal fibers belong to the corticospinal, corticonuclear, and corticopontile tracts. The dorsal or tegmental portion of the pons contains other tracts which are continued upward from the medulla oblongata. It includes the trapezoid body and everything between this and the fourth ventricle. The gray matter in the floor of the fourth ventricle contains the medial and lateral vestibular nuclei. The vestibular nerve can be seen along the ventromedial aspect of the inferior cerebellar peduncle. The spinal tract and nucleus of the trigeminal nerve are not so conspicuous as they were at lower levels, but can be distinguished. The nucleus of the facial nerve is a small, rounded area of gray matter situated in the ventrolateral part of the tegmental portion of the pons. Fibers which take origin in this nucleus can be seen passing dorsalward toward the floor of the fourth ventricle where at a higher level they form the genu of the facial nerve (see Fig. 177) and again pass ventralward. In this second part of their course they form a large and well defined bundle of fibers which can be seen in this section occupying a position ventromedial to the spinal tract of the trigeminal nerve. The rounded mass of gray matter ventral to the facial nucleus is the caudal end of the superior olivary nucleus. The thalamo-olivary tract is prominent just medial to the facial and olivary nuclei. The medial lemniscus is now a flattened band of fibers with its greatest dimension in a transverse direction. The medial longitudinal fasciculus has assumed a triangular shape and lies near the floor of the fourth ventricle close to the midline. The tectospinal tract lies ventral to it.

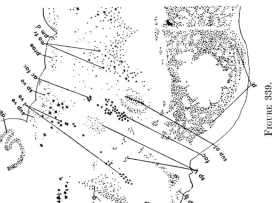

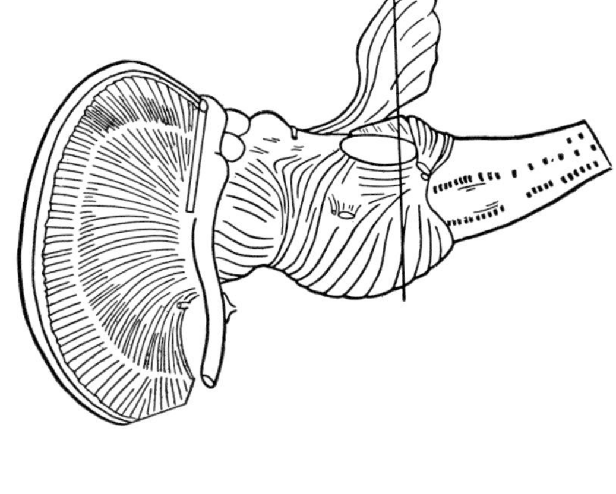

Figure 341.

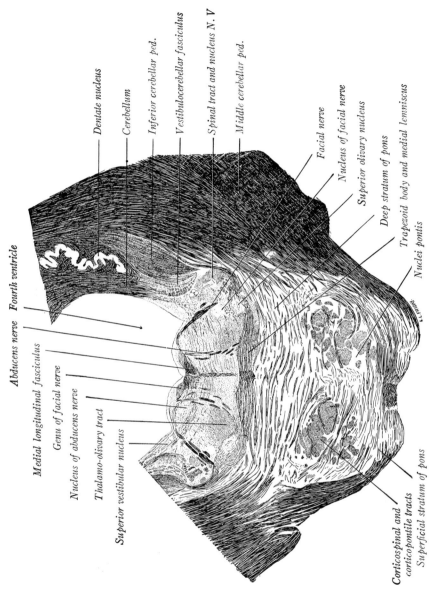

FIGURE 342. Section through the pons at the level of the facial colliculus in the plane indicated in Fig. 344. Magnification 3¾.

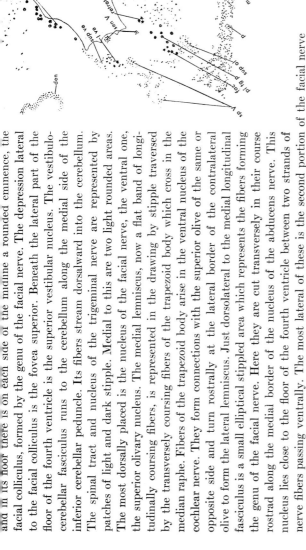

Figure 343.

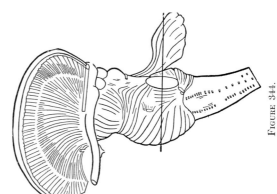

Figure 344.

and in its floor there is on each side of the midline a rounded eminence, the facial colliculus, formed by the genu of the facial nerve. The depression lateral to the facial colliculus is the fovea superior. Beneath the lateral part of the floor of the fourth ventricle is the superior vestibular nucleus. The vestibulo-cerebellar fasciculus runs to the cerebellum along the medial side of the inferior cerebellar peduncle. Its fibers stream dorsalward into the cerebellum. The spinal tract and nucleus of the trigeminal nerve are represented by patches of light and dark stipple. Medial to this are two light rounded areas. The most dorsally placed is the nucleus of the facial nerve, the ventral one, the superior olivary nucleus. The medial lemniscus, now a flat band of longitudinally coursing fibers, is represented in the drawing by stipple traversed by the transversely coursing fibers of the trapezoid body which cross in the median raphe. Fibers of the trapezoid body arise in the ventral nucleus of the cochlear nerve. They form connections with the superior olive of the same or opposite side and turn rostrally at the lateral border of the contralateral olive to form the lateral lemniscus. Just dorsolateral to the medial longitudinal fasciculus is a small elliptical stippled area which represents the fibers forming the genu of the facial nerve. Here they are cut transversely in their course rostrad along the medial border of the nucleus of the abducens nerve. This nucleus lies close to the floor of the fourth ventricle between two strands of nerve fibers passing ventrally. The most lateral of these is the second portion of the facial nerve passing ventrally, laterally, and caudally to make its exit from the brain stem. The more medial strand of fibers comes from the abducens nucleus and forms the abducens nerve. In the pontile nuclei the corticopontile fibers end and the transverse fibers take their origin. It is evident from the section that these transverse fibers are continued into and form the middle cerebellar peduncle.

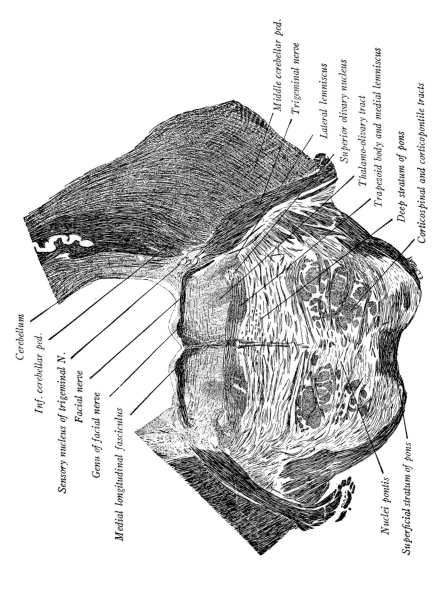

FIGURE 345.   Section through the pons at the level of the trigeminal nerve in the plane indicated in Fig. 347. Magnification 3¾.

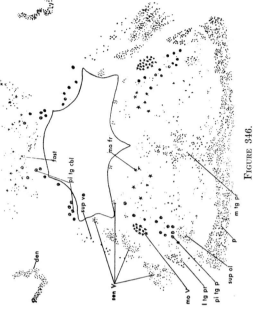

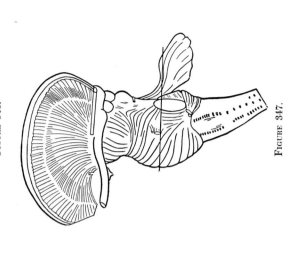

Figure 346.

Figure 347.

Figure 345 represents a section passing through the pons at the level of the trigeminal nerve. The facial colliculi are evident as elevations in the floor of the fourth ventricle. A lightly stippled area, the sensory nucleus of the trigeminal nerve, is a continuation of the column of gray matter which in the spinal cord was designated as the substantia gelatinosa Rolandi, and in the medulla was the nucleus of the spinal tract of the trigeminal nerve. Here it is cut at the point of transition between the spinal and main sensory nuclei. The trigeminal nerve can be seen cutting diagonally across the pons. Descending fibers from this nerve form the spinal tract of the fifth nerve which could be seen in all of the preceding sections. Medial to the nerve in the most ventral part of the reticular substance is the lateral lemniscus. It represents the continuation of the trapezoid body whose fibers turn rostrad along the lateral border of the superior olive. The superior olive, medial lemniscus, and trapezoid body appear very much as they did in the preceding section. Near the center of the tegmental portion of the pons is the thalamo-olivary tract. Beneath the facial colliculus is seen the rostral part of the genu of the facial nerve at the point where the fibers are beginning to turn lateralward. Fibers from the ascending part of the genu run lateralward beneath the floor of the fourth ventricle and then turn ventrally not far from the trigeminal nerve (see Fig. 177).

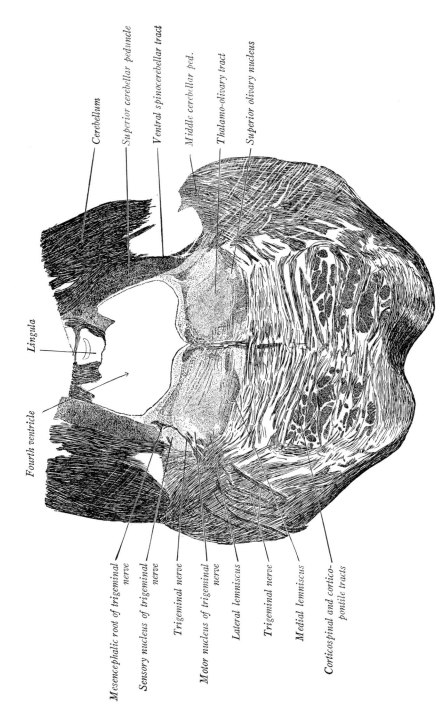

Cerebellum

Superior cerebellar peduncle

Ventral spinocerebellar tract

Middle cerebellar pd.

Thalamo-olivary tract

Superior olivary nucleus

Lingula

Fourth ventricle

Mesencephalic root of trigeminal nerve

Sensory nucleus of trigeminal nerve

Trigeminal nerve

Motor nucleus of trigeminal nerve

Lateral lemniscus

Trigeminal nerve

Medial lemniscus

Corticospinal and cortico-pontile tracts

FIGURE 348. Section through the pons at the level of the motor and main sensory nuclei of the trigeminal nerve in the plane indicated in Fig. 350. Magnification 3¾.

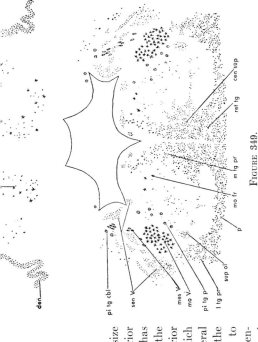

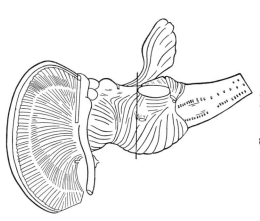

Figure 349.

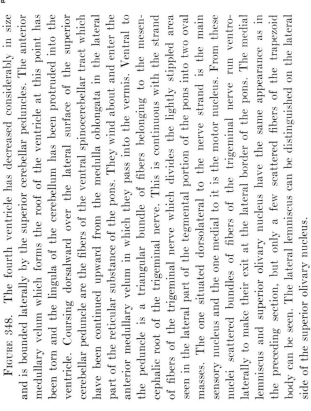

Figure 350.

Figure 348. The fourth ventricle has decreased considerably in size and is bounded laterally by the superior cerebellar peduncles. The anterior medullary velum which forms the roof of the ventricle at this point has been torn and the lingula of the cerebellum has been protruded into the ventricle. Coursing dorsalward over the lateral surface of the superior cerebellar peduncle are the fibers of the ventral spinocerebellar tract which have been continued upward from the medulla oblongata in the lateral part of the reticular substance of the pons. They wind about and enter the anterior medullary velum in which they pass into the vermis. Ventral to the peduncle is a triangular bundle of fibers belonging to the mesencephalic root of the trigeminal nerve. This is continuous with the strand of fibers of the trigeminal nerve which divides the lightly stippled area seen in the lateral part of the tegmental portion of the pons into two oval masses. The one situated dorsolateral to the nerve strand is the main sensory nucleus and the one medial to it is the motor nucleus. From these nuclei scattered bundles of fibers of the trigeminal nerve run ventrolaterally to make their exit at the lateral border of the pons. The medial lemniscus and superior olivary nucleus have the same appearance as in the preceding section, but only a few scattered fibers of the trapezoid body can be seen. The lateral lemniscus can be distinguished on the lateral side of the superior olivary nucleus.

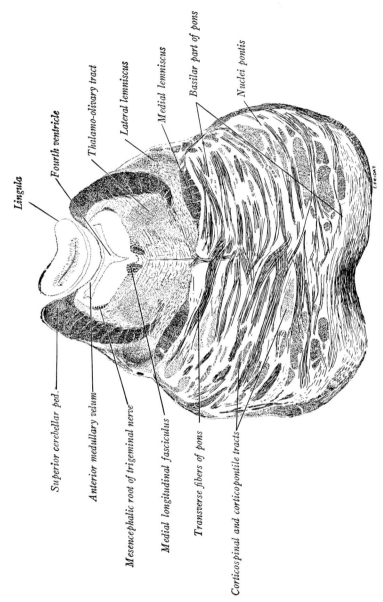

FIGURE 351.   Section through the rostral part of the pons in the plane indicated in Fig. 354. Magnification 4½.

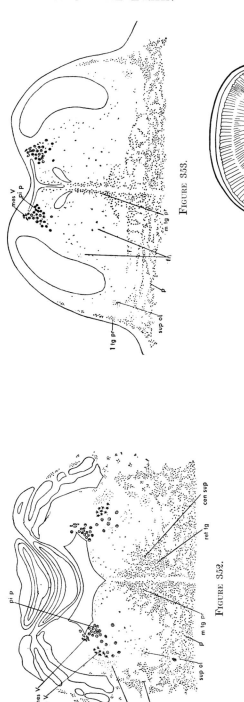

FIGURE 353.

FIGURE 354.

FIGURE 352.

FIGURE 351. The fourth ventricle is seen near its rostral extremity where it becomes narrow before it connects with the cerebral aqueduct. The lingula of the cerebellar vermis rests upon the dorsal surface of the anterior medullary velum, which joins the dorsal borders of the two superior cerebellar peduncles. At its ventral border some fibers can be seen streaming medialward toward the decussation illustrated in the next figure. At the lateral border of the central gray matter the mesencephalic root of the trigeminal nerve is represented as a small bundle of fibers cut transversely. On each side of the midline close to the floor of the fourth ventricle is seen the medial longitudinal fasciculus. The medial lemniscus has assumed a more lateral position than in the preceding sections. The lateral lemniscus has been displaced lateralward and dorsalward.

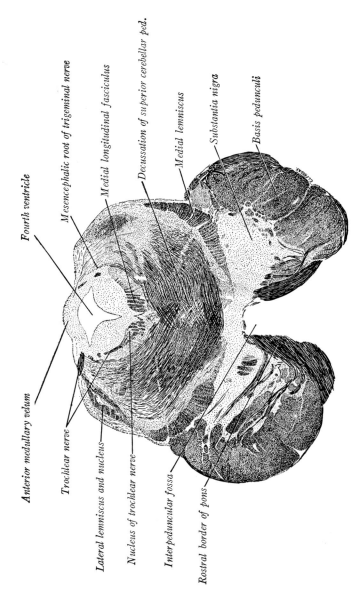

FIGURE 355. Section through the mesencephalon at the border of the pons in the plane indicated in Fig. 358. Magnification 4½.

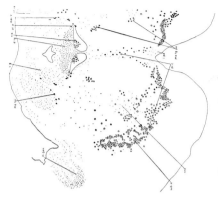

FIGURE 361.

FIGURE 360. Section through the mesencephalon at the level of the trochlear nucleus, showing the distribution of cell groups (Jacobsohn).

Figure 359 represents a section passing through the inferior colliculus. The tectum of the mesencephalon lies dorsal to the cerebral aqueduct. The ventral part of the section is formed by the cerebral peduncles in which there may be distinguished the tegmentum and basis pedunculi and between these parts the substantia nigra. The tegmentum is continuous across the midline, while the two bases pedunculi are separated by the interpeduncular fossa. The nucleus of the inferior colliculus is surrounded by a capsule of fibers derived from the lateral lemniscus. Lateral to this nucleus is the inferior quadrigeminal brachium which also consists of fibers derived from the lateral lemniscus. The corpus parabigeminum is a mass of gray matter situated ventrolateral to the nucleus of the inferior colliculus and in close relation to the dorsal extremity of the medial lemniscus. The trochlear nucleus is a well defined ovoid mass just dorsal to the medial longitudinal fasciculus. Lateral to it is the thalamo-olivary tract. Fibers belonging to the oculomotor nerve make their exit through the oculomotor sulcus. The substantia nigra has increased in extent. The gray matter forming the floor of the interpeduncular fossa at this level is known as the posterior perforated substance because it is perforated by numerous blood vessels.

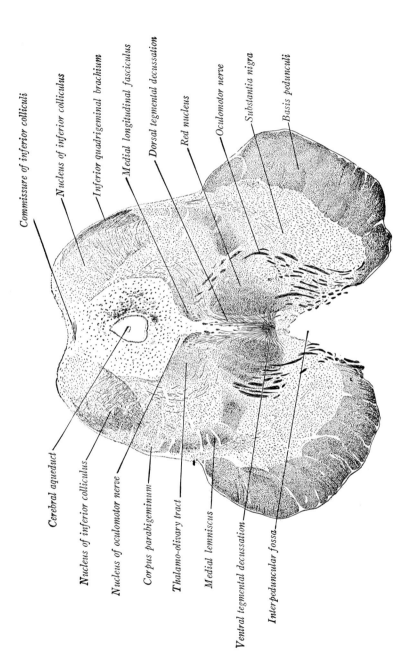

Commissure of inferior colliculi

Nucleus of inferior colliculus

Inferior quadrigeminal brachium

Medial longitudinal fasciculus

Dorsal tegmental decussation

Red nucleus

Oculomotor nerve

Substantia nigra

Basis pedunculi

Cerebral aqueduct

Nucleus of inferior colliculus

Nucleus of oculomotor nerve

Corpus parabigeminum

Thalamo-olivary tract

Medial lemniscus

Ventral tegmental decussation

Interpeduncular fossa

FIGURE 362.   Section through the mesencephalon at the level of the inferior colliculus in the plane indicated in Fig. 364. Magnification 4½.

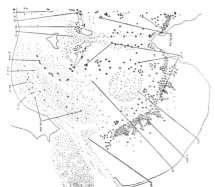

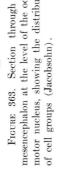

Figure 363. Section through the mesencephalon at the level of the oculomotor nucleus, showing the distribution of cell groups (Jacobsohn).

Figure 364.

Figure 362 represents a section passing through the mesencephalon at the level of the inferior colliculus and the fountain decussation. At this level most of the fibers of the lateral lemniscus have terminated in the colliculus, but many fibers can be seen along its lateral surface. Some of these belong to the inferior quadrigeminal brachium through which they run to the medial geniculate body. Between the red nuclei there are many decussating fibers. The fibers in the dorsal three-fourths of the field are arranged so that they resemble the spray of a fountain. These fibers come from the tectum and swing around the central gray stratum to the midline. After their decussation they form the tectospinal and tectobulbar tracts. In the ventral fourth of the field between the red nuclei are fibers which arise from these nuclei and cross in the midline. Their decussation is the ventral tegmental decussation or decussation of Forel. Fibers of the oculomotor nerve curve around the lateral part of the red nucleus, pass through the medial part of the substantia nigra and emerge through the oculomotor sulcus into the interpeduncular fossa. The substantia nigra, with the broad band of fibers of the basis pedunculi forming its ventrolateral boundary, appears much the same as it did in the previous section.

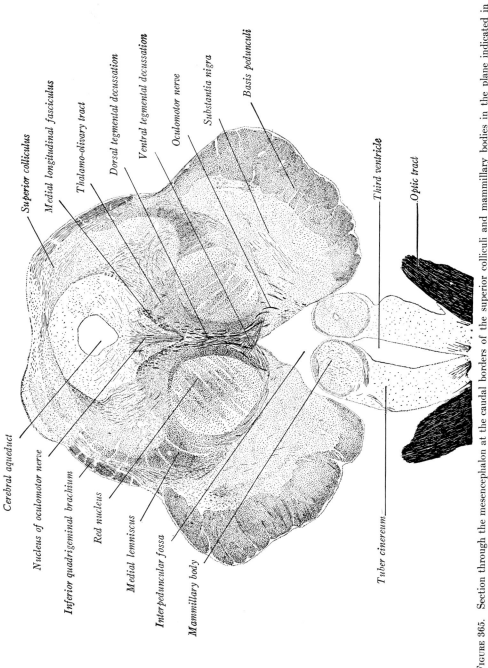

FIGURE 365. Section through the mesencephalon at the caudal borders of the superior colliculi and mammillary bodies in the plane indicated in Fig. 366. Magnification 4½.

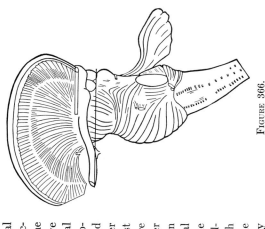

FIGURE 366.

Figure 365 represents a section passing through the mesencephalon at the level of the caudal borders of the superior colliculi and of the mammillary bodies. The inferior quadrigeminal brachium is well defined and is situated at the surface of the section between the superior colliculus and the basis pedunculi. Just medial to this and curving ventrally and medially to the lateral border of the red nucleus is the medial lemniscus. The nucleus of the oculomotor nerve now appears in three parts, paired lateral portions and an unpaired medial one. The medial longitudinal fasciculi have spread out in the form of a V along the lateral edges of the oculo-motor nuclei. The thalamo-olivary tract is seen lateral to the medial longitudinal fasciculus and dorsal to the red nucleus. The red nucleus in this section shows more gray matter and fewer fibers than in the preceding one. It is surrounded by a capsule of nerve fibers which is most dense on the medial side of the nucleus. Between the red nuclei two decussations of fibers are seen. The dorsal tegmental decussation is composed of fibers from the tectum which, after crossing, descend as the tectospinal and tectobulbar tracts. The ventral tegmental decussation is made up of fibers from the red nucleus. These cross and turn caudalward as the rubrospinal tract. The heavy strands of fibers coursing ventrally between the red nuclei belong to the oculomotor nerves. The substantia nigra and basis pedunculi have been displaced slightly lateral-ward by the widening of the interpeduncular fossa to receive the mammillary bodies which appear as two round masses lying between the peduncles. The very dark bundles of fibers in the most ventral part of the illustration are parts of the optic tracts. Ventral to the mammillary bodies a part of the third ventricle surrounded by the tuber cinereum may be seen.

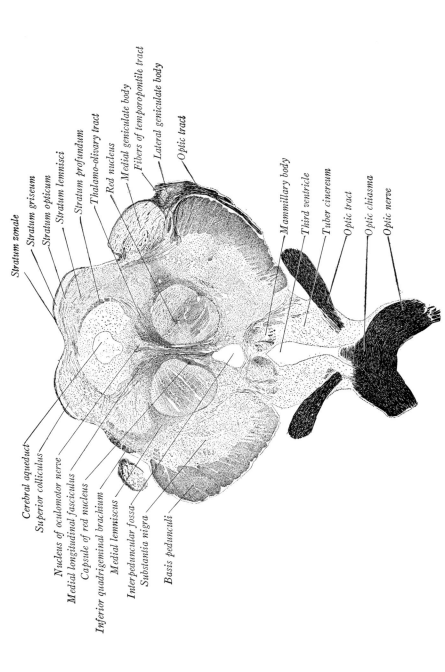

FIGURE 367. Section through the mesencephalon at the level of the superior colliculus and the optic chiasma in the plane indicated in Fig. 368.
Magnification 2¾.

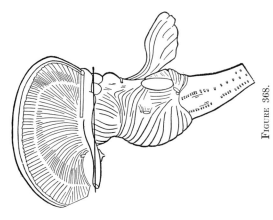

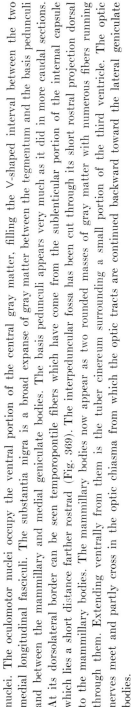

Figure 368.

Figure 367 represents a section passing through the mesencephalon at the level of the superior colliculi and the optic chiasma. The superior colliculi form the two rostral eminences in the lamina quadrigemina or tectum mesencephali. They are composed of several strata. There is a superficial thin layer of nerve fibers, the stratum zonale. Beneath this is a thicker layer, the stratum griseum, which contains few myelinated fibers and appears to be composed chiefly of gray matter. The next deeper layer, the stratum opticum, contains many fibers. Afferent fibers from the optic tract enter this layer by way of the superior quadrigeminal brachium. The stratum lemnisci lies just beneath the stratum opticum and is also rich in fibers. The thin layer of fibers next to the central gray matter is known as the stratum profundum. It is composed of tectospinal fibers which arise in the superior colliculus and cross the midline in the dorsal tegmental decussation. The inferior quadrigeminal brachium can be seen on the left side of the section. It terminates in the medial geniculate body. This is illustrated on the right side of the figure as a rounded body projecting lateralward from the tegmentum just dorsal to the dorsolateral border of the substantia nigra. The connection of the inferior quadrigeminal brachium with the medial geniculate body is illustrated in Fig. 147. The medial lemniscus is sharply curved with concavity directed dorsomedially. Its thickest portion lies near the lateral side of the red nucleus, but it extends laterally, and then dorsally in the tegmentum upon the medial side of the medial geniculate body and inferior quadrigeminal brachium. The thalamo-olivary tract lies dorsal to the red nucleus and lateral to the medial longitudinal fasciculus which extends as a flattened plate of dark fibers on each side of the oculomotor nuclei. The oculomotor nuclei occupy the ventral portion of the central gray matter, filling the V-shaped interval between the two medial longitudinal fasciculi. The substantia nigra is a broad expanse of gray matter between the tegmentum and the basis pedunculi and between the mammillary and medial geniculate bodies. The basis pedunculi appears very much as it did in more caudal sections. At its dorsolateral border can be seen temporopontile fibers which have come from the sublenticular portion of the internal capsule which lies a short distance farther rostrad (Fig. 369). The interpeduncular fossa has been cut through its short rostral projection dorsal to the mammillary bodies. The mammillary bodies now appear as two rounded masses of gray matter with numerous fibers running through them. Extending ventrally from them is the tuber cinereum surrounding a small portion of the third ventricle. The optic nerves meet and partly cross in the optic chiasma from which the optic tracts are continued backward toward the lateral geniculate bodies.

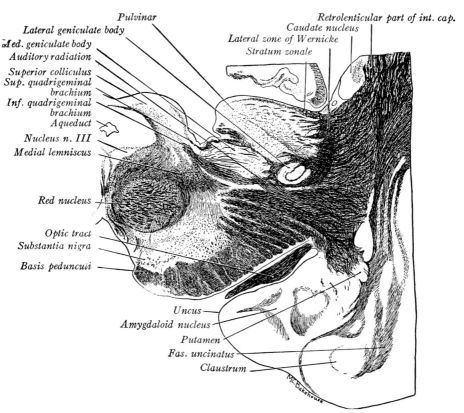

FIGURE 369. Section through the mesencephalon and internal capsule in the plane indicated by Figs. 370 and 371. (Redrawn from Déjerine.)

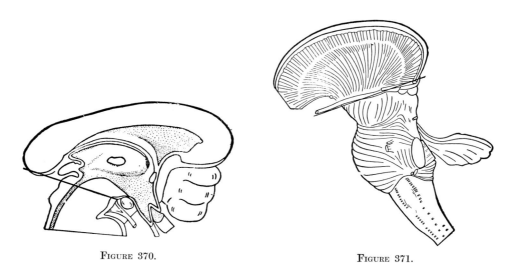

FIGURE 370.   FIGURE 371.

Oblique sections through the region of transition between midbrain and thalamus are represented by the following five illustrations. The oblique plane of section, indicated in the accompanying key figures, makes possible a clear display of the quadrigeminal brachia, fields of Forel, and the ansa lenticularis.

Figure 369 represents a section through the rostral part of the mesencephalon cut at a slightly different angle than the preceding section. It passes through the optic tract, sublenticular part of the internal capsule, and the

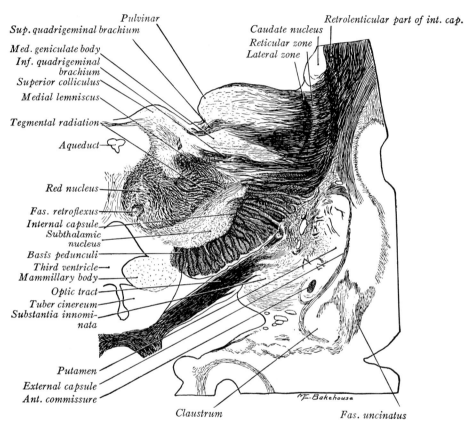

FIGURE 372. Section through the hypothalamus and internal capsule in the plane indicated by Fig. 373. (Redrawn from Déjerine.)

pulvinar of the thalamus (Fig. 372), and through the upper end of the mesencephalon (Fig. 370). Under cover of the pulvinar and resting upon the lateral surface of the mesencephalon are the rostral ends of the medial and lateral geniculate bodies. The lateral zone of Wernicke, shown better in Fig. 400, contains fibers from the optic tract and from the geniculocalcarine fasciculus. It is continuous with the stratum zonale on the dorsal surface, and the external medullary lamina on the lateral surface of the thalamus (Fig. 390). Fibers from the medial geniculate body, belonging to the auditory radiation, run lateralward into the sublenticular portion of the internal capsule where they become

lost among the temporopontile fibers. The temporopontile fibers may be traced
from the sublenticular portion of the internal capsule into the lateral part of
the basis pedunculi. The inferior quadrigeminal brachium is placed ventral to
the medial geniculate body and the superior quadrigeminal brachium dorsal
to it.

Figure 372 represents a section through the hypothalamus a short distance
rostral to the upper end of the mesencephalon. It passes through the optic

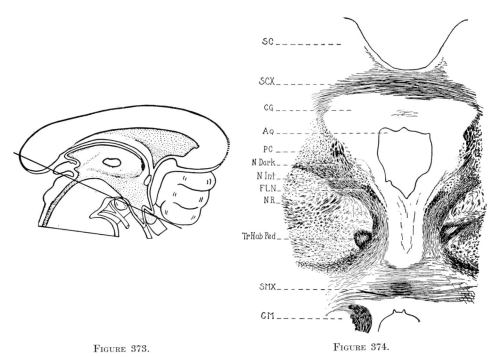

FIGURE 373.   FIGURE 374.

FIGURES 374, 377. Sections showing the nucleus of Darkschewitsch and the interstitial nucleus.
AQ, Aqueduct; *CG*, central gray; *CM*, mammillary body; *FLN*, medial longitudinal fasciculus;
N Dark, nucleus of Darkschewitsch; *N Int*, interstitial nucleus; *NR*, red nucleus; *PC*, posterior
commissure; *Pin*, pineal body; *SC*, superior colliculus; *SC X*, commissure of superior colliculus;
SM X, supramammillary decussation; *Tr Hab Ped*, tractus habenulopeduncularis; *Tr M T*, tractus
mammillothalamicus; *Vent 3*, third ventricle. Drawings by Ingram.

chiasma, tuber cinereum, mammillary body and superior colliculus of the
corpora quadrigemina (Fig. 373), and through the optic tract, retrolenticular
part of the internal capsule, and the pulvinar of the thalamus. Dorsal to the
optic tract is seen the highest part of the basis pedunculi. This is continuous
lateralward with the subthalamic portion of the internal capsule which is
situated between the lentiform nucleus and the subthalamus. The latter represents an upward continuation of the tegmentum of the mesencephalon which
it resembles somewhat in structure. The substantia nigra, which is well developed
in the preceding section, is replaced by the subthalamic nucleus of Luys. The
fasciculus retroflexus of Meynert is seen passing through the red nucleus.

Directed lateralward from this nucleus are coarse bundles of fibers belonging to the tegmental radiation through which the corticorubral tract makes its way from the internal capsule to the red nucleus. Dorsal to the tegmental radiation is the medial lemniscus, and dorsal to this, the inferior quadrigeminal brachium. This brachium is represented by a heavy bundle of fibers extending from the

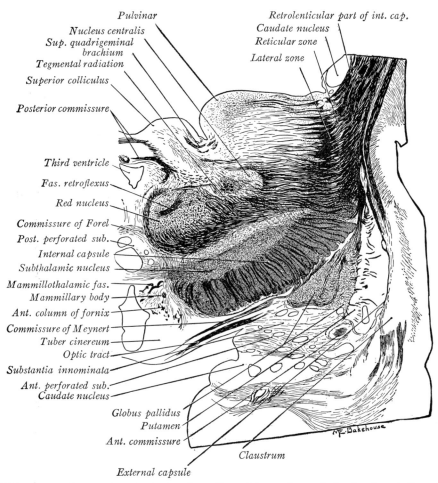

Figure 375. Section through the basal ganglia and internal capsule in the plane indicated by Fig. 376. (Redrawn from Déjerine.)

internal capsule along the ventral side of the medial geniculate body toward the inferior colliculus. It contains, in addition to the auditory fibers from the lateral lemniscus (Fig. 170), also cortical projection fibers from the sublenticular segment of the internal capsule. The medial geniculate body separates the two quadrigeminal brachia. The superior quadrigeminal brachium extends lateral-ward between the medial geniculate body and the pulvinar. In addition to fibers from the optic tract it contains projection fibers from the cerebral cortex.

These projection fibers come by way of the retrolenticular segment of the internal capsule and traverse the lateral zone of Wernicke and the superior quadrigeminal brachium to reach the superior colliculus. The lateral zone is well developed and is situated on the lateral side of the pulvinar, which it separates from the reticular zone and the internal capsule. Lateral to the optic tract are seen the substantia innominata, the anterior commissure, and the most ventral part of the lentiform nucleus. Lateral to these structures are the external capsule and claustrum.

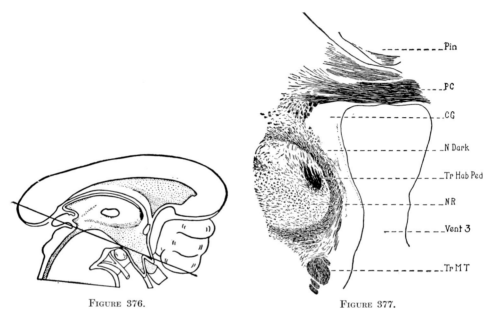

FIGURE 376.   FIGURE 377.

For description see Fig. 374.

Figure 375 represents a section through the hypothalamus and basal ganglia at a slightly higher level than the preceding one. It passes through the upper border of the optic tract and the retrolenticular part of the internal capsule and the pulvinar, and through the lamina terminalis, tuber cinereum, mammillary body, and posterior commissure (Fig. 376). The basis pedunculi is represented at this level by the subthalamic portion of the internal capsule with which it is directly continuous and by which the subthalamus is separated from the lentiform nucleus. The section passes above the level of the sublenticular part of the capsule and below the level of its anterior limb. Posteriorly the internal capsule is continuous through its retrolenticular portion with the internal sagittal stratum. Lateral to the optic tract is the substantia innominata, the anterior perforated substance, and the lowest part of the head of the caudate nucleus. Lateral to the internal capsule are the lentiform nucleus, external capsule, and claustrum. In the midline are seen the posterior perforated substance and the portion of the third ventricle that connects with the cavity of the infundibulum. Surrounding this portion of the ventricle are the tuber cinereum and mammillary body. The red nucleus is surrounded by a capsule formed chiefly by fibers of the brachium conjunctivum, and is pierced by the fasciculus retroflexus of Meynert. From the red nucleus the tegmental radiation streams lateralward. In the dorsal part of the section is the pulvinar of the thalamus with the lateral zone of Wernicke upon its lateral surface. This is separated by the reticular zone from the retrolenticular part of the internal capsule. The subthalamic nucleus is situated dorsal and medial to the internal

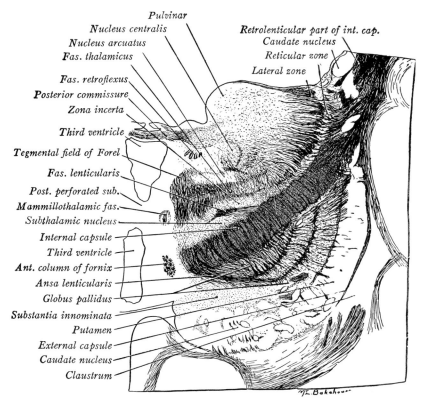

FIGURE 378. Section through the basal ganglia and internal capsule in the plane indicated by Figs. 379. and 380. (Redrawn from Déjerine.)

capsule. The mammillothalamic fasciculus and the anterior column of the fornix are cut across in the rostral part of the mammillary body.

Figure 378 was drawn from a section through the hypothalamus, thalamus, and lentiform nucleus. It passes through the internal capsule some distance below the anterior limb, cutting through the subthalamic and retrolenticular portions of the posterior limb (Fig. 380), and through the lamina terminalis and posterior commissure (Fig. 379.) The internal capsule forms a broad band of white matter separating the lentiform nucleus which lies upon its lateral aspect from the subthalamus and thalamus which lie medial to it. The lentiform nucleus is fused medially with the head of the caudate nucleus. Adjacent to

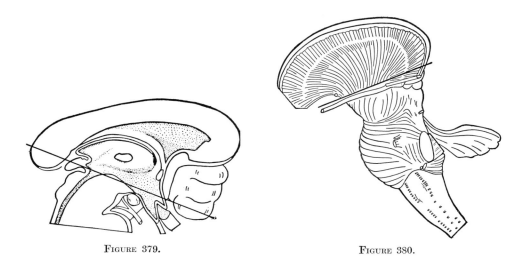

FIGURE 379.   FIGURE 380.

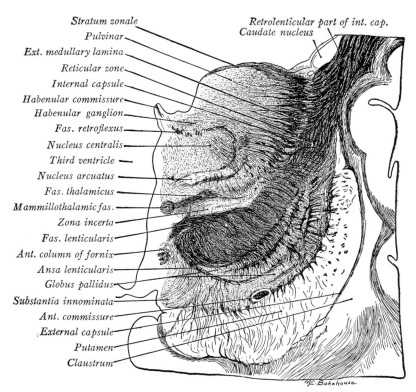

Stratum zonale
Pulvinar
Ext. medullary lamina
Reticular zone
Internal capsule
Habenular commissure
Habenular ganglion
Fas. retroflexus
Nucleus centralis
Third ventricle
Nucleus arcuatus
Fas. thalamicus
Mammillothalamic fas.
Zona incerta
Fas. lenticularis
Ant. column of fornix
Ansa lenticularis
Globus pallidus
Substantia innominata
Ant. commissure
External capsule
Putamen
Claustrum

Retrolenticular part of int. cap.
Caudate nucleus

FIGURE 381.   Section through the basal ganglia and internal capsule in the plane indicated by Figs.
382 and 383. (Redrawn from Déjerine.)

the gray matter surrounding the third ventricle are seen the anterior column of the fornix, the mammillothalamic fasciculus, and the fasciculus retroflexus of Meynert. The ansa lenticularis streams medially from the globus pallidus around the medial border of the internal capsule. Dorsal to the subthalamic nucleus is a field of myelinated fibers, the tegmental field (H) of Forel. It is prolonged laterward as the thalamic fasciculus (field H_1) of Forel. From the entire medial surface of the globus pallidus fibers pass backward through the internal capsule. They form the lenticular fasciculus (field H_2) and are continued medially into the tegmental field (H) of Forel. (See also Fig. 206.) Between the thalamic and lenticular fasciculi is a plate of gray matter, known as the zona incerta, which is continuous laterally with the reticular zone of

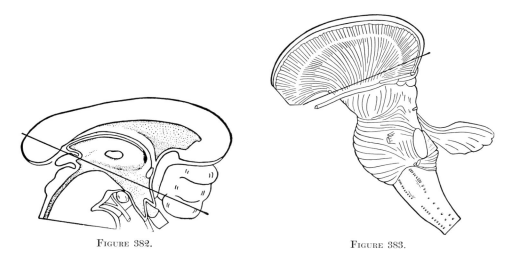

FIGURE 382.   FIGURE 383.

the thalamus. The reticular zone is a thin plate of gray matter separating the external medullary lamina of the thalamus from the internal capsule.

Figure 381 represents a section through the hypothalamus, thalamus, and lentiform nucleus slightly higher than the preceding one. It passes through the internal capsule immediately below its anterior limb and through the subthalamic, lenticulothalamic, and retrolenticular portions of the posterior limb (Fig. 383), and through the lamina terminalis and habenular commissure (Fig. 382). The retrolenticular part of the internal capsule separates the lentiform nucleus from the tail of the caudate nucleus. The lentiform nucleus lies on the ventrolateral side of the internal capsule and is composed of two parts, the globus pallidus and putamen. It is continuous medially with the caudate nucleus. The section was made below the level of the point where the anterior commissure crosses the midline, but cuts across the commissure as this curves under the lentiform nucleus. Medial to the internal capsule are seen the subthalamus and thalamus. Adjacent to the gray matter enclosing the third ventricle can be distinguished the anterior column of the fornix, the mammillothalamic fasciculus, and the fasciculus retroflexus. The latter is cut at the

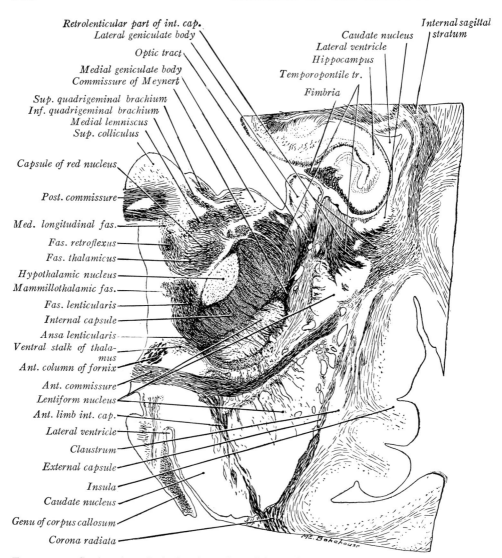

Retrolenticular part of int. cap.
Lateral geniculate body
Optic tract
Medial geniculate body
Commissure of Meynert
Sup. quadrigeminal brachium
Inf. quadrigeminal brachium
Medial lemniscus
Sup. colliculus
Capsule of red nucleus
Post. commissure
Med. longitudinal fas.
Fas. retroflexus
Fas. thalamicus
Hypothalamic nucleus
Mammillothalamic fas.
Fas. lenticularis
Internal capsule
Ansa lenticularis
Ventral stalk of thala-
mus
Ant. column of fornix
Ant. commissure
Lentiform nucleus
Ant. limb int. cap.
Lateral ventricle
Claustrum
External capsule
Insula
Caudate nucleus
Genu of corpus callosum
Corona radiata

Internal sagittal
stratum
Caudate nucleus
Lateral ventricle
Hippocampus
Temporopontile tr.
Fimbria

FIGURE 384. Section through the basal ganglia and internal capsule in the plane indicated by Figs. 385 and 386. (Redrawn from Déjerine.)

point where it enters the habenular ganglion. In the subthalamic region the fasciculus lenticularis rests upon the dorsomedial aspect of the internal capsule. It consists of fibers from the lentiform nucleus which have made their way through the internal capsule. Dorsal to it is the zona incerta and dorsal to that, the fasciculus thalamicus. The ansa lenticularis is seen coming from the globus pallidus. The origin of the ansa can be seen better in the preceding section. It winds around the medial border of the internal capsule and joins the fasciculus lenticularis in the subthalamus. Next to the internal capsule are the external medullary lamina and the reticular zone. The surface of the pulvinar is covered by the stratum zonale.

Horizontal sections through the internal capsule at three successive levels are represented in the accompanying illustrations. They show the subdivisions of the internal capsule and its relation to the subthalamus, thalamus, and corpus striatum.

Figure 384 represents a section through the internal capsule immediately above the sublenticular portion (Fig. 386), and through the anterior and posterior commissures (Fig. 385). The plane of this section makes an acute angle with those of the preceding sections. The inclination of the plane of section is such that it cuts through the lowermost fibers of the anterior limb

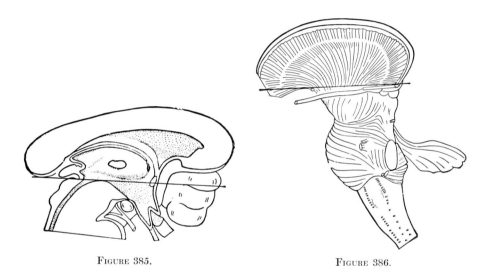

FIGURE 385.   FIGURE 386.

and the junction of the sublenticular with the retrolenticular portions of the internal capsule. Some temporopontile fibers belonging to the sublenticular portion are shown in the drawing and the continuity of the retrolenticular portion with the internal sagittal stratum is illustrated. The anterior limb separates the head of the caudate from the lentiform nucleus. The anterior commissure can be traced laterward and then somewhat backward under the lentiform nucleus. The external capsule separates the latter from the claustrum. In the subthalamus one sees the subthalamic nucleus upon the medial surface of the posterior limb of the internal capsule. In or near the gray matter bounding the third ventricle may be seen the anterior column of the fornix, the mammillothalamic fasciculus and the fasciculus retroflexus.

Figure 387 represents a typical horizontal section through the internal capsule. It was cut in a plane parallel to that of the preceding section and passes through the lower border of the interventricular foramen and through the habenular ganglion as indicated in Fig. 388, and through the anterior and posterior limbs, genu, and retrolenticular portion of the internal capsule as

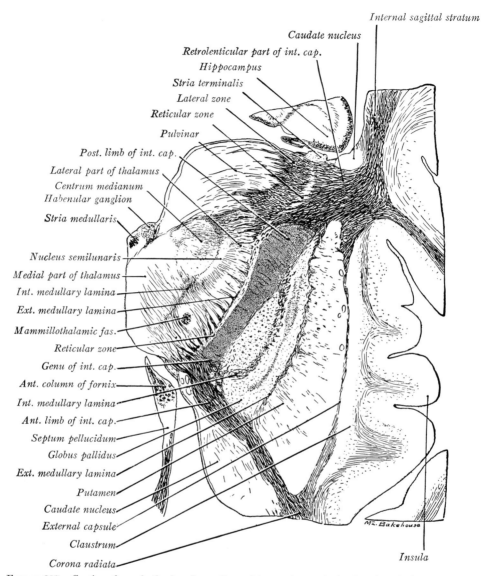

FIGURE 387.   Section through the basal ganglia and internal capsule in the plane indicated by Figs.
388 and 389.   (Redrawn from Déjerine.)

indicated in Fig. 389. The anterior limb consists of nearly horizontal fibers
which run in the plane of the section. It separates the head of the caudate
nucleus from the lentiform nucleus. The lenticulothalamic portion of the
posterior limb separates the lentiform nucleus from the thalamus. Its fibers
course vertically and are cut across in the section. The fibers of the retrolenticular portion are directed lateralward between the lentiform nucleus and
the tail of the caudate nucleus, on the lateral side of which the fibers turn

backward to join the internal sagittal stratum. The lentiform nucleus is divided
by medullary laminae into three segments, the outer of which is known as
the putamen and the two inner form the globus pallidus. The putamen is
separated from the claustrum by the external capsule and the claustrum lies
in contact with the white substance underlying the insula. Several parts of the
thalamus may be distinguished: namely, the pulvinar and the medial and
lateral parts of the thalamus, and, belonging to the ventral division of the
lateral part the centrum medianum and the semilunar nucleus, the latter
being known also as the posteromedial ventral nucleus. The medial and lateral
parts are separated by the internal medullary lamina, and on the lateral side
of the lateral part is the external medullary lamina. External to the pulvinar

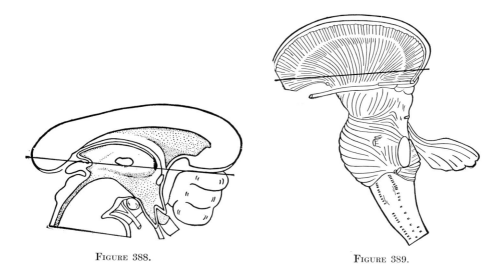

FIGURE 388.   FIGURE 389.

is the lateral zone of Wernicke. The external medullary lamina and the zone
of Wernicke are separated from the internal capsule by the reticular zone.

Figure 390 was drawn from a horizontal section passing through the highest
part of the interventricular foramen, and through the internal capsule a short
distance higher than the preceding section. In this as in the preceding section
the lentiform nucleus is coextensive with the insula, from which it is separated
by the external capsule and the claustrum. The internal capsule has the same
appearance as in the preceding section. In the thalamus one sees, in addition
to the pulvinar, the medial, lateral, and anterior parts. The latter is situated
at the anterior end of the thalamus near its dorsal (superior) surface wedged
in between the medial and lateral parts. The lateral zone of Wernicke is continuous with the stratum zonale, which covers the lateral surface of the
pulvinar, and with the external medullary lamina. The reticular zone forms a
thin plate of gray matter upon the medial surface of the internal capsule from
near the genu to the posterior extremity of its retrolenticular portion.

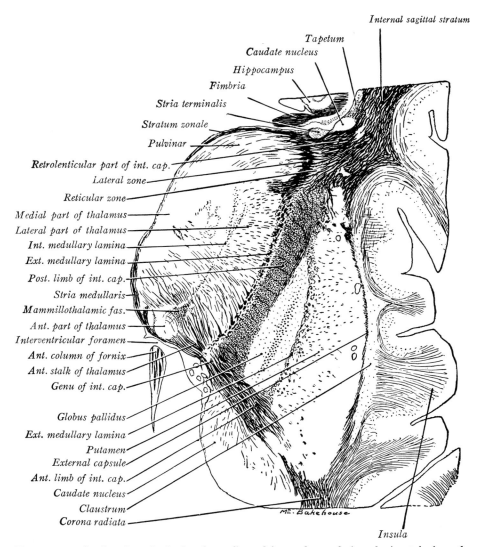

FIGURE 390. Section through the basal ganglia and internal capsule in a horizontal plane through the interventricular foramen. (Redrawn from Déjerine.)

Frontal sections through the cerebrum, stained by the Pal-Weigert method, have been reproduced from Jelgersma's atlas. These illustrations will be found useful in the study of gross sections through the cerebral hemisphere as well as in the study of stained preparations. Before the sections were made the brain stem had been cut away through the rostral end of the mesencephalon.

Figure 391 represents a frontal section of the cerebral hemisphere passing *through the genu of the corpus callosum.* The transversely directed fibers of the genu extend laterward into the radiation of the corpus callosum, which here is split into two parts that diverge to form the roof and floor of the anterior horn of the lateral ventricle. A little further rostrally these two limbs approach each other and meet where the callosal fibers enclose the end of the ventricle.

In the lateral wall of the ventricle is the head of the *caudate nucleus* which contains near its lateral margin some transversely cut bundles of fibers belonging to the *anterior limb of the internal capsule.* Laterally these bundles rest against the corona radiata. In the plane of this section and in others slightly more

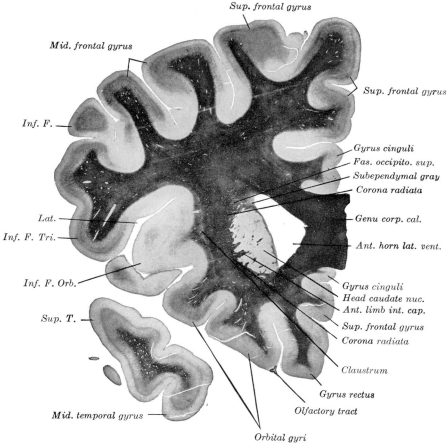

Sup. frontal gyrus
Mid. frontal gyrus
Sup. frontal gyrus
Inf. F.
Gyrus cinguli
Fas. occipito. sup.
Subependymal gray
Corona radiata
Lat.
Genu corp. cal.
Inf. F. Tri.
Ant. horn lat. vent.
Inf. F. Orb.
Gyrus cinguli
Head caudate nuc.
Ant. limb int. cap.
Sup. T.
Sup. frontal gyrus
Corona radiata
Claustrum
Gyrus rectus
Mid. temporal gyrus
Olfactory tract
Orbital gyri

FIGURE 391. From Atlas Anatomicum Cerebri Humani, by Prof. Dr. G. Jelgersma, Published by Messrs. Scheltema & Holkema; N. V. Amsterdam, Holland.

posterior, the horizontally coursing fiber bundles of the anterior limb of the internal capsule, which in Fig. 391 separate the caudate nucleus from the putamen, become incorporated in that portion of the corona radiata which is directed forward into the frontal lobe. The horizontal section represented in Fig. 387 illustrates how the anterior limb of the internal capsule, composed of horizontally coursing fibers, merges with the corona radiata rostral to the lentiform nucleus. A comparison of these two sections cut in planes approximately at right angles to each other makes it evident that that represented in Fig. 391 passes through the head of the caudate nucleus and the corona radiata rostral to the lentiform nucleus.

The *subependymal gray matter*, which forms a fairly thick layer covering the anterior end of the lateral ventricle and separates the ependyma from the radiation of the corpus callosum, is reduced in amount at the level of this section. But it is continued toward the occiput in this and succeeding sections as a column of gray matter along the dorsal border of the caudate nucleus. It is deeply stained in Weigert preparations because it contains large numbers of myelinated fibers, many of which are derived from the fasciculus occipito-frontalis superior (Fas. occipito. sup.) which lies just lateral to it.

In the isolated tip of the temporal lobe is seen the superior temporal gyrus (Sup. T.). Above the level of the lateral fissure (Lat.), the inferior frontal gyrus (Inf. F.) is subdivided into the triangular (Inf. F. Tri.) and orbital portions (Inf. F. Orb.).

Figure 392 represents a frontal section of the cerebral hemisphere cutting *through the rostrum of the corpus callosum*. The transversely directed fibers of the rostrum turn ventrally into the white matter overlying the orbital gyri. Between the rostrum and the body or trunk of the corpus callosum is stretched the septum pellucidum, one lamina of which has been largely torn away in this section. The radiation formed within the white center of the hemisphere by the transversely directed fibers of the corpus callosum intersects the corona radiata, the fibers of the two systems crossing and to some extent mingling. The corpus callosum can be followed back through the series of sections to the splenium in Fig. 402.

The head of the *caudate nucleus* is larger than in the preceding section and it is incompletely separated from the putamen by transversely cut bundles of fibers belonging to the anterior limb of the internal capsule. In this section the *putamen* rests upon the external capsule, which along with the claustrum separates it from the orbital gyri and the orbital portion of the inferior frontal gyrus. Between the plane of this section and the next the putamen and caudate nucleus fuse together beneath the anterior limb of the internal capsule and the combined nuclei come into contact with the anterior perforated substance (Figs. 32, 220).

As the *anterior limb of the internal capsule* is followed backward through the sections it becomes thicker (Figs. 393–395). It intervenes between the caudate and lentiform nuclei and consists of fibers which are directed forward and upward (Fig. 32). The lowest bundles are cut transversely in Fig. 392 and enter the corona radiata in Fig. 391. The remaining bundles are directed obliquely upward into the corona. The lenticulothalamic part of the posterior limb (Figs. 396–397) intervenes between the thalamus and lentiform nucleus and appears as a direct continuation of the basis pedunculi (Fig. 398). It is composed of fibers which course nearly vertically upward (Fig. 32). The retrolenticular part is molded upon the posterior part of the thalamus and its fibers are directed toward the occiput and somewhat laterad into the occipital portion of the corona radiata (Figs. 32, 400, 401). The sublenticular part of the posterior limb of the internal capsule is directed lateralward into the temporal lobe ventral to the posterior end of the lentiform nucleus (Figs. 228, 398). It helps to form the roof of the inferior horn of the lateral ventricle.

The section represented in Fig. 393 passes *through the anterior commissure*, where this crosses the midline and extends laterad beneath to the anterior limb of the internal capsule (Figs. 32, 229) and between the lentiform nucleus

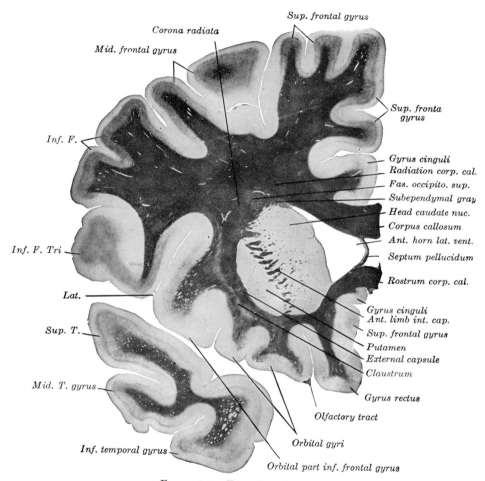

FIGURE 392.   From Jelgersma.

and the substantia perforata anterior. As it passes under the internal capsule it is bent somewhat downward. It then curves slightly toward the occiput as it passes under the lentiform nucleus and is directed into the white matter of the temporal lobe (Figs. 384, 394–396). In man the portion of the anterior commissure which unites the two olfactory bulbs is very inconspicuous and is not shown in this series of photographs.

The columns of the *fornix* are embedded in the ventral margins of the septal laminae (Fig. 393). From this position the fornix can be followed at first dorsally and then toward the occiput maintaining the same relation to the septum pellucidum (Figs. 393–399). It is separated from the thalamus by the interventricular foramen (Fig. 395) and the chorioidal fissure (Figs. 242, 396–399). The sections show clearly that the body of the fornix is composed of two lateral halves, which are continuous rostrally with the columns and toward

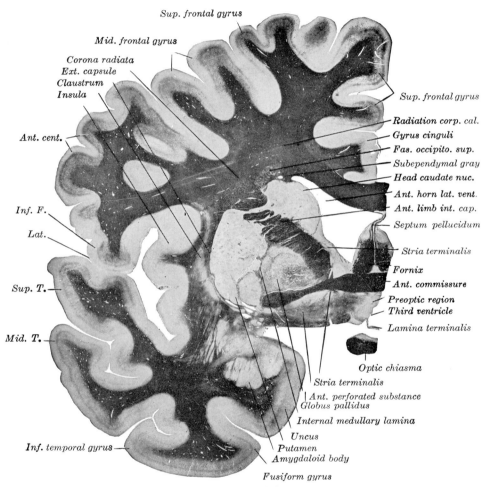

FIGURE 393.   From Jelgersma.

the occiput with the crura, which in turn are continuous with the fimbria of the fornix. Each lateral half has at first a somewhat rounded outline but becomes progressively more triangular as it is followed toward its junction with the crus. The crura and hippocampal commissure are not shown in this series of plates since they are present in the sections between those represented by Figs. 401 and 402. In Fig. 242 the crus can be traced into the fimbria which lies along the dorsomedial side of the hippocampus (Figs. 399, 401). The fimbria is continuous laterally with the alveus of the hippocampus and is bent sharply on itself so that its free margin, to which the chorioidal plexus is attached, is also directed laterally (Fig. 400). The chorioid fissure is closed by the chorioid plexus which is attached on the one hand to the fimbria of the hippocampus and on the other to the stria terminalis in the roof of the inferior horn of the lateral ventricle.

The rostral margin of the *optic chiasma* is included in the section represented in Fig. 393 as is also the lamina terminalis. The part of the third ventricle included in this and the next figure lies between the optic chiasma and the anterior commissure and represents the unevaginated part of the original telencephalic cavity. From the lateral margin of the chiasma the *optic tract* can be traced laterally and toward the occiput in the sulcus forming the lateral boundary of the hypothalamus (Fig. 395) and then along the side of the upper end of the basis pedunculi to the lateral geniculate body (Figs. 396–400).

Figure 394 represents a section which passes *through the optic chiasma* and the posterior border of the anterior commissure. The *caudate nucleus* lies on the medial side of the internal capsule in the angle formed by the intersection of the corona radiata and the radiation of the corpus callosum, from which intersection it is separated by the fasciculus occipitofrontalis superior and the subependymal gray matter. The head of the nucleus enters into the formation of the lateral wall and floor of the anterior horn of the lateral ventricle (Figs. 56, 391–395). It decreases rapidly in size as it is followed toward the occiput and becomes drawn out into a long slender curved tail, which forms the lateral part of the sloping floor of the central part of the lateral ventricle (Figs. 396–401) and curves downward into the roof of the inferior horn (Figs. 400–401). Here it becomes so small that it cannot be distinguished in some of the photographs (Figs. 398–399), but, nevertheless, it is continued forward in the roof of the ventricle to become continuous with the amygdaloid nucleus (Figs. 393–395).

The *amygdaloid nucleus* lies upon the dorsal surface of the uncus (Figs. 393–395), forms the roof of the anterior extremity of the inferior horn of the lateral ventricle (Fig. 395), and extends some little distance in the roof toward the occiput gradually decreasing in size (Fig. 396).

In frontal sections the *lentiform nucleus* has a triangular outline and is differentiated into an outer portion, the putamen, and an inner part, the globus pallidus. The globus pallidus is divided into two segments by an internal medullary lamina and is separated from the putamen by the external medullary lamina (Figs. 394–397). The dorsomedial boundary of the lentiform nucleus is formed by the internal capsule and its ventral surface rests on the anterior commissure (Figs. 393–395), the ansa lenticularis (Fig. 395) and the roof of the inferior horn of the lateral ventricle (Figs. 396–398). The putamen is much larger than the globus pallidus. It extends as a massive structure farther forward (Fig. 392) and as a thin and broken plate it spreads out toward the occiput (Fig. 399). The putamen is separated from the claustrum by the external capsule.

The *claustrum* is a thin plate of gray matter intervening between the external capsule and the white matter subjacent to the insular gyri. Its extent from before backward and from above downward corresponds with that of the putamen.

Figure 395 reproduces a frontal section through the cerebral hemisphere in a plane passing *through the anterior end of the thalamus*. The *insula* lies at

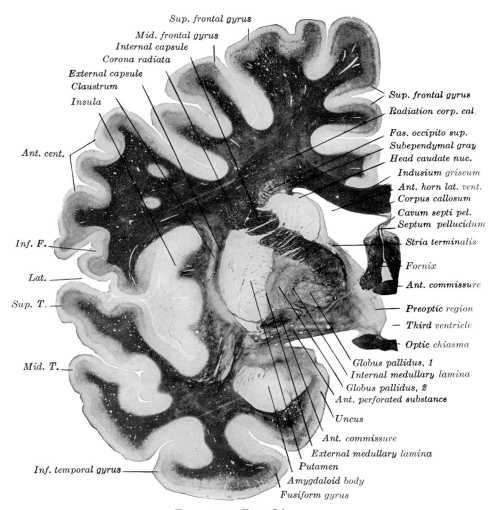

Sup. frontal gyrus
Mid. frontal gyrus
Internal capsule
Corona radiata
External capsule
Claustrum
Insula

Ant. cent.

Inf. F.

Lat.

Sup. T,

Mid. T.

Inf. temporal gyrus

Sup. frontal gyrus
Radiation corp. cal.
Fas. occipito sup.
Subependymal gray
Head caudate nuc.
Indusium griseum
Ant. horn lat. vent.
Corpus callosum
Cavum septi pel.
Septum pellucidum
Stria terminalis
Fornix
Ant. commissure
Preoptic region
Third ventricle
Optic chiasma
Globus pallidus, 1
Internal medullary lamina
Globus pallidus, 2
Ant. perforated substance
Uncus
Ant. commissure
External medullary lamina
Putamen
Amygdaloid body
Fusiform gyrus

FIGURE 394.   From Jelgersma.

the bottom of the lateral fissure and is closely related to the putamen from which it is separated by the claustrum and external capsule. The frontal, temporal, and parietal lobes project farther lateralward, forming the boundaries of the lateral fissure and overhanging the insula. The overhanging portions of these lobes form the opercula which have been cut away in Fig. 48. The temporal operculum (Figs 393–397) is separated by the deep lateral fissure from the frontal operculum (Figs. 393, 394) and from the parietal operculum (Figs. 395–399). At its bottom this fissure spreads out like a saucer, separating the opercula from the insula, and becomes continuous around the margins of the insula with the circular sulcus.

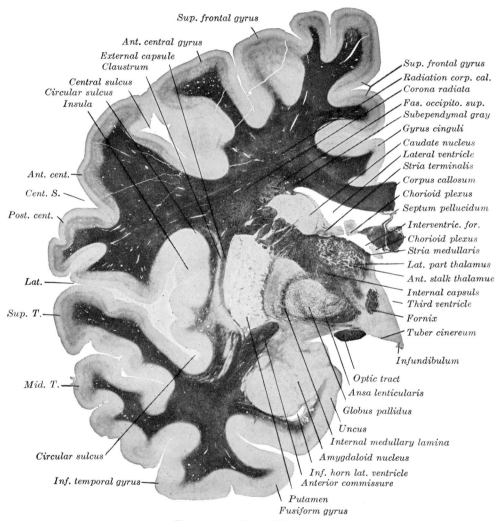

Sup. frontal gyrus
Ant. central gyrus
External capsule
Claustrum
Central sulcus
Circular sulcus
Insula
Ant. cent.
Cent. S.
Post. cent.
Lat.
Sup. T.
Mid. T.
Circular sulcus
Inf. temporal gyrus

Sup. frontal gyrus
Radiation corp. cal.
Corona radiata
Fas. occipito. sup.
Subependymal gray
Gyrus cinguli
Caudate nucleus
Lateral ventricle
Stria terminalis
Corpus callosum
Chorioid plexus
Septum pellucidum
Interventric. for.
Chorioid plexus
Stria medullaris
Lat. part thalamus
Ant. stalk thalamue
Internal capsuls
Third ventricle
Fornix
Tuber cinereum
Infundibulum
Optic tract
Ansa lenticularis
Globus pallidus
Uncus
Internal medullary lamina
Amygdaloid nucleus
Inf. horn lat. ventricle
Anterior commissure
Putamen
Fusiform gyrus

FIGURE 395.   From Jelgersma.

The *upper surface of the temporal lobe* also lies buried in the lateral fissure but can be exposed along with the insula by dissecting away the frontal and parietal lobes (Fig. 52). Upon this surface there can then be seen the anterior transverse temporal gyrus. It is continuous with the auditory receptive cortex at the junction of the superior and lateral surfaces of the temporal lobe (Figs. 259, 395) and from this point it extends obliquely backward and medialward

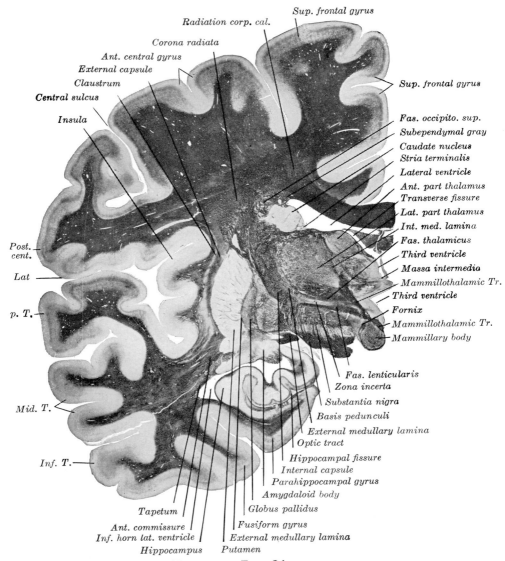

FIGURE 396. From Jelgersma.

in the depth of the lateral fissure (Figs. 52, 396–399). The cortex which covers it forms a part of the auditory receptive center.

Figure 396 represents a frontal section of the cerebral hemisphere cut in a plane passing *through the mammillary body. The dorsal thalamus* is divided into three parts: anterior, medial, and lateral. These subdivisions are incompletely separated by an internal medullary lamina. The massa intermedia joins the right and left sides together across the third ventricle. The anterior, medial, and lateral subdivisions can be distinguished in Figs. 396, 400.

In the *external medullary lamina* and between this and the internal capsule is the lateral reticular nucleus (Figs. 387, 396). The external medullary lamina can be followed through the series toward the occiput. In Fig. 400 its inferior margin is continuous with the lateral zone of Wernicke. At the anterior end of the thalamus fibers destined for the *anterior thalamic radiation* or anterior stalk of the thalamus run forward in heavy bundles through the anterior end of the lateral nucleus to enter the internal capsule (Fig. 395).

The *hypothalamus*, exclusive of the so-called pars optica hypothalami, lies in the interpeduncular fossa behind the optic chiasma (Fig. 31). The section

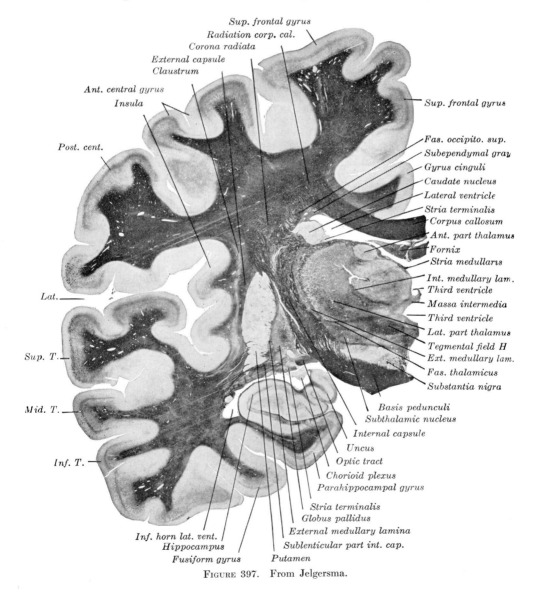

Sup. frontal gyrus
Radiation corp. cal.
Corona radiata
External capsule
Claustrum
Ant. central gyrus
Insula
Post. cent.
Lat.
Sup. T.
Mid. T.
Inf. T.
Inf. horn lat. vent.
Hippocampus
Fusiform gyrus

Sup. frontal gyrus
Fas. occipito. sup.
Subependymal gray
Gyrus cinguli
Caudate nucleus
Lateral ventricle
Stria terminalis
Corpus callosum
Ant. part thalamus
Fornix
Stria medullaris
Int. medullary lam.
Third ventricle
Massa intermedia
Third ventricle
Lat. part thalamus
Tegmental field H
Ext. medullary lam.
Fas. thalamicus
Substantia nigra
Basis pedunculi
Subthalamic nucleus
Internal capsule
Uncus
Optic tract
Chorioid plexus
Parahippocampal gyrus
Stria terminalis
Globus pallidus
External medullary lamina
Sublenticular part int. cap.
Putamen

FIGURE 397.   From Jelgersma.

represented in Fig. 395 cuts through the tuber cinereum and the infundibulum and that shown in Fig. 396 through the mammillary bodies. The column of the fornix having descended behind the anterior commissure (Fig. 394) runs downward and backward through the hypothalamus (Fig. 395) to reach the lateral side of the mammillary body (Fig. 396). From the mammillary body the mammillothalamic tract runs upward to the anterior division of the thalamus (Figs. 242, 396).

The *subthalamus* is interposed between the dorsal thalamus and basis pedunculi. Within it are included the rostral extremities of the red nucleus and substantia nigra (Figs. 398, 399) and also the subthalamic nucleus of Luys (Fig. 397) and the zona incerta (Fig. 396). Between the two latter the fasciculus lenticularis runs medialward to enter the field H of Forel (Figs. 349, 396). The fibers of this fasciculus come from the globus pallidus, passing more or less transversely through the internal capsule.

The *red nucleus* projects upward into the subthalamus where it is surrounded by a thick capsule from the side of which there extends lateralward the tegmental radiation (Figs. 346, 398, 399).

Figure 397 represents a frontal section of the cerebral hemisphere passing *through the cerebral peduncle behind the mammillary body.* Descriptions of the structures illustrated are given in connection with the other plates of this series.

Figure 398 represents a section passing *through the rostral end of the red nucleus.* The *third ventricle,* only one lateral half of which is represented, is here bounded laterally by the thalamus and ventrally by the subthalamus. Its membranous roof, which has been torn away, was attached along the taenia thalami to the stria medullaris thalami. Farther forward in a section passing through the mammillary body (Fig. 396) the massa intermedia forms a bridge of gray matter across the ventricle and joins the two lateral halves of the thalamus. Below it the cavity is bounded laterally by the subthalamus and hypothalamus. In the plane of the interventricular foramen (Fig. 395) the ventricle is a deep and rather narrow cleft with lateral boundaries formed chiefly by the hypothalamus. In a section passing through the optic chiasma and the posterior border of the anterior commissure the ventricle is bounded above and below by these structures and is reduced in height (Fig. 394). The gray matter forming its lateral wall at this point belongs to the telencephalon and differs functionally from the hypothalamus. It has been called the preoptic region. The cavity of the ventricle extends forward under the anterior commissure (Fig. 393) and forms the optic recess.

When, on the other hand, the third ventricle is followed toward the occiput, it becomes less deep as the striae medullares approach closer to the floor. In the plane represented by Fig. 400 the striae medullares are approached by the fasciculus retroflexus and both enter the habenular ganglion between the frontal planes represented by this and the next succeeding figure. The caudal border of this ganglion can be seen in Fig. 401 as can also the caudal border of the posterior commissure, which is separated by a fissure from the commissure of the superior colliculus.

The frontal section represented in Fig. 399 was cut in approximately the same plane as Fig. 207, from one lateral half of the cerebrum after the hind-brain and much of the midbrain had been removed by a section through the mesencephalon.

The posterior end of the putamen has become a flat plate, and, as it is followed farther toward the occiput, it becomes broken up into a series of small gray islands (Figs. 400, 401). The lateral surface of the lentiform nucleus is covered by the external capsule, the dorsal border of which fuses with the internal capsule along the line where this merges with the corona radiata. The *external and internal capsules taken together* form a white investment

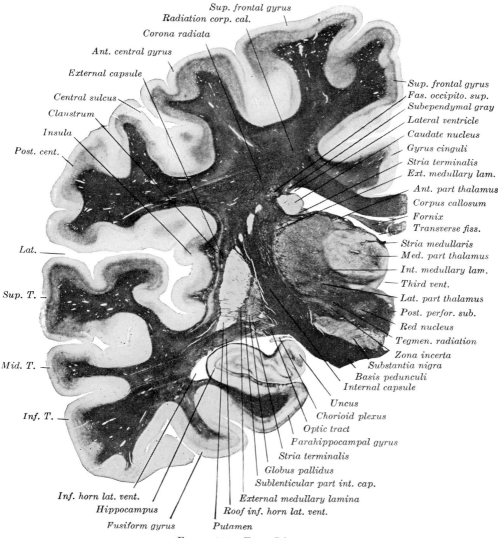

FIGURE 398. From Jelgersma.

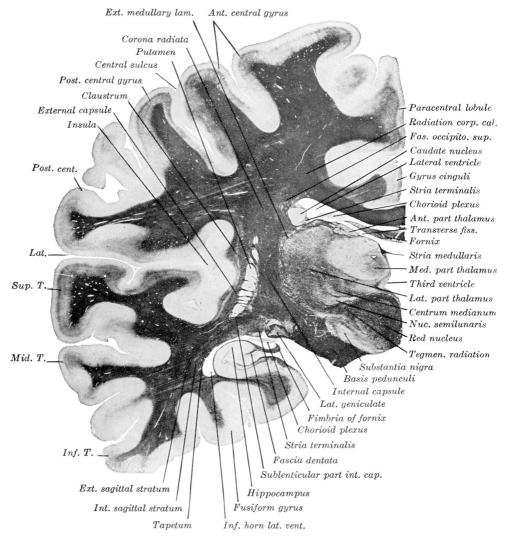

Ext. medullary lam.   *Ant. central gyrus*
Corona radiata
Putamen
Central sulcus
Post. central gyrus
Claustrum
External capsule
Insula
Post. cent.
Lat.
Sup. T.
Mid. T.
Inf. T.
Ext. sagittal stratum
Int. sagittal stratum
Tapetum

Paracentral lobule
Radiation corp. cal.
Fas. occipito. sup.
Caudate nucleus
Lateral ventricle
Gyrus cinguli
Stria terminalis
Chorioid plexus
Ant. part thalamus
Transverse fiss.
Fornix
Stria medullaris
Med. part thalamus
Third ventricle
Lat. part thalamus
Centrum medianum
Nuc. semilunaris
Red nucleus
Tegmen. radiation
Substantia nigra
Basis pedunculi
Internal capsule
Lat. geniculate
Fimbria of fornix
Chorioid plexus
Stria terminalis
Fascia dentata
Sublenticular part int. cap.
Hippocampus
Fusiform gyrus
Inf. horn lat. vent.

FIGURE 399. From Jelgersma.

for the lentiform nucleus, which is incomplete on the ventral side between the planes represented by Figs. 393 and 398. Here this nucleus is separated from the inferior horn of the lateral ventricle by such structures as the sublenticular part of the internal capsule and stria terminalis and from the anterior perforated substance by the anterior commissure.

The central sulcus and the anterior and posterior central gyri are cut obliquely in these frontal sections. The gyri of the temporal lobe, cut transversely, present a typical appearance and in order from above downward and medialward are the superior, middle, and inferior temporal, fusiform, and hippocampal gyri (Fig. 400). Somewhat farther anteriorly the uncus is also seen.

It is separated from the hippocampal gyrus by the rostral end of the hippocampal fissure (Fig. 397). Still farther anteriorly the uncus replaces the hippocampal gyrus and is closely related to the amygdaloid nucleus (Fig. 395).

Figure 400 represents a section passing *through the geniculate bodies*. These lie ventral to the thalamus and lateral to the zone of transition between the midbrain and thalamus. The *medial geniculate body* is surrounded on three sides by the mesencephalon, thalamus, and the lateral geniculate body. Its ventral surface projects as a slight eminence upon the basal surface of the brain. The *lateral geniculate body* consists of a series of superimposed curved lamellae. It lies ventral to the retrolenticular part of the internal capsule. On its dorsal surface is a thick curved band of deeply stained fibers, the lateral

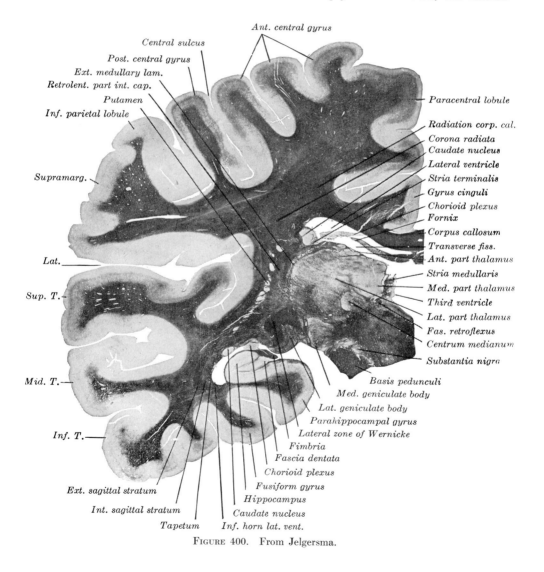

FIGURE 400. From Jelgersma.

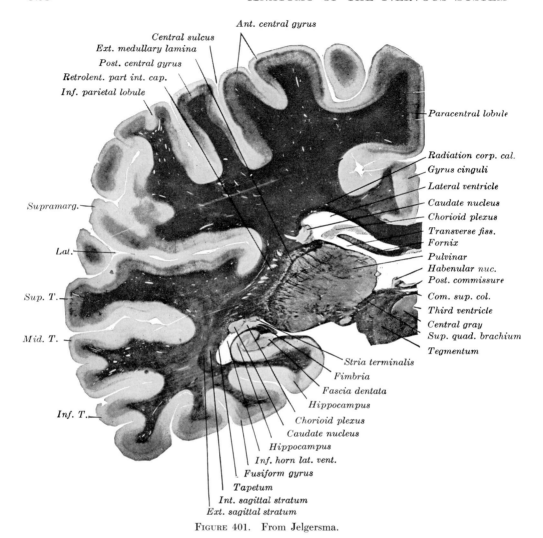

Ant. central gyrus
Central sulcus
Ext. medullary lamina
Post. central gyrus
Retrolent. part int. cap.
Inf. parietal lobule

Paracentral lobule

Radiation corp. cal.
Gyrus cinguli
Lateral ventricle
Caudate nucleus
Chorioid plexus
Transverse fiss.
Fornix
Pulvinar
Habenular nuc.
Post. commissure
Com. sup. col.
Third ventricle
Central gray
Sup. quad. brachium
Tegmentum

Supramarg.

Lat.

Sup. T.

Mid. T.

Stria terminalis
Fimbria
Fascia dentata
Hippocampus
Chorioid plexus
Caudate nucleus
Hippocampus
Inf. horn lat. vent.
Fusiform gyrus
Tapetum
Int. sagittal stratum
Ext. sagittal stratum

Inf. T.

FIGURE 401.   From Jelgersma.

zone of Wernicke, which is continuous dorsally and toward the occiput with the external medullary lamina of the thalamus (Figs. 369, 387). It is composed of fibers from the optic nerve and of others arising in the lateral geniculate body and belonging to the geniculocalcarine fasciculus.

The fibers of the *geniculocalcarine* fasciculus arise in the lateral geniculate body, curve forward and lateralward in the roof of the inferior horn of the lateral ventricle and, after completing their U-shaped bend, lie lateral to the inferior horn of the lateral ventricle in the external sagittal stratum of the temporal lobe (Figs. 192, 399–402). The *internal and external sagittal strata* are massive bundles of parallel anteroposteriorly directed fibers. The more internal of the two has been incorrectly called the optic radiation and the more external, which includes the geniculocalcarine tract, is often designated

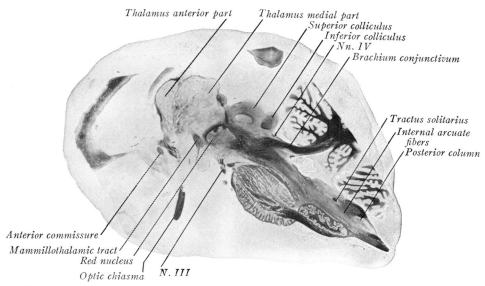

Thalamus anterior part *Thalamus medial part*
Superior colliculus
Inferior colliculus
Nn. IV
Brachium conjunctivum

Tractus solitarius
Internal arcuate fibers
Posterior column

Anterior commissure
Mammillothalamic tract
Red nucleus
Optic chiasma *N. III*

FIGURE 408. In this section the course of the brachium conjunctivum is shown. The third nerve is visible and only the edge of the pyramid is seen. The inferior olivary nucleus is cut through its longest diameter.

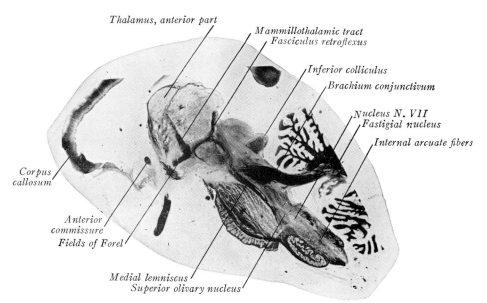

Thalamus, anterior part
Mammillothalamic tract
Fasciculus retroflexus

Inferior colliculus
Brachium conjunctivum

Nucleus N. VII
Fastigial nucleus

Internal arcuate fibers

Corpus callosum

Anterior commissure
Fields of Forel

Medial lemniscus
Superior olivary nucleus

FIGURE 409. In this section the fornix can be followed to the region of the mammillary body. The brachium conjunctivum is conspicuous, with part of the trigeminal nucleus lying just ventral to it in the midpontine region. The tractus solitarius is visible dorsally just opposite the cranial end of the inferior olivary nucleus. The optic chiasma appears large as the nerve and tract separate from it.

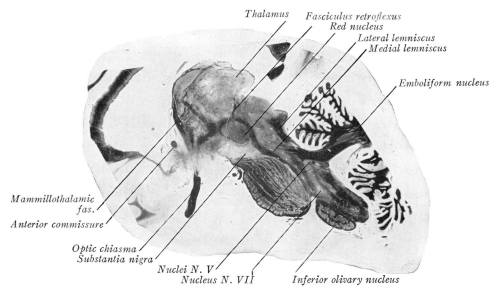

FIGURE 410. In this section the nuclei of the cerebellum are shown, and the lateral lemniscus, with the spinothalamic tracts, is conspicuous just caudal to the inferior colliculus. The basis pedunculi is partly shown, with the substantia nigra dorsal to it.

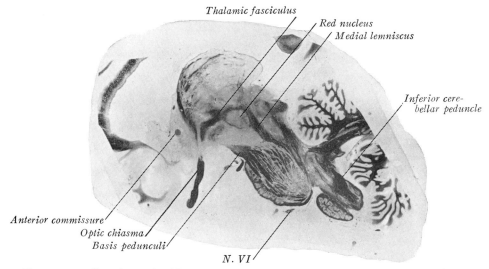

FIGURE 411. Conspicuous in this section is the restiform body forming largely from olivocerebellar fibers. The medial lemniscus is seen ascending toward the ventral part of the thalamus. Just above the red nucleus the clear area is the arcuate nucleus and above that the centrum medianum (or central nucleus), which may be followed in the next four illustrations.

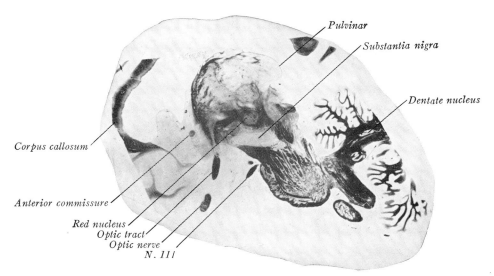

FIGURE 412. Divisions of the thalamus show well in this section, as does the substantia nigra, the guide line for which as it leaves the brain stem crosses the inferior quadrigeminal brachium carrying fibers of the auditory path past the inferior colliculus to the medial geniculate body seen in more lateral sections. Within the lateral ventricle near the anterior commissure is seen the edge of the caudate nucleus. The optic nerve and tract are shown as the section is lateral to the chiasma.

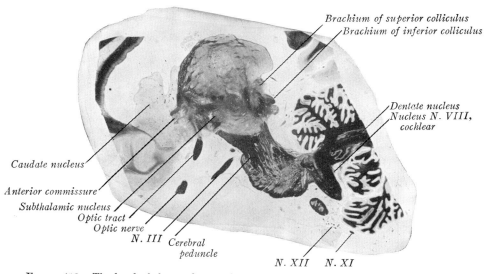

FIGURE 413. The head of the caudate nucleus has been cut in this section; the optic tract and nerve are well separated. The brachia of the two colliculi are shown and the restiform body is conspicuous.

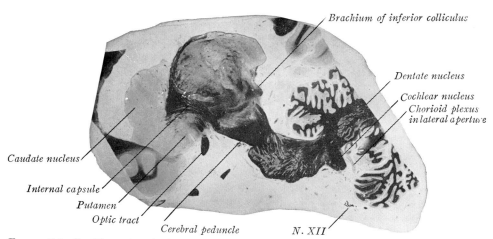

FIGURE 414.   In this section the internal capsule and its relations to caudate nucleus and thalamus are displayed. The mass of thalamic nuclei show subdivisions in this and the next section.

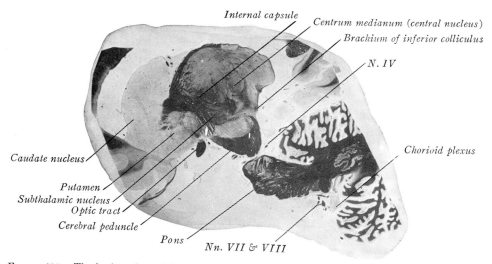

FIGURE 415.   The basis pedunculi has been cut through in this section and the optic nerve lies close to it; the lentiform nucleus is shown fused with the head of the caudate nucleus.

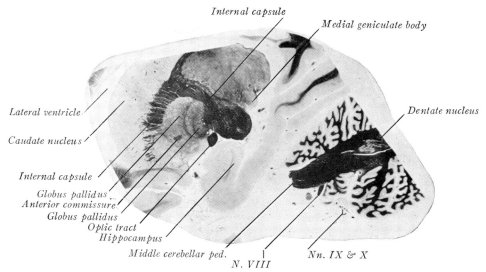

Internal capsule

Medial geniculate body

Lateral ventricle

Dentate nucleus

Caudate nucleus

Internal capsule

Globus pallidus
Anterior commissure
Globus pallidus
Optic tract
Hippocampus
Middle cerebellar ped.
N. VIII
Nn. IX & X

FIGURE 416. In this section relationship of the internal capsule, basal ganglia, and thalamus is well shown. The optic tract lies ventral to the basis pedunculi and the medial geniculate body just dorsal to it below the pulvinar.

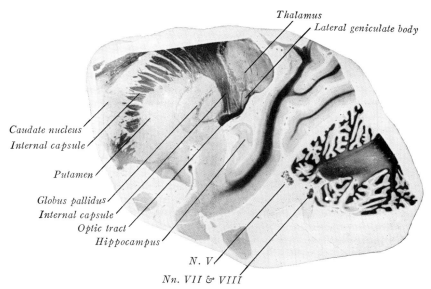

Thalamus
Lateral geniculate body

Caudate nucleus
Internal capsule

Putamen

Globus pallidus
Internal capsule
Optic tract
Hippocampus
N. V.
Nn. VII & VIII

FIGURE 417. In this section the optic tract has completed its course around the basis pedunculi and is shown entering the lateral geniculate body, only a small part of which is displayed. The lentiform nucleus is conspicuously large. The hippocampal gyrus lies in this section between optic tract and cerebellum. Compare with figures of gross brains (Figs. 49–51).

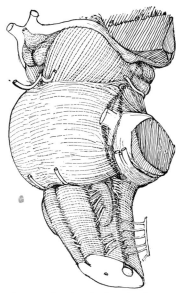

Figure 418. Oblique view of brainstem showing landmarks for use with sagittal sections. The dark band on the side is the column of nuclei belonging to the trigeminal nerve.

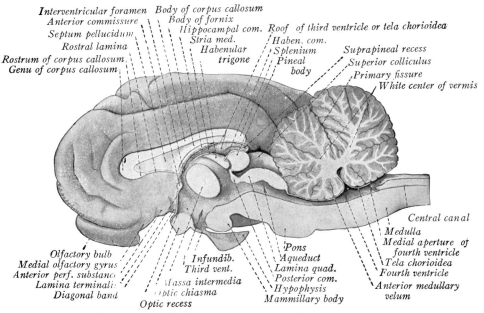

Interventricular foramen   Body of corpus callosum
Anterior commissure   Body of fornix
Septum pellucidum   Hippocampal com.   Roof of third ventricle or tela chorioidea
Rostral lamina   Stria med.   Haben. com.
Rostrum of corpus callosum   Habenular   Splenium   Suprapineal recess
Genu of corpus callosum   trigone   Pineal   Superior colliculus
   body   Primary fissure
   White center of vermis

Olfactory bulb   Central canal
Medial olfactory gyrus   Infundib.   Pons   Medulla
Anterior perf. substance   Third vent.   Aqueduct   Medial aperture of
Lamina terminalis   Lamina quad.   fourth ventricle
Diagonal band   Massa intermedia   Posterior com.   Tela chorioidea
   Optic chiasma   Hypophysis   Fourth ventricle
Optic recess   Mammillary body   Anterior medullary
   velum

Figure 419. Medial sagittal section of the sheep's brain.

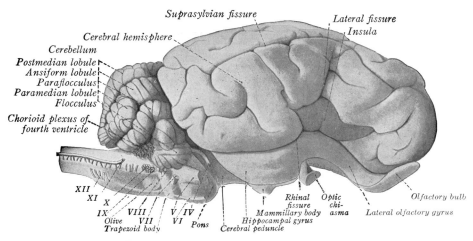

Suprasylvian fissure

Lateral fissure
Insula

Cerebral hemisphere
Cerebellum
Postmedian lobule
Ansiform lobule
Paraflocculus
Paramedian lobule
Flocculus

Chorioid plexus of
fourth ventricle

XII
XI
X
IX   VIII   V IV
Olive   VII   VI
Trapezoid body   Pons
Cerebral peduncle

Rhinal   Optic
fissure   chi-
Mammillary body   asma
Hippocampal gyrus

Olfactory bulb

Lateral olfactory gyrus

FIGURE 420.   Lateral view of the sheep's brain.

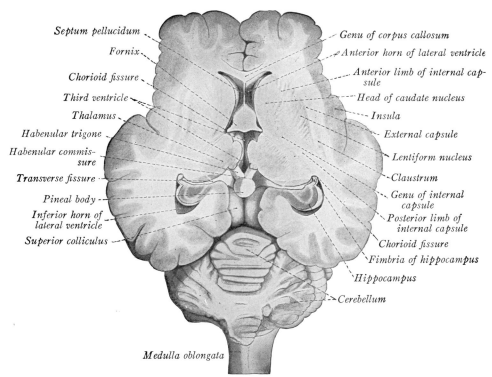

Septum pellucidum
Fornix
Chorioid fissure
Third ventricle
Thalamus
Habenular trigone
Habenular commis-
sure
Transverse fissure
Pineal body
Inferior horn of
lateral ventricle
Superior colliculus

Genu of corpus callosum
Anterior horn of lateral ventricle
Anterior limb of internal cap-
sule
Head of caudate nucleus
Insula
External capsule
Lentiform nucleus
Claustrum
Genu of internal
capsule
Posterior limb of
internal capsule
Chorioid fissure
Fimbria of hippocampus
Hippocampus
Cerebellum

Medulla oblongata

FIGURE 421.   Horizontal section through the sheep's brain, passing through the internal capsule
and corpus striatum.

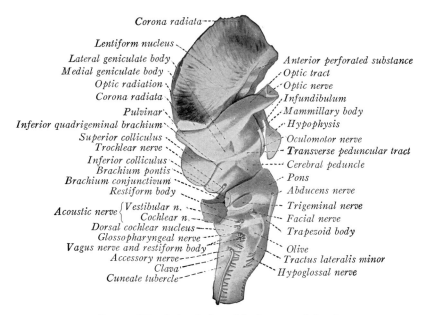

Corona radiata
Lentiform nucleus
Lateral geniculate body
Medial geniculate body
Optic radiation
Corona radiata
Pulvinar
Inferior quadrigeminal brachium
Superior colliculus
Trochlear nerve
Inferior colliculus
Brachium pontis
Brachium conjunctivum
Restiform body
Acoustic nerve { Vestibular n.
                 Cochlear n.
Dorsal cochlear nucleus
Glossopharyngeal nerve
Vagus nerve and restiform body
Accessory nerve
Clava
Cuneate tubercle

Anterior perforated substance
Optic tract
Optic nerve
Infundibulum
Mammillary body
Hypophysis
Oculomotor nerve
Transverse peduncular tract
Cerebral peduncle
Pons
Abducens nerve
Trigeminal nerve
Facial nerve
Trapezoid body
Olive
Tractus lateralis minor
Hypoglossal nerve

FIGURE 422.   Lateral view of brain stem of the sheep.

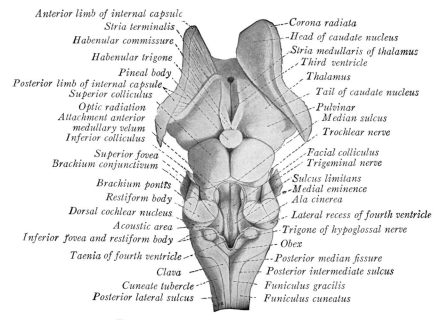

Anterior limb of internal capsule
Stria terminalis
Habenular commissure
Habenular trigone
Pineal body
Posterior limb of internal capsule
Superior colliculus
Optic radiation
Attachment anterior
  medullary velum
Inferior colliculus
Superior fovea
Brachium conjunctivum
Brachium pontis
Restiform body
Dorsal cochlear nucleus
Acoustic area
Inferior fovea and restiform body
Taenia of fourth ventricle
Clava
Cuneate tubercle
Posterior lateral sulcus

Corona radiata
Head of caudate nucleus
Stria medullaris of thalamus
Third ventricle
Thalamus
Tail of caudate nucleus
Pulvinar
Median sulcus
Trochlear nerve
Facial colliculus
Trigeminal nerve
Sulcus limitans
Medial eminence
Ala cinerea
Lateral recess of fourth ventricle
Trigone of hypoglossal nerve
Obex
Posterior median fissure
Posterior intermediate sulcus
Funiculus gracilis
Funiculus cuneatus

FIGURE 423.   Dorsal view of brain stem of sheep.

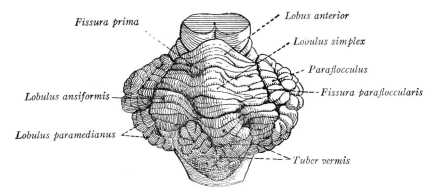

FIGURE 424. Cerebellum of the sheep, dorsorostral view.

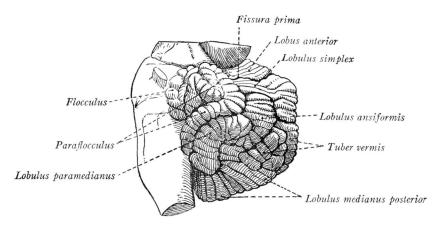

FIGURE 425. Cerebellum of the sheep, lateral view.

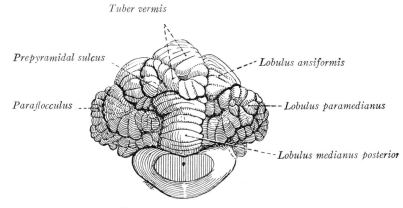

FIGURE 426. Cerebellum of the sheep, caudal view.

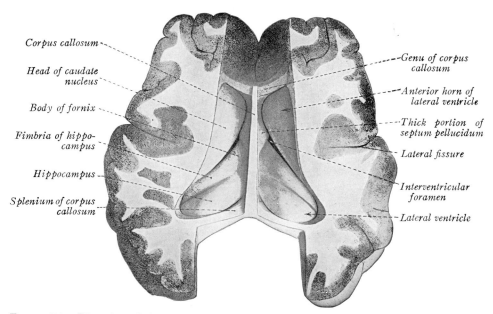

Corpus callosum

Head of caudate nucleus

Body of fornix

Fimbria of hippocampus

Hippocampus

Splenium of corpus callosum

Genu of corpus callosum

Anterior horn of lateral ventricle

Thick portion of septum pellucidum

Lateral fissure

Interventricular foramen

Lateral ventricle

FIGURE 427. Dissection of the telencephalon of the sheep to show the lateral ventricle and the structures which form its floor. Dorsal view.

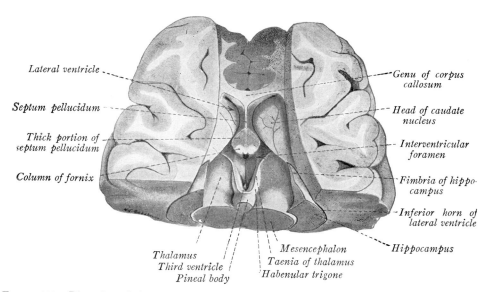

Lateral ventricle

Septum pellucidum

Thick portion of septum pellucidum

Column of fornix

Genu of corpus callosum

Head of caudate nucleus

Interventricular foramen

Fimbria of hippocampus

Inferior horn of lateral ventricle

Hippocampus

Thalamus
Third ventricle
Pineal body

Mesencephalon
Taenia of thalamus
Habenular trigone

FIGURE 428. Dissection of the rostral part of the sheep's brain to show the relation of the lateral ventricles, fornix, fimbria, and hippocampus to the thalamus and third ventricle. Dorsal view.

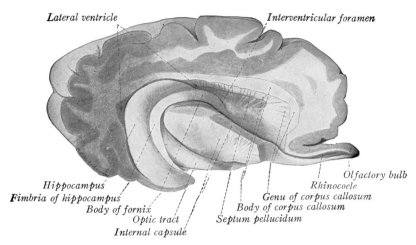

FIGURE 429.   Dissection of the cerebral hemisphere of the sheep to show the lateral ventricle. Lateral view.

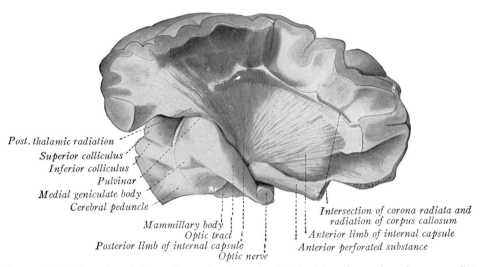

FIGURE 430.   Dissection of the cerebrum of a sheep showing the internal capsule and corona radiata. The lentiform nucleus has been removed.

remain colorless unless the preparation has been counterstained. The method is adapted for the study of the development and extent of myelination and for tracing myelinated fiber tracts. This method may also be used for a study of degenerated fiber tracts, which remain colorless in preparations in which the normal fiber tracts are well stained. Weil's method also stains myelin sheaths blue. The preparations are very similar to those made by the Weigert method.

28. The *Marchi method* is a differential stain for degenerating fibers. These contain droplets of chemically altered myelin. The tissue is fixed in a solution containing potassium bichromate (Müller's fluid). This treatment prevents the normal myelinated fibers from staining with osmic acid, but does not prevent the droplets of chemically altered myelin in the degenerated fiber from being stained black by this reagent. In a section prepared by this method the normal myelinated fibers are light yellow, while the degenerated fibers are represented by rows of black dots.

29. The *silver stains,* including the *Bodian, Cajal, Rasmussen,* and *Davenport methods* and the *pyridine-silver technique* of Ranson depend upon the special affinity for silver possessed by nerve cells and their processes. After treatment with silver the tissue is transferred to a solution of pyrogallic acid or hydroquinone which reduces the silver in the neurons. Nerve cells and their processes are stained yellow, brown, or black by these methods. Myelin sheaths remain unstained. The neurofibrils are stained somewhat more darkly than other parts of the cytoplasm. The Nauta technique stains degenerating terminals more darkly than normal fibers.

30. The *Golgi method* furnishes preparations which demonstrate the external form of the neurons, and make it possible to trace individual axons and dendrites for considerable distances. The method also stains neuroglia. It is selective and rather uncertain in its results, since only a small proportion of the nerve cells are impregnated in any preparation. The stain is due to the impregnation of the nerve cells and their processes with silver.

31. The best stains for demonstrating the tigroid masses or Nissl bodies are *toluidine blue, cresyl violet,* and *Nissl's methylene blue.* These are basic dyes, and in properly fixed nervous tissue they color the tigroid masses as well as the nuclear chromatin of nerve cells blue. Additional staining methods are available which act also as microchemical tests. The Prussian blue method reveals iron, the Feulgen method thymonucleic acid. By examination of the tissues in specific wave lengths of ultraviolet light, a distinction may be made between structures containing substances of different chemical composition (e.g. ribose and desoxyribose nucleic acid). This latter method is termed microspectrophotometry.

Further chemical examination of small portions of cells is possible by the freezing-drying method with application of chemical tests to the ashed remnants of a microscopic section after incineration on the prepared slide.

THE PERIPHERAL NERVOUS SYSTEM

32. *Spinal Nerves.* Study transverse sections of a cutaneous nerve stained with osmic acid and by the pyridine-silver method (see p. 133 and Fig. 106).

33. Study transverse sections of the ventral and dorsal roots of a spinal nerve stained with osmic acid and by the pyridine-silver method (see p. 134 and Fig. 107).

34. *Spinal Ganglia.* Study a longitudinal section of a spinal ganglion stained by the pyridine-silver method. The cells of the spinal ganglion and their axons have been described on pages 135–137 (Fig. 108). Observe the glomeruli at the beginning of the axons, and the nucleated capsules surrounding the cells and glomeruli. Myelinated axons are stained yellow and unmyelinated axons black by this method. Trace the unmyelinated axons of the small cells and the myelinated axons of the large cells toward the central fiber bundle of the ganglion. As these fibers enter this central bundle look for their bifurcation. A myelinated fiber bifurcates at a node of Ranvier where the axon is constricted,

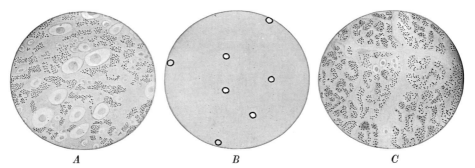

A   *B*   *C*

FIGURE 433. From sections of the vagus nerve of the dog: *A*, Below the level of the nodose ganglion, pyridine-silver stain; *B*, at the level of the esophageal plexus, osmic acid; *C*, at the level of the esophageal plexus, pyridine-silver stain.

but there is a slight triangular expansion at the point of bifurcation of an unmyelinated axon.

35. Study a section of a spinal ganglion stained with toluidine blue or cresyl violet. Note the variation in size of these ganglion cells. The arrangement of Nissl granules in the most numerous type of large cells is shown in Fig. 82, *B*, and in common types of small cells in Fig. 82, *D* and *E*. Nuclei associated with the capsules surrounding the ganglion cells are shown in Fig. 82, *G*.

36. *The Cranial Nerves.* These differ in structure depending on the types of fibers they contain. The olfactory nerves are unmyelinated. The majority of the fibers in the *vagus* are unmyelinated and this holds particularly true for the terminal portions of the nerve on the esophagus and stomach. The pharyngeal and superior laryngeal branches receive most of the large and medium sized fibers of the vagus so that below the level of the nodose ganglion it contains many more unmyelinated than myelinated fibers. These are represented by black dots in Fig. 433, *A*. The few large fibers that are present below the level of the nodose ganglion are given off in the recurrent laryngeal nerve, and most of the remaining small and medium sized myelinated fibers are given off to the pulmonary plexuses. At the level of the esophageal plexus the vagus contains a very few fine myelinated fibers (Fig. 433, *B*) and enormous numbers of unmyelinated axons (black dots in Fig. 433, *C*). Many of them are sensory

fibers arising from cells in the nodose ganglion. Others are preganglionic visceral efferent fibers which have either lost their sheaths during their course down the vagus or have come all the way from the medulla as unmyelinated fibers. Study cross-sections of the vagus nerve cut below the level of the nodose ganglion and at the level of the esophageal plexus. In the dog the vagus and the cervical sympathetic trunk run parallel in the neck and are enclosed in a common sheath. If a section of this vagosympathetic trunk, stained with osmic acid, is available for study, the vagus can be differentiated because its myelinated fibers vary in size, while those in the sympathetic trunk are all small and are more closely packed together.

37. *The Sympathetic Nervous System.* The structure of sympathetic nerves and ganglia has been described on pp. 153–155. They may be studied in the laboratory along with the rest of the peripheral nervous system but a consideration of the autonomic nervous system can be deferred until after a study of the cranial nerves and brain stem. Study sections of the cervical sympathetic trunk stained with osmic acid and with silver. It is composed of closely packed fine myelinated preganglionic fibers which are running from the upper thoracic white rami to the superior cervical sympathetic ganglion. With these there are associated a small number of unmyelinated fibers.

38. Study sections of the greater splanchnic nerve stained with osmic acid and with silver. The greater splanchnic nerve is composed of fibers from the lower thoracic white rami which have run for a longer or shorter distance through the sympathetic trunk. Some of these, including myelinated fibers of all sizes as well as unmyelinated axons, are visceral afferent fibers from the spinal ganglia; others are fine myelinated preganglionic fibers from the ventral roots. The greater splanchnic nerve, although much larger, has the same histologic structure as a white ramus. It is important to note that the white rami, sympathetic trunk, and greater splanchnic nerve are better myelinated than is the vagus nerve below the level of the nodose ganglion.

39. Study a section of the internal carotid nerve stained with osmic acid. The internal carotid nerve, like other branches from the sympathetic trunk to the blood vessels, is composed of postganglionic visceral efferent fibers most of which are unmyelinated.

40. Study a section of the human superior cervical sympathetic ganglion stained by the pyridine-silver method. Note multipolar ganglion cells, dendritic glomeruli, capsules surrounding cells and glomeruli, and intra- and extracapsular dendrites. It is difficult to distinguish between long dendrites and the axons of the sympathetic ganglion cells. These postganglionic axons are large and stain lightly in pyridine-silver preparations. Note the fine darkly-stained preganglionic fibers from the cervical sympathetic trunk which intertwine with the long dendrites in the intercellular plexus and penetrate the capsules to intertwine with the short dendrites within the glomeruli (Fig. 118).

THE SPINAL CORD

41. Review the development and *gross anatomy of the spinal cord* (pp. 12 and 21–28). Examine the demonstration preparations of the vertebral column,

showing the spinal cord exposed from the dorsal side. In these preparations study the meninges and ligamentum denticulatum, as well as the shape and size of the spinal cord. Note the level of the termination of the spinal cord, the level of the origin of the various nerve roots and of their exit from the vertebral canal, and the level of the various segments of the cord with reference to the vertebrae. Note the filum terminale and the cauda equina. Study the meninges and blood supply of the cord.

42. *The Spinal Cord in Section.* Examine the Pal-Weigert sections of the cervical, thoracic, lumbar, and sacral regions, and from them reconstruct a mental picture of the topography of the entire cord. How does it vary in shape and size at the different levels? Identify all the fissures, sulci, septa, funiculi, gray columns, commissures and nerve roots, the reticular formation, the substantia gelatinosa, and the caput, cervix, and apex of the posterior gray column. (See pp. 166–172.)

43. *The Microscopic Anatomy of the Spinal Cord.* Study all of the histologic preparations of the spinal cord which have been furnished you. (See pp. 172–174.) Study the neuroglia in Golgi preparations. Study the pia mater, septa, blood vessels, and ependyma in hematoxylin and eosin preparations. Study the nerve cells in Nissl, Golgi, and silver preparations. Study the myelinated fibers in Weigert preparations and both the myelinated and unmyelinated fibers in the silver preparations. Note the arrangement of each of these histologic elements and be sure that you understand the relations which they bear to each other.

44. *Draw* in outline, ventral side down, each of four Pal-Weigert sections taken, respectively, through the cervical, thoracic, lumbar, and sacral regions of the human spinal cord. Make the outlines very accurate in shape and size, with an enlargement of 8 times. Put in the outline of the gray columns, the central canal, and the substantia gelatinosa Rolandi. Put each outline on a separate sheet and do not ink the drawings at present.

45. Identify the various *cell columns* in the gray matter and note how they vary in the different levels of the cord (Nissl or counterstained Weigert preparations). (See pp. 169–178 and Figs. 135, 136.) Indicate these cell groups in their proper places in the four outline sketches of the spinal cord. What becomes of the axons arising from each group of cells? Why are the anterolateral and posterolateral cell groups seen only in the regions associated with the brachial and lumbosacral plexuses? The intermediolateral column only in the thoracic and highest lumbar segments? Why is the gray matter most abundant in the region of the intumescentiae and the white matter most abundant at the upper end of the spinal cord?

46. What elements are concerned in spinal reflexes? (See pp. 178–182.)

47. What connections do the fibers of the *spinal nerves* establish in the spinal cord? What is the origin and the peripheral termination of the somatic efferent fibers, of the visceral efferent fibers, of the somatic afferent fibers, and of the visceral afferent fibers of the spinal nerves? (See pp. 137–140 and Fig. 109.) What are the proprioceptive and exteroceptive fibers, and in what peripheral structures do they end? (See pp. 140–149.)

48. In a pyridine-silver preparation of the cervical spinal cord of a cat,

note that as the *dorsal root* enters the cord the unmyelinated fibers run through the lateral division of the root into the dorsolateral fasciculus (Fig. 143). The medial division of the root is formed of myelinated fibers which enter the posterior funiculus. Read about the intramedullary course of these fibers (pp. 183–187).

49. The *fiber tracts*, of which the white substance is composed, cannot be distinguished in the normal adult cord. They can be recognized from differences in the degree of their myelination in fetal cords and in preparations showing degeneration resulting from disease or injury in various parts of the nervous system (p. 194; Figs. 146, 147). From such preparations as are available for this purpose and from your reading (pp. 187–201) form a clear conception of the origin, course, and termination of each of the fiber tracts.

50. Indicate the location of each of these tracts in the outline drawing of the cervical portion of the spinal cord, entering the ascending tracts and the ventral corticospinal tract on the right side, and all of the descending tracts except the ventral corticospinal tract on the left side. Why should the ventral and lateral corticospinal tracts be indicated on opposite sides of the cord? Wax crayons should be used to give the several tracts a differential coloring. Use the following color scheme:

Somatic afferent tracts:
  Proprioceptive—yellow.
  Exteroceptive—blue.
Somatic motor tracts:
  Corticospinal tracts—red.
  Rubrospinal tract—brown.
All other tracts—black.

51. The fasciculus cuneatus and fasciculus gracilis should be colored yellow and then dotted over with blue to indicate that while the proprioceptive fibers predominate, there are also some exteroceptive fibers in these tracts.

52. Study the first five clinical illustrations (pp. 431–437) and write an explanation of the symptoms in terms of the locations of the lesions and the functions of the parts destroyed.

53. Now take the human brain and identify all of its principal divisions. Dissect out the *arterial circle of Willis,* and identify the branches of the internal carotid, vertebral, and basilar arteries and their branches (Figs. 65–67 and pp. 77–81).

54. Study the venous drainage of the brain (pp. 81–88).

55. Study the meninges and cerebrospinal fluid (pp. 71–77).

56. Identify all of the cranial nerves (Figs. 29, 31).

57. Locate the cerebellar peduncles. Examine demonstration preparations in which the three peduncles have been exposed by dissection (Fig. 32). Now remove the cerebellum from the previously intact brain. Cut through the peduncles on both sides of the brain as far as possible from the pons and medulla, sacrificing the cerebellum slightly if necessary in order to leave as much of the peduncles as possible attached to the brain stem.

58. Study the *roof of the fourth ventricle* (p. 41 and Figs. 30, 34, 40, 41).

Examine the chorioid plexus of the fourth ventricle. Note the line of attachment of the tela chorioidea. Tear this membrane away. The torn edge which remains attached to the medulla is the taenia of the fourth ventricle (Fig. 33). Study the attachments of the anterior medullary velum and the decussation of the trochlear nerve within the velum. Remove this membrane. The floor of the fourth ventricle is now fully exposed.

59. Remove the pia mater from the brain stem, carefully cutting around the roots of the cranial nerves with a sharp-pointed knife to prevent these nerves being torn away from the brain when this membrane is removed.

60. Carefully examine the *medulla, pons, floor of the fourth ventricle,* and the *mesencephalon,* observing all the details mentioned on pp. 35–43 and illustrated in Figs. 29, 30, 31, 33.

61. Take the transverse *sections through the human brain stem* which have been provided and, by comparison with the gross specimen, determine the level of each section. Draw in outline each of these transverse sections through the brain stem. Put each drawing on a separate page, ventral side down, with the transverse diameter corresponding to the longer dimension of the paper. Study each preparation in detail and identify all of the parts, indicating them lightly in pencil. Do not label the drawings at this time. Make sure that all proportions are correct. The sections through the medulla should be enlarged eight diameters, those through the pons and mesencephalon four diameters.

62. If the instructor feels that too much time would be occupied in making these drawing, the students may be allowed to study the preparations without drawing them at this time. In that case when the functional analysis of the brain stem is taken up, the colored record of that analysis can be made on sheets of tracing paper, covering Figs. 154, 155, 157, 159, 162, 163, 164, 168, 170. When this plan has been used it has saved a great deal of time and has resulted in a more satisfactory record of the functional analysis. Each sheet of tracing paper is pasted along its inner edge to the page carrying the figure to be analyzed. The outside outline of the figure is traced in black ink. After the nine figures have been covered and outlined in this way the various fiber tracts and nuclei can be entered in their proper colors and correct positions in these outlines as the various functional systems are studied in detail.

63. *Section Through the Decussation of the Pyramids.* Keep in mind the tracts which extend into the brain from the spinal cord and note the changes in their form and position. Identify the decussation of the pyramids, the nucleus gracilis and nucleus cuneatus, the spinal root of the trigeminal nerve and its nucleus, the reticular formation. Note the change in the form of the gray substance (Figs. 153, 154, 305, 307, 309, 311).

64. *Section Through the Decussation of the Lemniscus.* Note the rapid change in the form of the gray matter. Identify the internal and external arcuate fibers, the decussation of the lemniscus and the beginning of the medial lemniscus, as well as the structures continued up from the preceding level (Figs. 153, 155, 313, 316).

65. *Section Through the Olive and the Hypoglossal Nucleus.* At this level the central canal opens out into the fourth ventricle. The posterior funiculi

and their nuclei are disappearing or have disappeared. The dorsal spinocerebellar tract lies lateral to the spinal tract of the trigeminal nerve and is directed
obliquely backward toward the restiform body. Identify, in addition to those
structures which are continued from the preceding level, the inferior olivary
nucleus with the olivocerebellar fibers, the dorsal and medial accessory olivary
nuclei, the external arcuate fibers, the nucleus and fibers of the hypoglossal
nerve, the dorsal motor nucleus of the vagus, the tractus solitarius and its
nucleus, the nucleus ambiguus and the lateral reticular nucleus (Figs. 153, 157,
319, 322).

66. *Section Through the Inferior Cerebellar Peduncle.* The inferior cerebellar peduncle and the spinal tract of the fifth nerve are conspicuous in the
dorsolateral part of the section. In the floor of the fourth ventricle locate the
nucleus of the hypoglossal nerve, the dorsal motor nucleus of the vagus, the
medial and the spinal vestibular nuclei. The spinal tract of the fifth nerve and
its nucleus are deeply situated ventral to the restiform body and broken up by
the olivocerebellar fibers (Figs. 159, 326).

67. *Section Through the Lower Margin of the Pons.* Identify such portions
of the pons, brachium pontis, and cerebellum as are contained in the section.
Dorsolateral to the inferior cerebellar peduncle is the dorsal cochlear nucleus,
and ventrolateral to it the ventral cochlear nucleus. Identify the striae medullares and the medial and lateral vestibular nuclei (Figs. 162, 330, 334).

68. *Section Through the Facial Colliculus.* Differentiate between the ventral
and the dorsal portions of the pons, and in the ventral portion identify the
longitudinal fasciculi, transverse fibers, and the nuclei pontis. In the dorsal
part identify the nuclei and root fibers of the sixth and seventh nerves including
the genu of the seventh nerve. Locate the spinal tract of the fifth nerve and its
nucleus, the trapezoid body, and superior olivary nucleus (Figs. 163, 338, 342,
344).

69. *Section Through the Middle of the Pons Showing the Motor and Main
Sensory Nuclei of the Fifth Nerve.* In addition to these nuclei note the beginning
of the mesencephalic root of the fifth nerve. The superior cerebellar peduncle
makes its appearance in the dorsal part of the section (Figs. 164, 345, 348).

70. *Section Through the Inferior Colliculus.* Identify the basis pedunculi,
substantia nigra, medial and lateral lemnisci, cerebral aqueduct, central gray
matter, mesencephalic root of the fifth nerve, fasciculus longitudinalis medialis,
nucleus of the trochlear nerve, and the decussation of the superior cerebellar
peduncle (Figs. 167, 168, 359, 362).

71. *Section Through the Superior Colliculus.* Identify in addition to the
structures continued upward from lower levels, the red nucleus, the nucleus
of the third nerve, and the root fibers of that nerve, the ventral and dorsal
tegmental decussations, the inferior quadrigeminal brachium, and the medial
geniculate body (Figs. 170, 365, 367).

THE CEREBELLUM

72. On the cerebellum identify the vermis, hemispheres, lobules, and divided
peduncles (Figs. 36–40).

73. Divide the cerebellum in the median plane. In the medial sagittal section identify the white medullary body of the cerebellum, the arbor vitae, cerebellar cortex, folia, and sulci (Figs. 30, 195, *B*). Cut the right half into horizontal sections and the left into sagittal sections and study the medullary center and nuclei of the cerebellum (Figs. 195–197).

74. Study the histologic sections of the cerebellar cortex and master the details of its structure (Figs. 200, 201; pp. 282–285).

FUNCTIONAL ANALYSIS OF THE BRAIN STEM

75. Review the sections of the brain stem as directed in the following paragraphs, paying special attention to the functional significance of the various nuclei and fiber tracts as far as they can be followed in the series of sections. In general, the afferent tracts and nuclei should be entered in color on the right side of the drawings already made, and the efferent tracts and nuclei on the left side. But this order must be reversed in certain cases to allow for the decussation of the tracts. Label the various tracts and nuclei. Use the following color scheme:

Somatic afferent:
  Exteroceptive—blue.
  Proprioceptive—yellow.
Visceral afferent—orange.
Visceral efferent—purple.
Somatic efferent—red.
All cerebellar connections not strictly proprioceptive—brown.
Other tracts—black.

PROPRIOCEPTIVE PATHS AND CENTERS

76. The *cerebellum* is the chief proprioceptive correlation center, and the *restiform body* consists for the most part of proprioceptive afferent paths (Fig. 269). Note its shape, position, and connections in all the gross specimens.

77. Now take the sections of the medulla, locate the *dorsal spinocerebellar tract* in each, and indicate its position in yellow on the right side of your outlines. Locate the *external arcuate fibers*. From where do they come and where do they go? Draw in yellow those belonging to the right peduncle. Locate in your sections the *olivocerebellar tract*, and with brown indicate in your outline the fibers running into the right peduncle (Fig. 159).

78. From you text ascertain the course of the *ventral spinocerebellar tract* and indicate its position in yellow on the right side of the outlines (Fig. 198; p. 393).

79. *Proprioceptive Path to the Cerebral Cortex.* Indicate in yellow the terminal portion of the right *dorsal funiculi*, and with yellow stipple the right *nucleus gracilis* and *nucleus cuneatus* (Figs. 154, 155). Study the internal arcuate fibers and the medial lemniscus, drawing the internal arcuate fibers from right to left and the medial lemniscus on the left side (yellow). Where do the fibers of the medial lemniscus terminate? What is the source and what the destination

Van Rijnberk, G., 1908, 1912: Das Lokalizationsproblem im Kleinhirn, Ergebnisse der Physiol., Bd. vii, p. 653 and Bd. 12, p. 533.

———, 1931: Das Kleinhirn, Ergebnisse der Physiol., vol. 31, p. 592.

Van Valkenburg, C. T., 1913: Experimental and Pathologico-anatomical Researches on the Corpus Callosum, Brain, vol. 36, p. 119.

Verhaart, W. J. C., 1938: Comparison of the Corpus Striatum and the Red Nucleus as Subcortical Centra of the Cerebral Motor System, Psychiat. en Neurol., El. Amst. 42, pp. 676–737.

———, 1949: The Central Tegmental Tract, J. Comp. Neurol., vol. 90, pp. 173–192.

Vészi, J., 1918: Untersuchungen über die Erregungsleitung in Rückenmark, Ztschr. f. allg. Physiol., vol. 18, pp. 58–92.

Vogt, Cecile, 1909: La Myéloarchitecture du Thalamus du Ceropithèque, J. f. Psychol. u. Neurol., Leipzig, vol. 12, p. 285 (Ergänzungsheft).

Vonderahe, A. R., 1937: Anomalous Commissure of the Third Ventricle, Arch. Neurol. & Psychiat., vol. 37, pp. 1283–1288.

Walberg, Fred, 1952: The Lateral Reticular Nucleus of the Medulla Oblongata in Mammals. A Comparative-Anatomical Study, J. Comp. Neurol., vol. 96, pp. 283–343.

———, 1956: Descending Connections to the Inferior Olive. An Experimental Study in the Cat, J. Comp. Neurol., vol. 104, pp. 77–173.

Walberg, Fred, and A. Brodal, 1953: Spino-pontine Fibers in the Cat. An Experimental Study, J. Comp. Neurol., vol. 99, pp. 251–287.

———, 1953: Pyramidal Tract Fibers from Temporal and Occipital Lobes, Brain, vol. 76, pp. 491–508.

Walker, A. E., 1938: The Primate Thalamus, University of Chicago Press.

———, 1938: The Thalamus of the Chimpanzee, J. Anat., vol. 73, pp. 37–93.

———, 1940: The Spino-thalamic Tract in Man, Arch. Neurol. & Psychiat., vol. 43, pp. 284–298.

Wallenberg, A., 1905: Sekundäre Bahnen aus dem frontalen sensibeln Trigeminuskerne des Kaninchens, Anat. Anz., Bd. 26, p. 145.

Walshe, F. M. R., 1919: On the Genesis and Physiological Significance of Spasticity and Other Disorders of Motor Innervation, Brain, vol. 42, p. 1.

———, 1935: On the "Syndrome of the Premotor Cortex" (Fulton) and the Definition of the Terms "Premotor" and "Motor," Brain, vol. 58, p. 49.

———, 1942: Anatomy and Physiology of Cutaneous Sensibility; A Critical Review, Brain, vol. 65, pp. 48–112.

Wang, S. C., and S. W. Ranson, 1939: Autonomic Responses to Electrical Stimulation of the Lower Brain Stem, J. Comp. Neurol., vol. 71, pp. 437–455.

———, ———, 1939: Descending Pathways from the Hypothalamus to the Medulla and Spinal Cord. Observations on Blood Pressure and Bladder Responses, J. Comp. Neurol., vol. 71, pp. 457–472.

Ward, A. A., 1948: The Cingular Gyrus: Area 24, J. Neurophysiol., vol. 11, pp. 13–24.

Ward, J. W., 1936: A Histological Study of Transplanted Sympathetic Ganglia, Am. J. Anat., vol. 58, pp. 147–177.

———, 1938: The Influence of Posture on Responses Elicitable from the Cortex Cerebri of Cats, J. Neurophysiol., vol. 1, pp. 463–475.

———, 1952: Motor phenomena elicited in the unanesthetized animal by electrical stimulation of the cerebral cortex, A. Res. Nerv. & Ment. Dis., Proc., vol. 30, pp. 223–237.

Warwick, R., 1953: Representation of the Extra-ocular Muscles in the Oculomotor Nuclei of the Monkey, J. Comp. Neurol., vol. 98, pp. 449–503.

Weddell, A., L. Guttmann, and E. Gutman, 1941: Local Extension of Nerve Fibers into Denervated Areas of Skin, J. Neurol. & Psychiat., vol. 4, pp. 206–225.

Weddell, G., and J. A. Harpman, 1940: The Neurohistological Basis for the Sensation of Pain Provoked from Deep Fascia, Tendon, and Periosteum, J. Neurol. & Psychiat., vol. 3, pp. 319–328.

Weddell, G., D. C. Sinclair, and W. H. Feindel, 1948: An Anatomical Basis for Alterations in Quality of Pain Sensibility, J. Neurophysiol., vol. 11, pp. 99–110.

Weed, L. H., 1914: A Reconstruction of the Nuclear Masses in the Lower Portion of the Human Brain-stem, Publications of the Carnegie Institution of Washington, 1914.

———, 1914: Observations Upon Decerebrate Rigidity, J. Physiol., vol. 48, p. 205.

Weil, A., and A. Lassek, 1929: The Quantitative Distribution of the Pyramidal Tract in Man, Arch. Neurol. & Psychiat., vol. 22, pp. 495–510.

Weinberger, L. M., and F. C. Grant, 1942: Experiences with Intramedullary Tractotomy; Studies in Sensation, Arch. Neurol. & Psychiat., vol. 48, pp. 355–381.

Weisenburg, T. H., 1934: A Study of Aphasia, Arch. Neurol. & Psychiat., vol. 31, p. 1.

Weisenburg, T. H., and S. S. Stack, 1923: Central Pain from Lesions of the Pons, Arch. Neurol. & Psychiat., vol. 10, pp. 500–511.

Weiss, P., 1945: Experiments on Cell and Axon Orientation in Vitro: The Role of Colloidal Exudates in Tissue Organization, J. Exper. Zool., vol. 100, pp. 353–386.

Weiss, P. and H. B. Hiscoe, 1948: Experiments on the Mechanism of Nerve Growth, J. Exper. Zool., vol. 107, pp. 315–395.

Weiss, P., and H. Wang, 1936: Neurofibrils in Living Ganglion Cells of the Chick, Cultivated in Vitro, Anat. Rec., vol. 67, pp. 105–117.

Weiss, P., and Mac V. Edds, Jr., 1945: Sensory-Motor Nerve Crosses in the Rat, J. Neurophysiol., vol. 8, pp. 173–194.

Welch, W. K., and M. Kennard, 1944: Paralysis in Flexion and Tremor in Monkey Following Cortical Ablations, J. Neurosurg., vol. 1, pp. 258–264.

White, J. C., and R. H. Smithwick, 1941: The Autonomic Nervous System, The Macmillan Company, New York.

Whitlock, D. G., and W. J. H. Nauta, 1956: Subcortical Projections from the Temporal Neocortex in Macaca Mulatta, J. Comp. Neurol., vol. 106, pp. 183–212.

Wilkinson, H. J., 1927: The Argyll-Robertson Pupil, Med. J. Australia, vol. 1, pp. 267–272.

————, 1929: The Innervation of Striated Muscle, Med. J. Australia, vol. 2, pp. 768–793.

Willard, W. A., 1915: The Cranial Nerves of Anolis Carolinensis, Bull. Museum Comp. Zoöl., Harvard, vol. 59, p. 17.

Willems, E., 1911: Les noyaux masticateurs et mésencéphaliques du trigemeau, Le Névraxe, vol. 12, p. 7.

Williams, D. R., and P. Teitelbaum, 1956: Control of Drinking Behavior by Means of an Operant-Conditioning Technique, Science, vol. 124, pp. 1294–1296.

Wilson, J. G., 1905: The Structure and Function of the Taste-buds of the Larynx, Brain, vol. 28, p. 339.

Wilson, J. G., and F. H. Pike, 1915: The Mechanism of Labyrinthine Nystagmus, Arch. Int. Med., vol. 15, p. 31.

Wilson, S. A. K., 1912: Progressive Lenticular Degeneration, Brain, vol. 34, p. 295.

————, 1914: An Experimental Research into the Anatomy and Physiology of the Corpus Striatum, Brain, vol. 36, p. 427.

Wilson, W. C., and H. W. Magoun, 1945: The Functional Significance of the Inferior Olive in the Cat, J. Comp. Neurol., vol. 83, pp. 69–77.

Windle, W. F., 1926: Non-bifurcating Nerve Fibers of the Trigeminal Nerve, J. Comp. Neurol., vol. 40, p. 229.

————, 1934: Correlation Between the Development of Local Reflexes and Reflex Arcs in the Spinal Cord of Cat Embryos, J. Comp. Neurol., vol. 59, p. 487.

————, 1940: Physiology of the Fetus, W. B. Saunders Company, Philadelphia.

————, 1955: Regeneration in the Central Nervous System, Charles C Thomas, Springfield, Ill.

Windle, W. F., and W. W. Chambers, 1950: Regeneration in the Spinal Cord of the Cat and Dog, J. Comp. Neurol., vol. 93, pp. 241–257.

Windle, W. F., J. E. O'Donnell, and E. E. Glasshagle, 1933: The Early Development of Spontaneous and Reflex Behavior in Cat Embryos and Fetuses, Physiol. Zoöl., vol. 6, p. 521.

Wislocki, G. B., and E. W. Dempsey, 1948: The Chemical Cytology of the Chorioid Plexus and Blood Brain Barrier of the Rhesus Monkey (Macaca Mulatta), J. Comp. Neurol., vol. 88, pp. 319–345.

Wislocki, G. B., and E. M. K. Geiling, 1936: The Anatomy of the Hypophysis of Whales, Anat. Rec., vol. 66, pp. 17–41.

Wislocki, G. B., and E. H. Leduc, 1954: The Cytology of the Subcommissural Organ, Reissner's Fiber, Periventricular Glial Cells and Posterior Collicular Recess of the Rat's Brain, J. Comp. Neurol., vol. 101, pp. 283–309.

————, ————, 1956: On the Ending of Reissner's Fiber in the Filum Terminale of the Spinal Cord, J. Comp. Neurol., vol. 104, pp. 493–517.

Woldring, S., and M. N. J. Dirken, 1951: Site and Extension of Bulbar Respiratory Center, J. Neurophysiol., vol. 14, pp. 227–242.

Wolf, G. A., Jr., 1941: The Ratio of Preganglionic Neurons to Postganglionic Neurons in the Visceral Nervous System, J. Comp. Neurol., vol. 75, pp. 235–243.

Wolff, H. G., 1938: The Cerebral Blood Vessels—Anatomical Principles, A. Res. Nerv. & Ment. Dis., Proc., vol. 18, pp. 29–68.

————, 1943: Pain, A. Res. Nerv. & Ment. Dis., Proc., vol. 23.

Wolff, H. G., and J. D. Hardy, 1947: On the Nature of Pain, Physiol. Rev., vol. 27, pp. 167–199.

Wolff, H. G., and S. Wolf, 1948: Pain, American Lecture Series, Charles C Thomas, Springfield, Ill.

Woolsey, C. N., 1943: Second Somatic Receiving Areas in the Cerebral Cortex of Cat, Dog and Monkey, Fed. Proc. Am. Soc. Exper. Biol., vol. 2, p. 55.

Woolsey, C. N., P. H. Settlege, D. R. Meyer, W. Spencer, T. P. Hamuy, and A. M. Travis, 1952: Patterns of Localization in Precentral and "Supplementary" Motor Areas and Their Relation to the Concept of a Premotor Area, ARNMD, vol. 30, pp. 238–266.

Yagita, K. von, 1906: Ueber die Veränderung der Medulla oblongata nach einseitiger Zerstörung des Strickkörpers nebst einem Beitrag zur Anatomie des Seitenstrangkernes, Okayama Igakwai-Zassi, 1906, p. 201.

Yntema, C. L., 1944: Experiments on the Origin of the Sensory Ganglia of the Facial Nerve in the Chick, J. Comp. Neurol., vol. 81, pp. 147–167.

Yntema, C. L., and W. S. Hammond, 1945: Depletions and Abnormalities in the Cervical Sympathetic System of the Chick Following Extirpation of the Neural Crest, J. Exper. Zool., vol. 100, pp. 237–264.

——, ——, 1954: The Origin of Intrinsic Ganglia of Trunk Viscera from Vagal Neural Crest in the Chick Embryo, J. Comp. Neurol., vol. 101, pp. 515–541.

——, ——, 1955: Experiments on the Origin and Development of the Sacral Autonomic Nerves in the Chick Embryo, J. Exper. Zool., vol. 129, pp. 375–413.

Yoss, R. E., 1953: Studies of the Spinal Cord. Part II. Topographic Localization Within the Ventral Spino-cerebellar Tract in the Macaque, J. Comp. Neurol., vol. 99, pp. 613–638.

Yuasa, R., T. Ban and T. Kurotsu, 1957: Studies on the Electrocardiographic Changes during the Electrical Stimulation of the Hypothalamus of Rabbits, Med. J. Osaka Univ., vol. 8, pp. 141–158.

Index

The numbers in *italics* refer to the pages on which the structures are illustrated.

Gombault and Philippe, triangle of, 197
Gower's tract, 189
Granular corpuscles, compound, 127
    layer of cerebellum, 283
        of cerebral cortex, 351
Granule cells of cerebellar cortex, 283, 285
        of cerebral cortex, 349
        of fascia dentata, 334
        of olfactory bulb, 342
Granules, Nissl. See *Nissl bodies.*
    neurosecretory, 107, 283, 311
    pigment, in cytoplasm, 107
Gray column, dorsal, 166
        of spinal cord, cells of, 166, 174
        ventral, 168
    commissure, 168
    matter, 20, 166, 173
        central, 168, 293
        microscopic structure of, 173
        of spinal cord, 166, 173
            development, 96
        subependymal, 515
    rami communicantes, 159
Groove. See also *Sulcus* and *Fissure.*
    neural, 11
Ground bundle. See *Fasciculus proprius.*
Growth of axon, 92, 118, 123
Gudden, bundle of. See *Tract, mammilloteg-
        mental.*
    commissure of, 267
Gustatory apparatus, 252, 372
    area in cerebral cortex, 372
Gyrus (or Gyri), *31*, 56, *60*, 61
    angular, *58*
    annectent, 56
    callosal. See *Gyrus cinguli.*
    centralis anterior, 57, *526*, *528*
        posterior, 58
    cinguli, 62, 366, 373, *525*
    dentatus. See *Fascia dentata.*
    effects of stimulus, 367
    fornicatus, 62, *62*
    frontal, ascending. See *Gyrus centralis anterior.*
        inferior, 57
        middle, 57
        superior, 57
        transverse, 58
    fusiform, 62, *526*
    hippocampal, 61, *332*, *522*
    insulae, 59
    on lateral aspect of cerebral hemisphere, 55, 56
    limbic. See *Lobe, limbic.*
    lingual, 60, 61, *61*, 369
    marginalis. See *Gyrus, frontal, superior.*
    olfactory, lateral, 331, 332, *332*
        medial, 331
    orbital, *31*, 62, *517*
    postcentral. See *Gyrus centralis posterior.*
    precentral. See *Gyrus centralis anterior.*
    rectus, 62
    subcallosal, *332*, *332*

Gyrus (or Gyri), supracallosal, 65, *528*. See also
        Indusium griseum.
    supramarginal, 58
    temporal, 57
        transverse, 58, 370
    uncinatus. See *Gyrus, hippocampal.*

H, H₁, H₂ fields of Forel, *300*, *304*, 316, *317*, *508*,
        523
Habenular commissure, 302
    ganglion, 302
    nucleus, 10, *294*, *302*, *528*
    trigone, 302
Habenulopeduncular tract, 302, *345*, *533*
Habit formation and cortex, 376
Hair follicles, nerve endings in, 145
Hallucinations, olfactory, 346
Head, innervation of, autonomic, *158*, 160, *415*
Headache, and referred pain, 427, 430
    from intracranial lesion, 442
Hearing. See also under *Auditory.*
    neural mechanism for, 388
Heart, innervation of, 416, 428
Heat, conduction of sensation of, 190
Heat-conservation pathway, 309
Heat-loss pathway, 309
Hemianopsia, 267, 430, *431*, 442
Hemiballismus, 424
Hemiplegia, 423
Hemisection of spinal cord, effect of, 201
Hemispheres. See *Cerebellar* and *Cerebral.*
Hemoencephalic barrier, 74
Hemorrhage, artery of cerebral, 81
    of internal capsule, 442
Hereditary pattern of structure, 123
Herpes zoster and dermatomes, 130
Heschl's convolution, 58. See *Gyrus, temporal,
        transverse.*
Hillock, axon, 100
Hindbrain, 17. See *Metencephalon* and *Rhom-
        bencephalon.*
Hippocampal commissure. See *Commissure of
        fornix.*
    digitations, *334*
    fissure, *63*
    gyrus. See *Parahippocampal gyrus.*
    paths, 336
    rudiment, 65, 332, *332*
Hippocampus, 70, 80, 334, *334*, 342, *343*, *510*
    efferent fibers from, 344
    fimbria of, 70, 334
    functions of, 335
    molecular layer of, 342
Histogenesis of nervous system, 89–97
Homonymous hemianopsia, 268, 430, 442
Horizontal cells of Cajal, *349*, *350*, 351
Hormone, antidiuretic, 210
Horn, Ammon's. See *Hippocampus.*
Humoral substances, 157, 210
Hypogastric plexus, 162